IAP Handbook of
Developmental and Behavioral Pediatrics

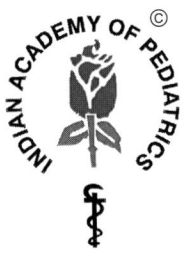

IAP Handbook of
Developmental and Behavioral Pediatrics

Editor-in-Chief
Samir H Dalwai
Developmental Behavioral Pediatrician
New Horizons Child Development Centre and Research Foundation
National Coordinator, IAP Fellowship in Developmental and Behavioral Pediatrics
Nanavati Max Superspecialty Hospital, Mumbai, Maharashtra, India

Chief Academic Editors

Jeeson C Unni	**Shabina Ahmed**
Senior Associate Consultant	Founder Director
Aster Medcity	Assam Autism Foundation
Kochi, Kerala, India	Guwahati, Assam, India
Editor-in-Chief, IAP Drug Formulary	

Academic Editors

Kawaljit Singh Multani
Consultant Pediatrician
11 Air Force Hospital
Ghaziabad, Uttar Pradesh, India

Leena Deshpande	**Leena Srivastava**
Developmental and Behavioral Pediatrician	Head, Division of Developmental and Behavioral Pediatrics
iCAN Child Development Centre	Department of Pediatrics
MGM Hospital, Apollo Hospital	Bharati Vidyapeeth Medical College and Hospital
Navi Mumbai, Maharashtra, India	Visiting Consultant, Developmental Pediatrics, CloudNine Hospital and LMCCH
	Pune, Maharashtra, India

Forewords

MKC Nair	Remesh Kumar R	Upendra Kinjawadekar
Piyush Gupta	Bakul Jayant Parekh	Vineet Saxena

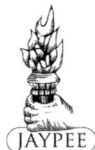

JAYPEE BROTHERS MEDICAL PUBLISHERS
The Health Sciences Publisher
New Delhi | London

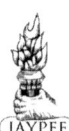 **Jaypee Brothers Medical Publishers (P) Ltd**

Headquarters
Jaypee Brothers Medical Publishers (P) Ltd
EMCA House, 23/23-B
Ansari Road, Daryaganj
New Delhi 110 002, India
Landline: +91-11-23272143, +91-11-23272703
+91-11-23282021, +91-11-23245672
Email: jaypee@jaypeebrothers.com

Corporate Office
Jaypee Brothers Medical Publishers (P) Ltd
4838/24, Ansari Road, Daryaganj
New Delhi 110 002, India
Phone: +91-11-43574357
Fax: +91-11-43574314
Email: jaypee@jaypeebrothers.com

Overseas Office
JP Medical Ltd.
83 Victoria Street, London
SW1H 0HW (UK)
Phone: +44 20 3170 8910
Fax: +44 (0)20 3008 6180
Email: info@jpmedpub.com

Website: www.jaypeebrothers.com
Website: www.jaypeedigital.com

© 2022, Indian Academy of Pediatrics

The views and opinions expressed in this book are solely those of the original contributor(s)/author(s) and do not necessarily represent those of editor(s) of the book.

All rights reserved. No part of this publication may be reproduced, stored or transmitted in any form or by any means, electronic, mechanical, photocopying, recording or otherwise, without the prior permission in writing of the publishers.

All brand names and product names used in this book are trade names, service marks, trademarks or registered trademarks of their respective owners. The publisher is not associated with any product or vendor mentioned in this book.

Medical knowledge and practice change constantly. This book is designed to provide accurate, authoritative information about the subject matter in question. However, readers are advised to check the most current information available on procedures included and check information from the manufacturer of each product to be administered, to verify the recommended dose, formula, method and duration of administration, adverse effects and contraindications. It is the responsibility of the practitioner to take all appropriate safety precautions. Neither the publisher nor the author(s)/editor(s) assume any liability for any injury and/or damage to persons or property arising from or related to use of material in this book.

This book is sold on the understanding that the publisher is not engaged in providing professional medical services. If such advice or services are required, the services of a competent medical professional should be sought.

Every effort has been made where necessary to contact holders of copyright to obtain permission to reproduce copyright material. If any have been inadvertently overlooked, the publisher will be pleased to make the necessary arrangements at the first opportunity. The **CD/DVD-ROM** (if any) provided in the sealed envelope with this book is complimentary and free of cost. **Not meant for sale.**

Inquiries for bulk sales may be solicited at: jaypee@jaypeebrothers.com

IAP Handbook of Developmental and Behavioral Pediatrics

First Edition: **2022**

ISBN: 978-93-89776-48-5

Printed at

Dedication
This book is dedicated to our parents and teachers who by their wisdom and patience continue to help us develop far beyond our childhood years and to our little patients who are the reason for the spring in our step every morning!

Contributors

A Somasundaram
Co-Founder and
Developmental Pediatrician
D'Soul Child Development Centre
Chennai, Tamil Nadu, India

Abhishek R Jain
Consultant Pediatric Neurologist
Rainbow Children's Hospital
Hyderabad, Telangana, India

Abraham K Paul
Consultant Pediatrician and Convener
Newborn Hearing Screening
Programme—IAP
Cochin Hospital
Kochi, Kerala, India

Alka A Subramanyam
Associate Professor
Department of Psychiatry
TNMC and BYL Nair Charitable Hospital
Mumbai, Maharashtra, India

Ami Shah
Consultant Clinical Geneticist
Genetic Clinic
Department of Pediatrics
Nanavati Superspecialty Hospital
Mumbai, Maharashtra, India

Anaita Udwadia-Hegde
Consultant Pediatric Neurologist
Jaslok Hospital and Research Center
SRCC Narayana Health Children's Hospital
Breach Candy Hospital Trust
Wadia Children's Hospital
Mumbai, Maharashtra, India

Anjan Bhattacharya
Senior Consultant Developmental
Pediatrician and Head
Child Development Centre
Apollo Multispecialty Hospital, Kolkata
Director
Nabajatak Child Development Center
Kolkata, West Bengal, India

Ann M Neumeyer
Child Neurologist
Assistant Professor
Harvard Medical School
Medical Director, Lurie Center for Autism/
MassGeneral Hospital for Children
Boston, Massachusetts, USA

Aradhana Rohil
Fellowship in Developmental and
Behavioral Pediatrics
New Horizons Child Development Centre
and Research Foundation
Mumbai, Maharashtra, India

B Yambao-Dela Cruz
UC Davis MIND Institute
UC Davis Health
California, San Francisco, USA

Barkha Chawla
Developmental Pediatrician
New Horizons Child Development Centre
and Research Foundation
Mumbai, Maharashtra, India

Dilip R Patel
Professor
Pediatrics and Adolescent Medicine
Department of Pediatric and Adolescent
Medicine
Western Michigan University Homer
Stryker MD School of Medicine
Kalamazoo, Michigan, USA

Hilla Sukhadwala
Fellowship in Developmental and
Behavioral Pediatrics
New Horizons Child Development Centre
and Research Foundation
Mumbai, Maharashtra, India

Jeeson C Unni
Senior Associate Consultant
Aster Medcity
Kochi, Kerala, India
Editor-in-Chief, IAP Drug Formulary

Contributors

Jyoti Bhatia
Senior Consultant (Developmental and Behavioral Pediatrics)
Department of Pediatrics
Max Superspecialty Hospital, Patparganj
New Delhi, India

Kawaljit Singh Multani
Consultant Pediatrician
11 Air Force Hospital
Ghaziabad, Uttar Pradesh, India

Kaye M Napalinga
Consultant Pediatrician
MedMom Institute for Human Development
Pasig City, Philippines

Kersi Chavda
Consultant Psychiatrist
Department of Psychiatry
Hinduja Hospital and Sir HN Hospital
Mumbai, Maharashtra, India

Lata Bhat
Developmental and Behavioral Pediatrician
Indraprastha Apollo Hospital
New Delhi, India

Lavanya Iyer
Counseling Psychologist and Remedial Educator
iCAN Child Development Centre
Navi Mumbai, Maharashtra, India

Leena Deshpande
Developmental and
Behavioral Pediatrician
iCAN Child Development Centre
MGM Hospital, Apollo Hospital
Navi Mumbai, Maharashtra, India

Leena Srivastava
Head, Division of Developmental and Behavioral Pediatrics
Department of Pediatrics
Bharati Vidyapeeth Medical College and Hospital
Visiting Consultant, Developmental Pediatrics, CloudNine Hospital and LMCCH
Pune, Maharashtra, India

Lokesh Lingappa
Senior Consultant Pediatric Neurologist
Rainbow Children's Hospital
Hyderabad, Telangana, India

MA Florita
UC Davis MIND Institute
UC Davis Health
California, San Francisco, USA

Manju George Elenjickal
Associate Professor and In-Charge
Child Development Centre
Department of Pediatrics
Pushpagiri Medical College Hospital
Thiruvalla, Kerala, India

Manoj Bhatawdekar
Consulting Psychiatrist
Bhatawdekars' Clinic
Mumbai, Maharashtra, India

Naveen Jain
Coordinator and Senior Consultant
Department of Neonatology
Kerala Institute of Medical Sciences
Thiruvananthapuram, Kerala, India

Neelkamal Soares
Professor of Pediatric and Adolescent Medicine
Western Michigan University Homer Stryker MD School of Medicine
Kalamazoo, Michigan, USA

Neepa Thacker Dave
Pediatric Ophthalmologist and Strabismologist
Kids Eye Clinic
Mumbai, Maharashtra, India

Neethu Mary Mathew
Audiologist and
Speech Language Pathologist
Pratheeksha Child Development Centre
Department of Pediatrics
Pushpagiri Medical College Hospital
Thiruvalla, Kerala, India

Omkar Pradip Hajirnis
Consultant Pediatric Neurologist
Synapses Child Neurology and
Development Centre
Jupiter Hospital, Bhaktivedanta Hospital
and Research Centre
Thane, Maharashtra, India

Patricia Osbourn
Deputy Director
University of New Mexico
Pediatrics Center for Development and
Disability
Albuquerque, New Mexico

Prameela Joji
Consultant Pediatric ICU and ER
Kerala Institute of Medical Sciences
Thiruvananthapuram, Kerala, India

Randi J Hagerman
UC Davis MIND Institute
UC Davis Health
California, San Francisco, USA

Rashid Merchant
Senior Consultant Pediatrician
Nanavati Superspecialty Hospital
Mumbai, Maharashtra, India

Rhishikesh Thakre
Director and Chief Neonatologist
Neo Clinic and Hospital
Aurangabad, Maharashtra, India

Samir H Dalwai
Developmental Behavioral Pediatrician
New Horizons Child Development Centre
and Research Foundation
National Coordinator, IAP Fellowship in
Developmental and Behavioral Pediatrics
Nanavati Max Superspecialty Hospital
Mumbai, Maharashtra, India

Santhosh Rajagopal
Developmental Pediatrician
Rio Hospital for Women and Children
Madurai, Tamil Nadu, India

Sarbani Raha
Child Neurologist
Child Neurology and Epilepsy Clinic
Vadodara, Gujarat, India

Shabina Ahmed
Founder Director
Assam Autism Foundation
Guwahati, Assam, India

Shambhavi Seth
Developmental Pediatrician
Director, Bright Beginnings Child
Development Centre, New Delhi
Senior Consultant, Max Hospital Saket
and Gurugram
BLK Superspecialty Hospital
New Delhi, India

Shekhar Patil
Consultant
Department of Pediatric Neurology
Apollo Hospital
Navi Mumbai, Maharashtra, India

Shibani Kanungo
Associate Professor of Pediatric and
Adolescent Medicine
Western Michigan University Homer
Stryker MD School of Medicine
Kalamazoo, Michigan, USA

Snehal Mallakmir
Consultant Clinical Geneticist
Genetic Clinic
Department of Pediatrics
Nanavati Superspecialty Hospital
Mumbai, Maharashtra, India

SS Kamath
Consultant Pediatrician
Indira Gandhi Co-Operative Hospital
Kochi, Kerala, India

Swati Y Bhave
Adjunct Professor
Department of Adolescent Medicine
Dr DY Patil Medical College and Dr DY
Patil Vidyapeeth, Pune
Senior Consultant in Adolescent
Pediatrics
Head and In-Charge of Adolescent
Wellness Clinic, Jehangir Hospital
Pune, Maharashtra, India
Executive Director AACCI, Mumbai
(Association of Adolescent and Child Care
in India)

Vasudha N Rao
Consultant Pediatric Oncology
Rainbow Children's Hospital
Bengaluru, Karnataka, India

Vrajesh Udani
Child Neurologist and Epileptologist
PD Hinduja Hospital
Mumbai, Maharashtra, India

Waheeda Pagarkar
Consultant in
Audiovestibular Medicine
Great Ormond Street Hospital for
Children, London, UK
University College London Hospitals NHS
Foundation Trust, London, UK
New Horizons Audiology and Hearing
AIDS Centre for Adults and Children
Mumbai, Maharashtra, India

Yamini Jagannath Howe
Developmental and Behavioral Pediatrician
Instructor, Harvard Medical School
Lurie Center for Autism/MassGeneral
Hospital for Children
Boston, Massachusetts, USA

YK Amdekar
Former Medical Director
BJ Wadia Children's Hospital
Mumbai, Maharashtra, India

Z Bassi
Consultant in Pediatric
Neurodevelopment and Neurodisability
Department of Development Pediatrics
Alder Hey Children's Hospital
Liverpool, UK

Zafar Mahmood Meenai
Director, Ummeid Group of Child
Development Centers
Bhopal and Nagpur
Advisor and International Advocacy
Group Member of American Academy of
Cerebral Palsy and Developmental
Medicine (AACPDM) and Past Chair of
International Affairs Committee

Foreword

I am happy to know that the IAP Chapter of Neurodevelopmental Pediatrics is publishing a *Handbook of Developmental and Behavioral Pediatrics* with contributions from eminent developmental pediatricians across the country and abroad. This comprehensive handbook covers all essential topics in the subject in 60 chapters. This handbook has come at a critical time, when we are looking for a simple user-friendly handbook for the personnel of District Early Intervention Centres under Rshtriya Bal Swasthya Karyakram (RBSK).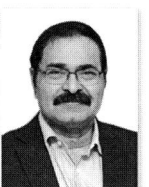

I do hope that this handbook would serve to initiate students of pediatrics into the field of developmental and behavioral pediatrics. It would also serve as a handy reference not only for practicing pediatricians but also for the developmental behavioral pediatricians—Developmental Therapist team at all levels. The DEIC therapy team of physiotherapists, occupational therapist, speech therapist, child psychologists, and special educators may find it handy. It could also be a textbook on Developmental Behavioral Pediatrics for the large number of community health personnel both in government and in private sector.

MKC Nair
DSc PhD MD MMedSc (NewCastle) MBA MA (Philosophy)
MA (MC&J) FNNF FIAP FIACAM FAMS
Fomer Vice Chancellor and Professor Emeritus-Research
Kerala University of Health Sciences
Founder Director and Professor Emeritus in Developmental
Behavioral and Adolescent Pediatrics, CDC Kerala
Director, NIMS-Spectrum-Child Development Research Centre
Editor, IAP Textbook of Pediatrics and High-risk Newborn
Editor, Illingworth's The Development of the
Infant and the Young Child (11th Edn)
E-mail: *cdcmkc@gmail.com*

Foreword

I am very much privileged to present the foreword for the *Handbook of Developmental and Behavioral Pediatrics*, which is being published by IAP to better equip practicing pediatricians to understand and assess developmental and behavioral problems in children. This book is a step forward in IAP's mission to continuously enlarge its scope to cover the entire spectrum of child health and child care. It is a 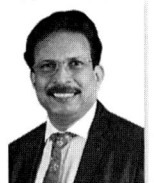 comprehensive compilation of valuable information for the early detection of developmental and behavioral disorders in children, along with providing remedial measures.

Research into adult health issues and behavioral disorders clearly indicate that many such problems originate in childhood. It logically follows that these could have been better resolved with early intervention. As the saying goes, "Prevention is better than cure." Hence, developmental and behavioral pediatrics has a special role to play in heralding a healthy society. This stream focuses on scientifically evaluating the child's physical, emotional and cognitive development to identify problem areas and prescribe corrective measures, which are designed to enable a transition to healthy adulthood. Judging by the important role this plays in child health, there can be no doubt that this domain of pediatrics will eventually take center stage in our profession.

Conventional wisdom holds that "Happy childhood leads to happy life". However, with the advent of developmental pediatrics, we can confidently rephrase this as "Healthy childhood leads to healthy life". However, as this his domain deals with the intangible "gray areas" of life, practitioners of this craft will need special qualities like sensitivity, observation, empathy and a helping nature to derive the best results. This handbook introduces the clinician to the fundamentals of developmental and behavioral issues and acquaints oneself to the new doors that are being opened in the field of pediatrics.

I congratulate the editorial team comprising Dr Samir H Dalwai as the Editor-in-Chief, Dr Jeeson Unni and Dr Shabina Ahmed as Chief Academic Editors, Dr Kawaljit Singh Multani, Dr Leena Srivastav and Dr Leena Deshpande as Academic Editors. They have taken pains to access the best brains in the field from across the country and abroad to produce an authoritative high quality publication which is worthy of the reader's attention. I wish them success in this venture and hope that the reader response will motivate them to continue updating this book with further inputs in the years to come.

Remesh Kumar R
National President 2022
Indian Academy of Pediatrics

Foreword

I am extremely happy to know that IAP has taken a very important initiative and is publishing a *Handbook of Developmental and Behavioral Pediatrics*. Neurodevelopmental disorders have a diverse influence on function, development, learning, behavior, mental health, and the child's capacity to meet the range of age-based expectations across a variety of settings.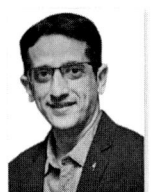

What happens to children in the earliest years of their lives has a great impact on their immediate well-being and their future. Similarly, what does not happen for a child in their early years can be an impediment to their well-being and entire future. Any significant deviation in the behavior or the development of the child needs to be detected and addressed in the most comprehensive way. I am sure that this handbook will provide a collegiate and supportive structure for pediatricians and other medically trained professionals who work with children and families affected by eurodevelopmental and behavioral disorders, and share similar professional and related personal challenges.

In the last two years of the pandemic, while the entire medical fraternity irrespective of the field of their expertise was busy concentrating on prevention, control and cure of COVID-19, sadly, too many children around the world were denied the right to reach their full potential. And every year, some of them are held back, deprived, in one way or another, of the love, care, nurturing, health, nutrition and protection that they need to survive, grow and develop resulting in some behavioral and neurodevelopmental challenges.

The editorial team under the leadership of very talented Dr Samir H Dalwai and comprising of great academicians with huge experience in the field across the country like Dr Jeeson Unni, Dr Shabina Ahmed, Dr KS Multani, Dr Leena Shrivastava, Dr Leena Deshpande are aware about the advances in the field as well as the ground reality in regard to the current understanding of general pediatricians of behavioral and developmental pediatrics.

In acknowledgment of the complexity and uncertainty inherent to this area of developmental and behavioral pediatrics, the editors value the sharing of knowledge and experience towards the development of good clinical judgment. They have addressed dual goals of alleviating current distress, and working towards optimal outcomes, considering the fact that there is no magic bullet to treat or cure many of these disorders. This handbook has kept a highly practical focus, emphasizing evaluation, counseling, medical treatment, and follow-up with a single aim to promote and support the development of excellence in the practice of Neurodevelopmental and Behavioral Pediatrics.

I am sure this handbook will be a permanent companion of every medical practitioner working in the field of child health.

Best Wishes

Upendra Kinjawadekar
National President Elect 2022
Indian Academy of Pediatrics

Foreword

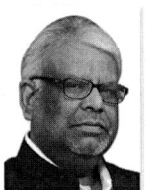

I am very happy to know that the Indian Academy of Pediatrics is coming out with the first *Handbook of Developmental and Behavioral Pediatrics*!

Developmental and Behavioral Pediatrics has traditionally been a subject, which has not received its due importance in the medical curriculum. Infectious diseases, intensive care, even growth and nutrition have been accorded much higher significance. However, as times have changed and pediatricians are faced with a larger proportion of concerns in the field of development and behavior in their practice, it is imperative for the practicing pediatrician to be well versed with basic clinical manifestations as well as primary intervention on these topics.

Indeed, the Indian Academy of Pediatrics has launched one of its most significant programs on Nurturing Care for Early Childhood Development; development and behavior is a very important component of the same. I am glad that this handbook is being released during these times, as this will add to the overall knowledge and practice of early child development.

I congratulate the Editor-in-Chief, Dr Samir Dalwai, the Chief Academic Editors, Dr Shabina Ahmed and Dr Jeeson Unni as well as the Academic Editors, Dr Leena Deshpande, Dr Leena Srivastava and Dr Kawaljit Singh Multani as well as all the esteemed authors who have contributed to this handbook.

I am sure this handbook will serve as an import source of knowledge to clinicians and academicians alike as well as residents and students and will stimulate a holistic interest in the subject.

Piyush Gupta MD FIAP FNNF FAMS
President, Indian Academy of Pediatrics, 2021

Foreword

Dear friends,
Greetings from the Indian Academy of Pediatrics!

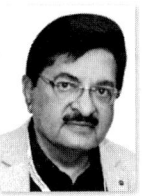

In today's era, where the competition among children is rising at a fierce pace – a time when children are scoring more than 90 percent, the most common complaint heard from the parents are a few rather simple questions – Why is my child not able to study well? What is wrong with my child? Why is my child not attentive in class? Why is the teacher always complaining about my child? Why does my child get low marks in a certain subject, but excel in others? This has become more common today because of the COVID-19 pandemic scenario, wherein the schools were completely shut for more than a year. Unfortunately, the answer to these questions is not that simple, but the best person who can answer is from a comparatively new and upcoming field—Developmental and Behavioral Pediatrician.

Developmental and Behavioral Pediatrics is a specialized branch of pediatrics that deals with evaluation, counseling as well as providing treatment for children, adolescents, and their families with a wide range of developmental and behavioral difficulties including learning disorders, writing difficulties, math disorders, attention deficit/hyperactivity disorder, habit disorders, etc. to name a few. Unfortunately, the very mention of a behavioral and developmental pediatrician requirement often makes the parent rather defensive. They cannot accept that anything could be wrong with their child. However, we—the general pediatricians—can help the situation easily. By having a basic knowledge about the different issues, we can be the first point of contact and help in the correct diagnosis.

Since it is a specialized science, not all of us are trained in proper detection of the various scenarios that may lead to an actual visit to the specialist. This is where this book proves its usefulness. By having several problems faced by parents explained in a simple and lucid language, I am sure that it will help us in early and easy detection and provide the correct way forward. This book fills a void, which was felt regarding this specialized area of expertise, and I am certain that it will be very well received by all our colleagues.

With the schools on the verge of reopening once again and the concerns of parents regarding their child's scholastic performance, this handbook which was actually conceived pre-pandemic in 2020 and has dealt extensively with these topics as well, will aid the common pediatrician to guide the parents carefully in such situations. The book is very aptly named *Handbook of Developmental and Behavioral Pediatrics*. This handbook covers the most essential questions that have been asked by several parents during our practice and has been written by stalwarts in the field of Developmental and Behavioral Pediatrics. Since it is written by pediatricians, you can be assured that the contents are hundred percent proper and applicable in your day-to-day lives.

I would like to take this opportunity to thank all the editors and contributors in general and Dr Samir Dalwai in particular who have burnt the midnight oil and made the dream of mine and all pediatricians come true. It is without doubt an amazing handbook worth recommendation to be there in every parent and pediatrician's bookshelf. I am certain that the timing for the book and its contents could not have been better in any manner. Keep up the great work. Kudos to the entire team who has worked diligently on this project throughout the pandemic while fulfilling their duties at the same time.

Happy Reading!

Bakul Jayant Parekh
President, Indian Academy of Pediatrics, 2020

Foreword

Dear Friends,

It gives me immense pleasure to introduce the '*Handbook of Developmental and Behavioral Pediatrics*' by IAP. As we all know that Growth, Development and Behavioral Pediatrics is the most intriguing, interesting and unique aspect of our specialty. It is the real Pediatrics, which sets it apart from Medicine. It starts right from the time when the fetus is formed and especially how a newborn baby grows into a mature human being, passing through various milestones one after the other.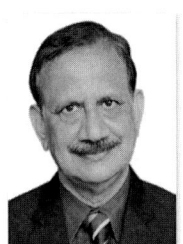

Even at the first glance, an astute pediatrician knows whether the baby is growing normally or if there is something amiss. Despite this skill which every pediatrician possesses by virtue of his/her training, it always needs to be honed and sharpened and approached in a systematic manner. I am sure that this handy book by IAP will stand out among all the available books on the subject of Development and Behavioral Pediatrics.

Each one of us needs to go through this book again and again so that the benefit of this fantastic book reaches to its final target—the little babies. Their growth and developmental assessment is our primary responsibility after all. Given the expertise of the Editorial Team and contributors, it will serve to be an indispensible tool for practicing pediatricians and postgraduates.

No words of appreciation are enough for Dr Jeeson Unni and Dr Shabina Ahmed who have worked so hard as Chief Academic Editors, and Dr Kawaljit Singh Multani, Dr Leena Srivastava and Dr Leena Deshpande, who have taken the responsibility of Academic Co-Editors and Dr Samir H Dalwai the Editor-in-Chief who has taken the mantle upon himself to bring out this gem for IAP. IAP is thankful to their yeoman service for the children as well as pediatricians.

Vineet Saxena
Honorary Secretary General
Indian Academy of Pediatrics 2022-23

Preface

Over the past decade, interest in Developmental and Behavioral Pediatrics has shown a remarkable surge. A steady decline in infectious disorders, increased survival of high-risk neonates, smaller families, rising incomes and an overall increase in aspiration about the quality of life for the family has contributed to increasing awareness and increased care seeking for children and adolescents with neurodevelopmental and behavioral problems. The pediatrician who was content with a cursory look at motor milestones and weight gain is now being asked probing questions about the child's development and behavior. "Wait and watch", worse—"Nothing can be done"—the earlier answers for most cases, is now neither acceptable assurance nor scientifically correct advice. A spiraling increase in autism and other neurobehavioral problems, coupled with insistence from schools, and indeed society, for perfection to fit the curriculum and expected norms are leading to increased consultancy for these issues.

The Indian Academy of Pediatrics has been at the forefront of training and coaching more than 30,000 pediatrician members to equip them with clinical skills. The demand for training on developmental and behavioral problems in children and adolescents has led to many of us having overbooked calendars. Often, the way this subject is practiced in the western world is far removed from the limitations and advantages of our family-oriented culture; teachers and authors that adapt with this important aspect are oft sought after. The IAP Fellowship in Developmental and Behavioral Pediatrics is now into its sixth successful year with an increased demand from Fellows for content of Indian origin. The thirst for such knowledge, albeit in a palatable dosage, has led to the birth of the first such *Handbook of Developmental and Behavioral Pediatrics*.

This handbook is organized into chapters that deal with basics of developmental and behavioral pediatrics and chapters that offer some in-depth knowledge about individual conditions. There are chapters on therapeutics as well various social aspects like digital exposure and medicolegal aspects, as well as a peek into the history of this subject. Each chapter has a brief introduction about the topic followed by simple to grasp clinical features often with key questions and a succinctly presented management of the condition. As such, the handbook can be read across at one go (for an examination, perhaps!) or can be used as a ready reference in the busy clinic. The authors have been invited nationally as well as overseas to present a swathe of clinical and academic aspects of the above. We are sure this will spur the uninitiated—the students and residents—into the subject, as well as the practicing pediatricians to spend a little more time with their patients with neurodevelopmental and behavioral disorders. Serious students of this subject will have to wait a little longer for a detailed textbook to follow this handbook soon. Meanwhile, if even a few families seen by each pediatrician receive a longer interaction about their child's concerns, we will be both delighted and relieved to have pulled off a difficult job well.

We will be happy to receive constructive criticism and suggestions about this handbook as we are sure it will help us "develop" the next edition better (Developmental Behavioral Pediatricians are an optimistic lot!). As blessed practitioners of this enchanting field, we are gratified by the fact that pursuit of no other subject or practice helps the practitioner to develop the self as much as this subject does. To this, we owe our emancipation! Long live the practice of Developmental Behavioral Pediatrics!

The despondency of earlier years where neurodevelopmental disorders were relegated to optional short notes in theory examinations and to asylums in real life gave way to Tennyson's "Tis better to have loved and lost than never to have loved at all" approach, when our earlier generation attempted forays into offering a more humane life to those affected. We hope coming generations of pediatricians will rather see most of these "disorders" for what they are in Ghalib's words, *"Meherbaan ho ke bula lo mujhe chaho jis waqt, Main gaya waqt nahin hoon ke phir aa bhi na sakun!"* (Your benevolent intervention is all that I seek for my resurrection; I am not time that I may never return once it passes.)

It is never too late. It is only needed that we try!

Samir H Dalwai
Jeeson C Unni
Shabina Ahmed
Leena Deshpande
Leena Srivastava
Kawaljit Singh Multani

Acknowledgments

We wish to thank the Indian Academy of Pediatrics for the opportunity to contribute this handbook, which will serve to increase the knowledge of developmental and behavioral pediatrics.

We wish to thank the authors who have contributed their knowledge in a simple and lucid manner and complied with the (various) timelines.

We wish to thank our families who supported us through hours of being locked away in front of a screen interspersed with late night frantic phone discussions.

We wish to thank our individual staff and teams who accommodated our absence from our regular clinics.

We wish to thank Dr Bakul Parekh, who encouraged us when the idea for such a text was floated way back in 2020, Dr Piyush Gupta who helped us keep the momentum going through the COVID year, Dr Remesh Kumar R for always supporting us with this academic venture as well as our teachers, Dr YK Amdekar, Dr MKC Nair, Dr Rashid H Merchant and Dr Swati Bhave for their presence in this handbook.

We wish to thank Dr Waheeda Pagarkar, Dr Dilip R Patel, Dr Randi J Hagerman, Dr Ann M Neumeyer, Dr Patricia Osbourn, Dr Yamini Jagannath Howe, Dr MA Florita, Dr B Yambao-Dela Cruz, Dr Kaye M Napalinga, Dr Zahabiyah Bassi, Dr Shibani Kanungo and Dr Neelkamal Soares for their distinguished contribution in this field as well as adding an international flavor to this handbook.

We are forever grateful to our mentors Dr Sachidanand S Kamath and Dr Abraham K Paul for their guidance.

We are thankful to Shri Jitendar P Vij (Group Chairman), Mr. Ankit Vij (Managing Director), Ms Chetna Malhotra Vohra (Associate Director—Content Strategy) and Dr Rajul Jain (Development Editor) of Jaypee Brothers Medical Publishers (P) Ltd, New Delhi for their constant help in publishing the book.

Finally, we wish to formally thank each other—the editors! One remembers the concluding lines from the legendary Robbins and Kumar's Textbook of Pathology—"It is not that we always thought alike, but we were always happy to acknowledge each other's thoughts."

We thank each other and all the authors for standing by us through all the unforeseen difficulties. This book is a conception of the COVID years as much a child of our years of study and work in this field.

Finally, we wish to thank the innumerable children and adolescents and their families who across the decades have taught us not just what little we know about this subject, but what it means to be human. We are but a product of their chisel.

Contents

1. **A History of Developmental Behavioral Pediatrics: An Idea whose Time has Come** 1
   Samir H Dalwai

2. **Normal Development and Behavior** 6
   Kawaljit Singh Multani

3. **Theories of Normal Development and Behavior** 13
   Kawaljit Singh Multani

4. **Developmental Concerns in Pediatric Practice** 21
   YK Amdekar

5. **Developmental Surveillance and Screening** 24
   Leena Deshpande

6. **Approach to Global Developmental Delay** 28
   Leena Srivastava

7. **Developmentally Supportive Care** 35
   Naveen Jain

8. **Follow-up of the High-risk Newborn** 40
   Rhishikesh Thakre

9. **Genetics and Neurodevelopmental Disorders** 48
   Rashid Merchant, Snehal Mallakmir, Ami Shah

10. **Intellectual Disability** 54
    Samir H Dalwai, Aradhana Rohil

11. **Multiple Disabilities** 59
    Leena Deshpande

12. **Down Syndrome** 62
    A Somasundaram

13. **Turner Syndrome** 70
    Shambhavi Seth

14. **Noonan Syndrome** 74
    Kawaljit Singh Multani

15. **Fragile X Syndrome** 81
    MA Florita, B Yambao-Dela Cruz, Kaye M Napalinga, Randi J Hagerman

16. **Klinefelter Syndrome** 85
   Kawaljit Singh Multani

17. **Prader-Labhart-Willi Syndrome** 89
   Manju George Elenjickal, Neethu Mary Mathew

18. **Angelman Syndrome** 92
   Shabina Ahmed

19. **Williams Syndrome** 95
   Jyoti Bhatia

20. **Neurofibromatosis** 99
   Z Bassi

21. **Tuberous Sclerosis** 104
   Z Bassi

22. **Mucopolysaccharidosis: Developmental and
    Behavioral Outcomes** 109
   Shibani Kanungo, Neelkamal Soares

23. **Rett Syndrome** 115
   Leena Srivastava

24. **Sleep Disorders** 120
   Leena Srivastava, Kawaljit Singh Multani

25. **Feeding Disorders** 128
   Leena Deshpande

26. **Elimination Disorders** 132
   Kawaljit Singh Multani

27. **Seizures and Epilepsy** 137
   Sarbani Raha, Vrajesh Udani

28. **Cerebral Palsy** 143
   Anaita Udwadia-Hegde, Omkar Pradip Hajirnis

29. **Movement Disorders in Children with
    Neurodevelopmental Disorders** 147
   Abhishek R Jain, Lokesh Lingappa

30. **Neuroregressive Disorders** 154
   Shekhar Patil

31. **Inborn Errors of Metabolism: Developmental and
    Behavioral Outcomes** 158
   Shibani Kanungo, Neelkamal Soares

32. Traumatic Brain Injury 162
    Prameela Joji

33. Neuromalignancies and Developmental Outcomes......................166
    Vasudha N Rao, Samir H Dalwai

34. Attention Deficit Hyperactivity Disorder 170
    Samir H Dalwai, Hilla Sukhadwala

35. Disruptive Behavior Disorders 175
    Leena Deshpande

36. Anxiety..180
    Manoj Bhatawdekar

37. Depressive Disorders...185
    Kersi Chavda, Alka A Subramanyam

38. Tics..190
    Kawaljit Singh Multani

39. Hearing Abnormalities in Children:
    Assessment and Management...195
    Abraham K Paul

40. Visual Impairment 202
    Neepa Thackar Dave

41. Balance Disorders and Dizziness in Children............................205
    Waheeda Pagarkar

42. Developmental Coordination Disorder 211
    Leena Deshpande

43. Sensory Processing Disorders: Developmental Aspects............215
    Leena Deshpande

44. Language and Speech Disorders..220
    Patricia Osbourn

45. Selective Mutism 223
    Samir H Dalwai

46. Medical Comorbidities in Autism Spectrum Disorder 227
    Yamini Jagannath Howe, Ann M Neumeyer

47. Autism Spectrum Disorder 231
    Samir H Dalwai

48. Scholastic Backwardness 239
    SS Kamath, Kawaljit Singh Multani

49. Development Behavioral Disorders in Adolescence 243
    Dilip R Patel, Swati Y Bhave

50. Specific Learning Disability 248
    Samir H Dalwai, Hilla Sukhadwala

51. Child Abuse 253
    Shabina Ahmed

52. Role of Evaluation in Developmental Behavioral Pediatrics 256
    Anjan Bhattacharya

53. Early Intervention 261
    Zafar Mahmood Meenai

54. Therapies and Interventions 266
    Lata Bhat

55. Principles of Pharmacotherapy in Developmental and
    Behavioral Pedaitrics 272
    Jeeson C Unni

56. Counseling 276
    Leena Deshpande, Lavanya Iyer

57. Electronic Media and Gadgets 281
    Samir H Dalwai, Barkha Chawla

58. Technology in Practice 287
    Kawaljit Singh Multani

59. Complementary and Alternative Medicine in
    Developmental Pediatrics 291
    Shambhavi Seth

60. Medicolegal Issues in Developmental and
    Behavioral Pediatrics 294
    Santhosh Rajagopal

Index *299*

Chapter 1

A History of Developmental Behavioral Pediatrics: An Idea whose Time has Come

Samir H Dalwai

"Men are haunted by the vastness of eternity. And so we ask ourselves: will our actions echo across the centuries? Will strangers hear our names long after we are gone, and wonder who we were, how bravely we fought, how fiercely we loved?"

David Benioff, Original Screenplay, Troy

"In the history of medicine, it is not always the great scientist or the learned doctor who goes forward to discover new fields, new avenues, and new ideas."

Elizabeth Kenny

INTRODUCTION

The major religions of the world have all advocated a progressive and inclusive outlook toward people with disability. In reality, for much of recorded history, disability was regarded as the result of evil spirits, the devil, witchcraft, or God's displeasure. History is rife with illustrations of the inhumane and shameful treatment of people with disabilities.

Gradually, "the doctor and the scientist replaced the priest as custodian of societal values and curing processes." Institutions for the disabled were established to allow other family members to meet work obligations and also to train the former for some vocational productive activity. The goal of interventions was to provide the person with the appropriate skills to rehabilitate or deal with it.

According to Jayne Clapton and Jennifer Fitzgerald, "Institutions became the instruments for the facilitation of exclusion and social death." In recent times, the notion of "disability" is seen from a rights-based sociopolitical assertion. The focus has moved away from exclusion and dependence (state-run institutions) to inclusion and independence (community-based facilities and care); countries have enacted legislation, which seeks to address issues of social justice and discrimination.

The history of developmental behavioral pediatrics is the story of pediatricians taking disability away from these rigid frameworks into a promotive as well as a healing positive space. This is the story of their emerging interest and expertise in developmental psychology and behavioral psychology: and the combination of both disciplines to shape this interdisciplinary field, and ultimately making its own space within general pediatrics to become a subspecialty.

William Healy, a Chicago physician, in 1909, setup the first child guidance clinic to deal with children exhibiting antisocial behavior, thus attempting to separate delinquency from the criminal justice system and establishing the role of personality that lay behind much of their behavioral problems. His pioneering work to separate behavioral psychology from the justice system has its roots in early theories of child development that have thereafter shaped modern theories of developmental behavioral pediatrics.

Since the late 1800s, the field of human development is a field devoted to identifying and explaining changes in behavior, abilities, and attributes that individuals experience throughout their lives. Charles Darwin's *A Biological Sketch of an Infant*, and more significantly, his famed *theory of evolution* was the driving force behind the discipline of developmental psychology and inspired many. Among them, G Stanley Hall considered to be the founder of American developmental psychology, believed that human development follows a course similar to that of the evolution of the species. His mentee at Clark University, Sigmund Freud proposed that development occurs through the resolution of conflict between what a person wants to do versus what the person *should* do. This notion formed the basis of Freud's *theory of psychosexual development*. Freud's *interactionist* perspective believed that both, biological and environmental factors, influenced human development (although he believed that environmental factors, such as parenting, were far more impactful). In contrast, the *maturational theory* of Arnold Gesell represents the biological theory that child development is a naturally unfolding progression that occurs according to some internal biological timetable and learning and teaching cannot override this timetable. Gesell held that children are "self-regulating" and develop only as they are ready to do so. He established the statistical norms to describe this sequence, as well as the age range within which each early behavior normally appears updated versions of which are still in use as general guidelines for normal development. He was the first to capture children's observations on film and also pioneered the use of one-way viewing screens.

Gesell's work on similarities across children's development and his focus on patterns of behavior set the stage for Jean Piaget. Unlike Gesell's method, in which the researcher stood apart from his objects of study, Piaget developed a research technique known as the *clinical method.* He worked on the study of the nature of knowledge in young children, as well as how it changes as they grow older. He termed this area of study *genetic epistemology*. According to his *cognitive-developmental theory*, children universally progress through a series of stages: the *sensorimotor stage* (birth to age 2 years), the *preoperational stage* (ages 2–7 years), the *concrete operational stage* (ages 7–11 years), and the *formal operational stage* (ages 11 years and beyond). He emphasized that children play an active role in their own development. This contribution laid the foundation for behavioral genetics.

Piaget's theory was at variance with Lev Vygotsky's *sociocultural* perspective, which emphasized the role of social interactions in cognitive development. According to Vygotsky, cognitive development occurs when children incorporate and internalize feedback from adults, parents, and teachers.

Pediatrics with its charter for preventive as well as curative care of children during their entire childhood (from birth to adulthood) was the natural specialty of medicine to see the developmental and behavioral problems first and try to manage them. Bronson Crothers, an eminent pediatric neurologist at Boston Children's Hospital, posited that ideally the pediatrician was in the best position to deal with children's behavior in the context of the family with emphasis on prevention and early diagnosis.

Thus, the basis for this subspecialty lay in the work of many pioneers in the early part of the last century that emphasized the common interests of psychology, psychiatry, and pediatrics. In 1970, Stanford Friedman was perhaps the first to use the term "behavioral pediatrics"; he defined behavioral pediatrics as "an area within pediatrics which focuses on the psychological, social, and learning problems of children and adolescents." He later added that in addition to "problem oriented" aspects of pediatrics, behavioral pediatrics also included prevention, advocacy, ward and clinic management, and the interdisciplinary delivery of health care.

In the 1975 special issue of Pediatric Clinics of North America, Julius Richmond titled his article *"An Idea Whose Time Has Come".* The other articles in this issue defined the different areas of behavioral pediatrics by major early investigators in the field and the list of chapter headings in the issue is an interesting way to gauge the field at that point of time.

In May 1982, Esther Wender and colleagues in the United States proposed the development of a permanent academic organization for sharing research findings in behavioral pediatrics and child development, to promote its teaching in pediatric residency programs, and act as a resource and advocacy group to promote mental health needs of children. As happens in a vibrant academic environment, after considerable ado over challenges to name and domain (and turf), this organization is what we are today know as Society for Developmental and Behavioral Pediatrics—thus formally bringing together the two streams of developmental medicine and behavioral psychology.

One of the leading lights of this movement, Melvine Levine extolled how we are "inextricably bound to general pediatric primary care" as one of the attributes that define us, along with "functioning at the tight junctions between psyche and soma, between the indigenous forces of nature and the shaping powers of nurture."

The initiative of pioneers like Marvin Gottlieb led to the publication of the Journal of Developmental and Behavioral Pediatrics (JDBP), in March of 1980.

Thus, though developmental behavioral pediatrics has strong roots going back to the 1920s; the reality in clinical practice was summarized, amusingly, in 1985 by Stanford Friedman as "those aspects of pediatrics generally ignored by most pediatric training programs." This was the beginning of incorporating developmental behavioral pediatrics as a subspecialty in pediatrics residency programs and also establishing subspecialty certification in developmental behavioral pediatrics.

THE INDIA STORY

According to Janeway, the course taken by most subspecialty areas of pediatrics traverses thus—"A small group of innovative pioneers develops new skills (both clinical and research), they come together at meetings and found their own society, train successors, publish a scientific journal, and finally obtain subspecialty certification. This whole process usually takes 20–30 years." The Indian Academy of Pediatrics (IAP) played a stellar role by offering a platform for developmental behavioral pediatrics in India. Publication of the first National Consensus Guidelines for Autism, attention deficit hyperactivity disorder (ADHD), learning disability and newborn hearing screening in 2017, establishment of the IAP fellowship for developmental and behavioral pediatrics and now the first official handbook representing a nationwide and beyond repertoire of authors has firmly established this subspecialty in India. The author acknowledges the support of innumerable stalwarts from IAP in this pioneering effort.

THE FUTURE

The number and quality of conferences and training programs has significantly increased and spread across the country, especially with the digital format post the coronavirus disease-2019 (COVID-19) lockdown and the emergence of dIAP (digital IAP). However, the real success of this movement will be judged more by how well this research and training involves general pediatricians and their practices. This needs to result in improving the developmental and behavioral health of children in the country. Considering the huge numbers needing help, there will never be enough specialists and it is left to a collaboration between general pediatricians and developmental behavioral pediatricians to care for every child needing these services.

Sharing the views of Ruth Stein, "The early workers recognized that the longitudinal process of child development distinguishes pediatric medicine from all other medical specialties, and child development and behavior have an impact on every pediatric healthcare encounter. This fascination drew many general pediatricians who saw development and behavior as the foundation of pediatrics and involved themselves with clinical care, teaching, and research activities of development and behavior as a general pediatrician. They saw development and behavior as so fundamental to all clinical pediatrics that it was hard to segregate it as a subspecialty. Hence, in the words of Haggerty and Richmond, we must hold forth that "Child development is a basic science of pediatrics and must be a central part of the skills of all pediatricians. The task now for developmental behavioral pediatrics is to complete the circle by finding ways to train pediatricians in the treatment and prevention of the large numbers of children with developmental, behavioral, and educational problems and not to become an isolated silo of expertise."

It now devolves upon the present generation of pediatricians and developmental behavioral pediatricians to make these dreams a reality.

FURTHER READING

1. Crothers B. A Pediatrician in Search of Mental Hygiene. The Commonwealth Fund. New York: London Oxford Press; 1937.
2. Friedman SB. Introduction: Behavioral Pediatrics. Pediatr Clin N Am. 1975;22:55.
3. Haggerty RJ, Friedman SB. History of developmental-behavioral pediatrics. J Dev Behav Pediatr. 2003;24(1):S1-18.
4. Hansen RL. Magical history tour of the Society for Developmental and Behavioral Pediatrics: Reflections on deletions, slashes, hyphens, and developmental context. Dev Behav Pediatr. 2010;31(5):441-8.
5. Holmbeck G, Jandasek B, Sparks C, Zukerman JM, Zurenda L. Theoretical Foundations of Developmental-Behavioral Pediatrics, Developmental-Behavioral Pediatrics. Elsevier Inc.; 2008.
6. Janeway CA. Growth and development of academic pediatrics in North America. Pediatr Res. 1971;5:560.
7. Richmond JB: Child development: A basic science of pediatrics. Pediatrics. 1967;39(5):649-58.
8. Stein REK. Are we on the right track? Examining the role of developmental behavioral pediatrics. Pediatrics. 2015;135(4):589-91.
9. The History of Disability: A History of 'Otherness'. [online] Available from: http://www.ru.org/index.php/human-rights/315-the-history-of-disability-a-history-of-otherness (Last accessed December, 2021).
10. Wender EH, Friedman SB. Proceedings of the National Conference on Behavioral Pediatrics, March 3-5, 1985, Easton, Maryland. J Dev Behav Pediatr. 1985;6:179.

Chapter 2

Normal Development and Behavior

Kawaljit Singh Multani

"If we want children to move mountains, we first have to let them get out of chairs."

Nicolette Sowder

INTRODUCTION

Development is defined as the acquisition of new skills and new functions and refers to the qualitative changes occurring in a child over time as he grows into an adult. Development is closely linked to maturation of the central nervous system (CNS) which is developing at a very fast rate in utero and early years of life. It is a continuous, orderly process that follows a certain set of principles which are discussed later. Development of a child is classically understood using the maturational-developmental theory of Arnold Gesell **(Fig. 1)** which describes growth as a cyclical spiral starting from conception till adulthood which consists of six turns. As the spiral grows, its speed slows and it widens

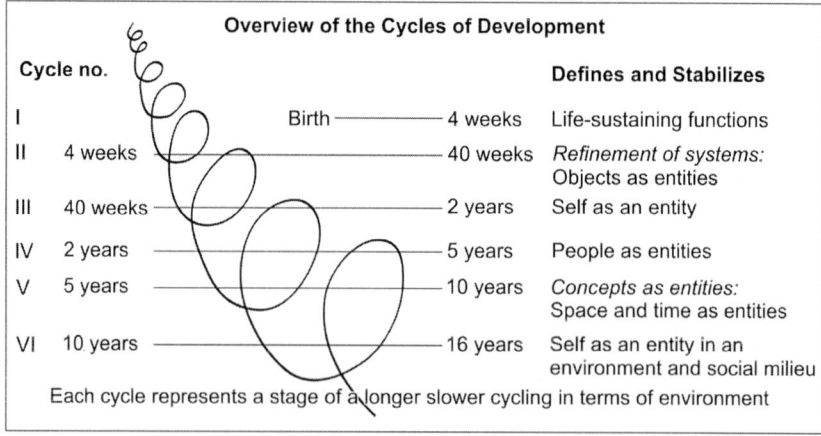

Cycle no.			Defines and Stabilizes
I		Birth — 4 weeks	Life-sustaining functions
II	4 weeks	— 40 weeks	*Refinement of systems: Objects as entities*
III	40 weeks	— 2 years	Self as an entity
IV	2 years	— 5 years	People as entities
V	5 years	— 10 years	*Concepts as entities: Space and time as entities*
VI	10 years	— 16 years	Self as an entity in an environment and social milieu

Overview of the Cycles of Development

Each cycle represents a stage of a longer slower cycling in terms of environment

Fig. 1: Gesell's spiral.

thereby widening and opening up as age advances. Each turn/cycle of spiral has six stages—smooth, breakup, sorting out, inwardizing, expanding, and "neurotic" fitting together which keep recurring throughout life. Gesell's research established normative trends for child development milestones in four areas, namely (1) motor, (2) adaptive (cognitive), (3) language, and (4) personal-social, which was originally published in 1925. His maturational theory lays a lot of emphasis on maturation of CNS and does not take into account the effect of external factors like environment of the child. There are many other theories of child development which will be discussed in the subsequent chapter.

PRINCIPLES OF DEVELOPMENT

Development of the child is guided by certain principles which are as under:
- Development is a dynamic process and the pattern of development is similar in all children.
- General behavior/responses are replaced by specific behavior/responses with time. The general movements of fetus and neonate are replaced by goal-directed movements in early infancy.
- Development can be divided into stages/periods with each stage having its own characteristics. Stages of development can be broadly divided into:
  - Prenatal period (from conception to birth)
  - Neonatal period (first month of life)
  - Infancy (1 month to 1 year)
  - Early childhood (1-6 years)
  - Late childhood (6-13 years)
  - Adolescence (>13 years)
  - Adulthood
- Development follows two sequences in the body: Cephalocaudal and proximodistal. First, the head stabilizes and then the trunk followed by the limbs. Proximal limb movement control appears first followed by more refined distal movements especially in upper limbs.
- In case of CNS, the development of function follows the pattern of myelination, i.e., from hind brain toward forebrain and from occipital lobe toward frontal lobe. This pattern is fixed but the rate varies between individuals.
- Each child has its own rate of development which is predictable.
- Primitive reflexes, e.g., Moro's reflex, have to be lost or modified in order to learn more complex motor behavior(s).
- There exist critical/sensitive periods in human development during which the child is most responsive to stimulation (biological and/or environmental). The best example for this is the hearing and language

development which has been extensively studied and researched. Children with hearing problems picked up early in life develop the maximum in the language domain; hence, the 1-3-6 approach in hearing screening of neonates advocated by Indian Academy of Pediatrics (IAP) which is discussed in a later chapter.

Measuring Development

Measurement of a child's development is a complex task that involves historical inputs from parents as well as measuring child's abilities using standardized tests and comparing the results with available standards for children of same age. Developmental evaluation of children is divided into four major domains—Physical/motor, social, cognitive, and language. Each domain has age-specific milestones and these form the basis of developmental surveillance and screening. Milestones of development in the four domains are represented based on the normative data of population with most children achieving the milestone by the end of the upper limit of age provided for the milestone being evaluated. Atypical development can be in the form of developmental delay (single domain or global if there is more than one domain affected), deviation (out of sequence development), dissociation (significant differences in rates of development in different domains) or regression (loss of previously-acquired milestones).

Many tests are available for developmental testing which may take few minutes to few hours. A simple convenient Indian test for office use is Trivandrum development screening chart (TDSC) which was initially designed for children up to 2 years of age and later updated to include children up to 6 year of age **(Figs. 2, 3, and 4)**. A detailed discussion on

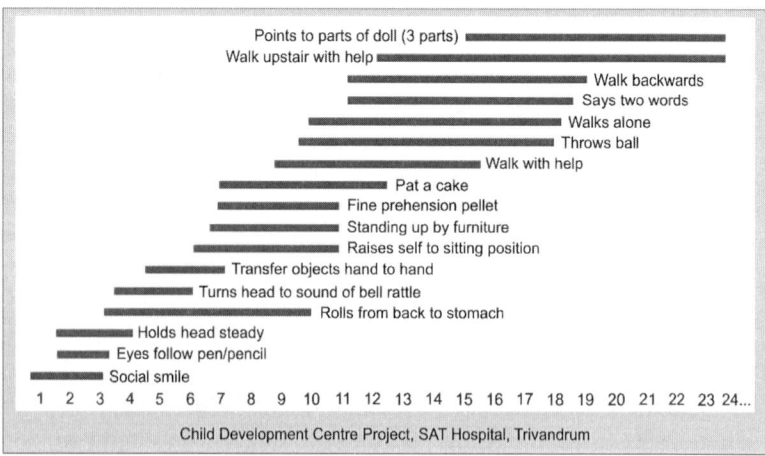

Fig. 2: Trivandrum developmental screening chart (TDSC).

Normal Development and Behavior 9

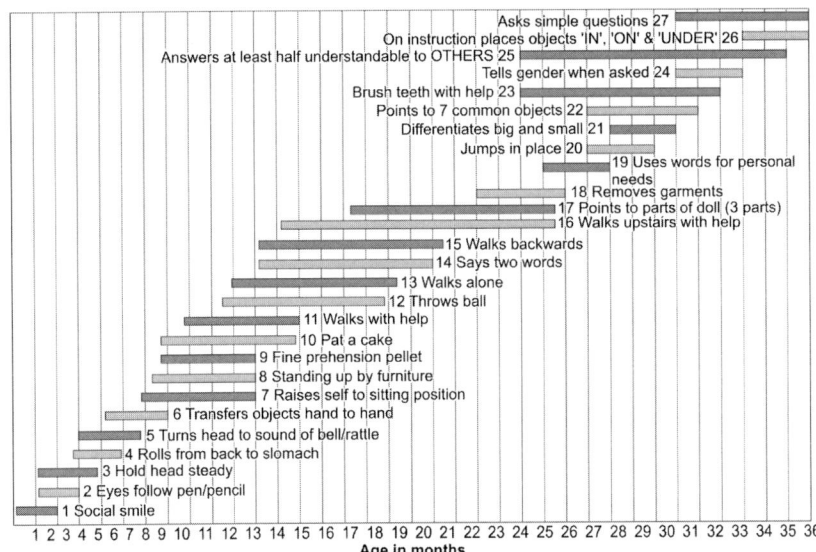

Fig. 3: Trivandrum Developmental Screening Chart (TDSC) (0–3 years).

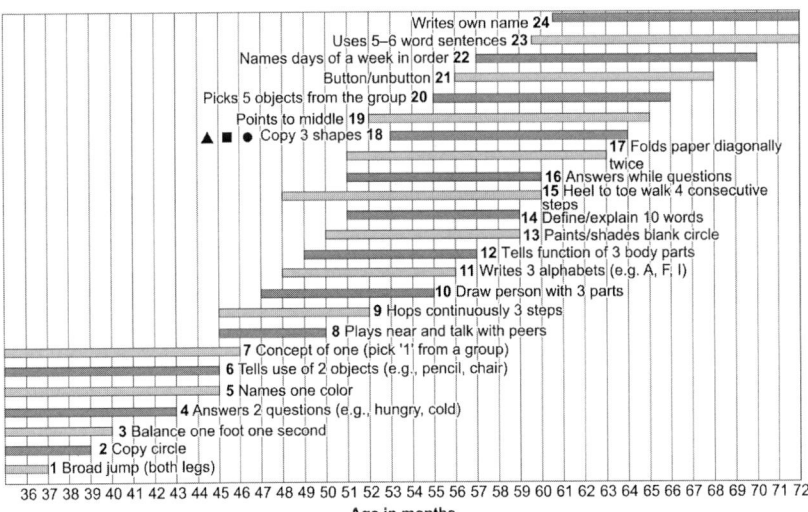

Fig. 4: Trivandrum developmental screening chart (TDSC) 3–6 years.

developmental testing is done in a later chapter. Children up to 6 years are tested using developmental quotient (DQ) which is derived using the formula: [developmental age (DA)/chronological age (CA)] × 100. For children above 6 years of age, multiple tests of intelligence are available and the results of

Normal Development and Behavior

Table 1: Key developmental milestones at 3, 6, 9, 18 and 24 months.

Age/Domain	Gross motor	Fine motor	Language	Personal-social
3 months	Neck control+	Hand regard+	Cooing+	Social smile+
6 months	Rolls over	Immature grasp	Monosyllables	Stranger anxiety+
9 months	Sits without support	Pincer grasp	Bisyllables	Separation anxiety+
18 months	Walks independently	Four cube tower	10–25 words	Pretend play+
24 months	Climbs stairs	Train of cubes	2–3 word sentences	Parallel play+

intelligence testing are labelled as intelligence quotient (IQ). A score of 70 or less in DQ or IQ is taken as abnormal and requires further evaluation and intervention in some form.

Developmental Milestones

The first few years of a child are crucial as they form the base for learning and development later in life. Research on child development has generated lot of interest in the area of early identification and intervention. Developmental milestones in different domains have been identified with upper limits of age for achieving the milestones. Some key developmental milestones at 3, 6, 9, 18, and 24 months are listed in **Table 1**.

Issues with Preterm Babies/Neonatal Intensive Care Unit Graduates

Every year, a large number of preterm babies are born whose survival rates are increasing with each passing year due to advances in neonatal care. The incidence of neurodevelopmental disabilities is higher in these children as compared to children born at term. The development pattern in these cases needs to be assessed after taking into account the extent of prematurity of the child. Corrected age [age of child based on expected delivery date (EDD) of the mother than actual delivery date of the child] should be used while assessing the developmental status of the child. This concession of corrected age to preterm babies is given till 24 months of age for "catching up" on development though there are no consensus guidelines for this. Preterm babies also have a higher incidence of issues in visual, hearing, language, and social domains in addition to motor domain and should be kept under follow up as they are likely to have behavioral issues and learning disabilities later in life.

Chapter 3

Theories of Normal Development and Behavior

Kawaljit Singh Multani

"The lengthy development process that humans experience are a "luxury" and we know that things evolve in a certain way because there is an advantage to it."

Marianella Casasola

INTRODUCTION

Human beings differ from most other animal species on the planet as they are the only species whose offspring continue to remain dependent on the parents and other caregivers for a prolonged period of time. In studies of comparative cognitive development among different species, it has been seen that this provides them longer periods for complex skill acquisition.

Historically, nativist theorists such as Plato and Descartes have been of the view that all characteristics and behavior of a person are as a result of inheritance and there is little role of one's environment; while those favoring the environmental influences on child development and behavior believe that all learning and behavior are a result of conditioning. The 20th century saw a surge in the research in the field of child development and behavior and many theories have been proposed by different scientists and researchers. Some of these theories are outlined here based on their main themes:

THEORIES ON CHILD DEVELOPMENT

- Psychoanalytical theories
  - Psychosexual: Sigmund Freud (1959) **(Fig. 1)**
  - Psychosocial: Erik Erikson (1980) **(Fig. 2)**
- Behavioral and behaviorism
  - Classical conditioning: John Watson (1928) **(Fig. 3)**
  - Operant conditioning: BF Skinner (1953) **(Fig. 4)**
- Social learning theories
  - Social learning: Albert Bandura (1977) **(Fig. 5)**

14 Theories of Normal Development and Behavior

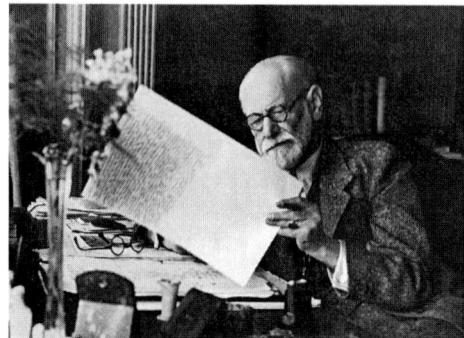

Fig. 1: Sigmund Freud.

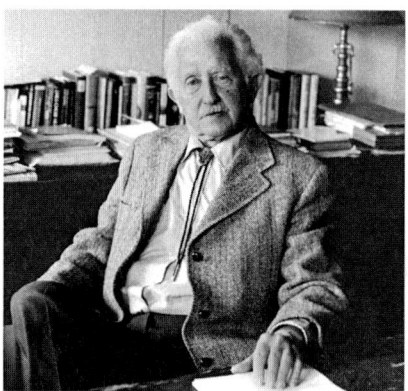

Fig. 2: Erik Erikson.

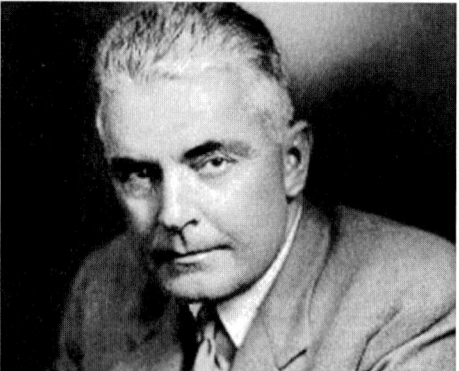

Fig. 3: John Watson.

- Biological theories
  - Maturationism: G Stanley Hall **(Fig. 6)** and Arnold Gesell (1950) **(Fig. 7)**
  - Ethology: Konrad Lorenz **(Fig. 8)**
  - Attachment: John Bowlby

Red Flags

Red flags in developmental context refer to critical milestones which if missed by a child should alert the parents or the clinician and the child should undergo a detailed developmental evaluation and if required, be started on early intervention programme. Children having red flags in language domain should also be evaluated for autism spectrum disorders.

Behavior and Temperament

Behavior is the response of an individual to his/her environment. Behavior is affected by one's feelings, needs, and emotions. It is closely linked to one's temperament. A child's temperament develops early in life and is influenced by biology and experiences. Rothbart and Bates qualify a person's temperamental differences based on three "A's"—differences in an individual's affective (emotional response), activational (physical energy) and attentive cores (concentration). These temperamental differences affect the behavior in everyday life and hence, some children are easy going while some are difficult to handle. Knowledge of a child's behavior and temperament is helpful for parents and teachers to deal with issues at home and school in order to avoid conflicts. Behavior of a person changes with time and can be modified while temperament may not. Many developmental theories are based on evolution of human behavior and will be discussed in the next chapter. As a child grows and learns, he picks up different behaviors based on multiple factors around him. Some behaviors are considered good while some are problematic either for the parents or society and are often a cause of concern for the parents. Multiple methods are available for assessing behavior and behavioral issues in children and commonly used ones include case history method, behavior rating scales, checklist, and questionnaire methods.

Early Intervention

Early identification and early intervention in cases with suspected/confirmed developmental delay has been found to have the best outcome in many observational studies. Targeted early intervention services like physical therapy, speech and language therapy, occupational therapy, and special education can work wonders and intervention plan should be preferably individualized for every child, if possible.

"The moment I decided to follow instead of lead, I discovered the joys of becoming part of a small child's world."

Janet Gonzalez-Mena

FURTHER READING

1. Berk LE. Child Development. 9th Edition. Boston, Massachusetts: Pearson; 2017.
2. Gesell A, Ilg FL. Child development: An introduction to the study of human growth. New York, Harper; 1949.
3. Illingworth RS. The development of infant and young child: Normal and abnormal, 10th Edition. London: Churchill Livingstone; 2013.
4. Nair MK, Nair GS, George B, Suma N, Neethu C, Leena ML, et al. Development and validation of Trivandrum Development Screening Chart for children aged 0-6 years. Indian J Pediatr. 2013;80:S248-55.
5. Scharf RJ, Scharf GJ, Stroustrup A. Developmental milestones. Pediatr Rev. 2016;37(1):25-37.

Theories of Normal Development and Behavior 15

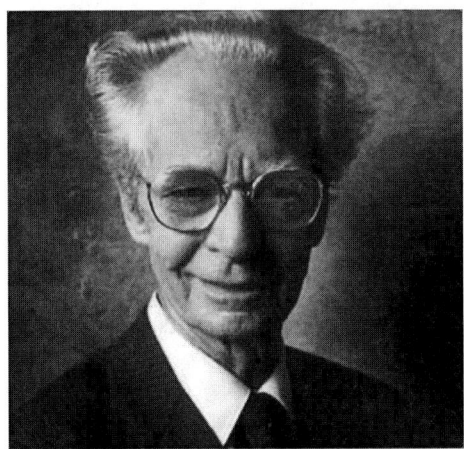

Fig. 4: BF Skinner.

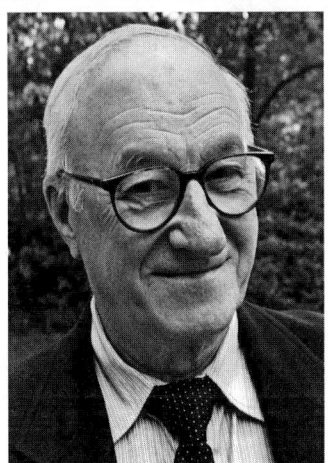

Fig. 5: Albert Bandura.

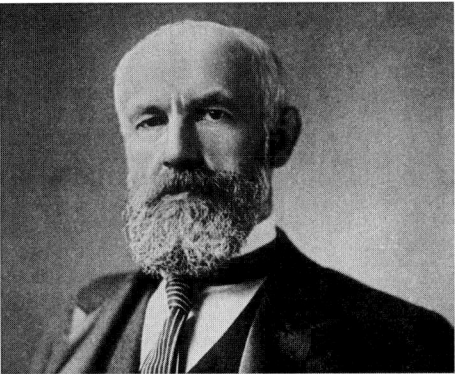

Fig. 6: G Stanley Hall.

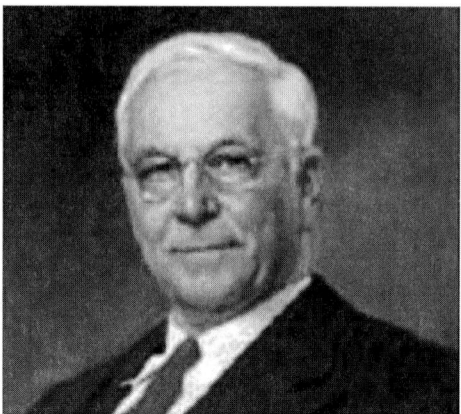

Fig. 7: Arnold Gessel.

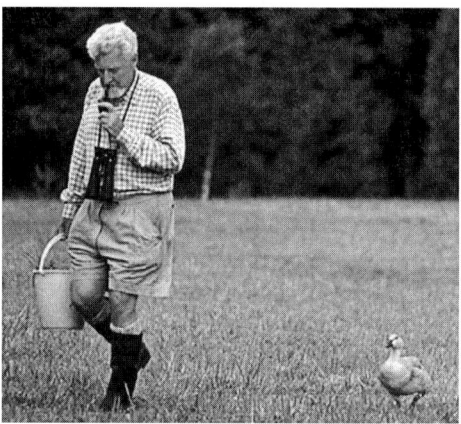

Fig. 8: Konard Lorenz.

- Cognitive theories
  - Cognitive development: Jean Piaget (1952) **(Fig. 9)**
  - Sociocultural: Lev Vygotsky (1978) **(Fig. 10)**
  - Information processing theory: George A Miller (1954)
  - Theory of multiple intelligences: Howard Gardener (1983)
- Systems theories
  - Ecological systems: Urie Bronfenbrenner (1977) **(Fig. 11)**

According to the psychoanalytical theories, a child's development and behavior is a result of conflicts between biological drives and societal expectations as the child moves through different stages in life. Freud highlighted the role of parents on the formation of the child's personality (psychosexual development) as he manages his sexual and aggressive drives. Erikson focused on the role of social influences on child's personality

Theories of Normal Development and Behavior 17

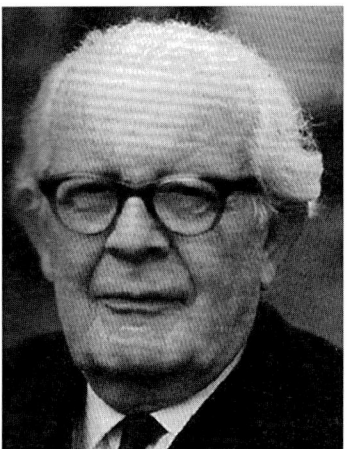
Fig. 9: Jean Piaget.

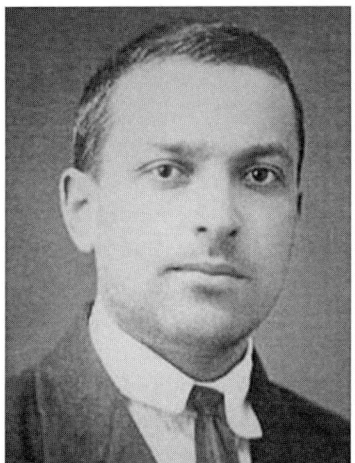
Fig. 10: Lev Vygotsky.

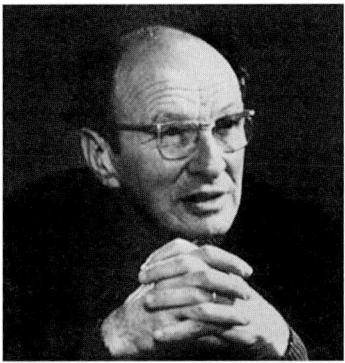
Fig. 11: Urie Bronfenbrenner.

(psychosocial development) while expanding on Freud's work and added that development is a lifelong continuous process.

The behavioral theories proposed that children are passive beings, like clay, and can be molded by their experiences, thereby highlighting the role of environment and nurture in a child's development. John Watson is considered the "father of American behaviorist theory" and most of his work is based on the famous works of Pavlov with dogs. Skinner introduced the term "operant conditioning" to highlight the role of the environment in learning and repetition of the same response to promote a certain behavior. Skinner believed that learning can be broken into small tasks and offering small rewards for accomplishing individual tasks will promote learning. There are four types of operant conditioning: positive reinforcement, negative reinforcement, punishment, and extinction. The first two strengthen behavior while the other two weaken behavior. These theories form the basis of various forms of behavior therapies in vogue today as well as guiding parents and teachers in handling children.

According to the social learning theory of Albert Bandura, children learn by observation and imitation. With time, children become selective in what they imitate. In his famous Bobo doll experiment, Bandura demonstrated that children can learn aggressive behaviors by simply observing another person acting aggressively.

According to the biological theories, development is based on heredity and it is the innate biological processes that govern growth and development. In their theory of maturationism, G Stanley Hall and Arnold Gessell proposed that there is a predetermined biological time table—"milestones of development" and proposed a normative approach to study of child development using age averages for defining what is normal versus abnormal. The theory, though widely popular, suffers from the issue of oversimplification and its disregard of the environmental influences on development and behavior. Konrad Lorenz, also known for his work on imprinting, in his theory of Ethology describes how behavior of a species is affected by its need for survival and describes critical and sensitive periods of learning which has its roots in Darwin's research on evolution. John Bowlby applied the ethological principles to his theory of attachment to describe how a child's attachment to its mother and caregivers can ensure the child's survival.

Cognitive development theories primarily focus on the learning of children and how they learn. Piaget's cognitive development theory believed that the child's development is guided by self-centered, focused activities which are the result of interaction of the child with his/her environment as he/she matures into an adult. It divides the child's life into four stages of development—(1) sensorimotor stage (birth–2 years), (2) preoperational stage (2–7 years), (3) concrete-operational stage (7–11 years), and (4) formal

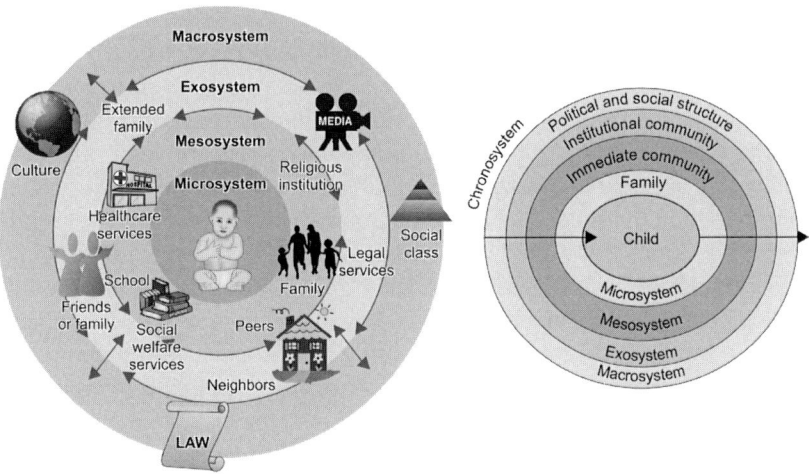

Fig. 12: Systems theory—the old and the new.

operational stage (11 years and beyond). Vygotsky in his sociocultural theory added the concept of "zone of proximal learning" and the role of family and society in a child's learning. He maintained that a child is a social being and his cognitive development is due to social interactions and highlighted the importance of language and culture. Miller, in his information processing theory, equates the human brain to a computer and how the brain responds/learns to/from the various inputs/interactions over a period of time; thereby highlighting the continuous pattern of development. He introduced the concepts of chunking, magic number "7" and TOTE (test-operate-test-exit). Gardener, in his theory of multiple intelligences, proposed that each individual has seven types of intelligences: linguistic, musical, logical-mathematical, spatial, body-kinesthetic, intrapersonal (insight), and interpersonal (social skills) and this provides a framework for different methods for teaching and assessment methods for children.

According to the bioecological systems model by Bronfenbrenner, the child's development is governed by the different systems in a child's environment, like a set of Russian dolls and the inter-relationships between these systems. The systems of a child are divided into microsystem, mesosystem, exosystem, and macrosystem, as shown in the picture; later, the concept of time was added to these as a new system called chronosystem which highlights the effects of reciprocal interaction between the child and his systems over a period of time. As the child develops, his zone of interaction expands and the interactions become more and more complex. The theory has four main components—person, processes (proximal and distal), context, and time. These components are intertwined at multiple levels and they play a major role in our understanding of human development **(Fig. 12)**.

CONCLUSION

The nature versus nurture debate on child development has been ongoing for many decades. The child develops as the central nervous system matures with time in an orderly fashion (nature) while the environment plays a crucial role as it provides the child the mould to grow and learn (nurture). Today, it is reasonable to assume that both nature and nurture are intricately intertwined in the process of child development and a bioecological model of child development should be the basis of all future research in the field as well as for formulating plans for enriching child development. These theories have guided us in understanding child development as well as formulating policies and guidelines for child development and education programs. In view of existing research and knowledge, it is safe to say that the earlier rigid views of stages of development are giving way to a more flexible and constantly changing view with a more balanced approach to human development which gives equal importance to the genetic, critical periods of development as well as environmental factors.

"No significant learning occurs without a significant relationship."

James Comer

"Do not limit a child to your own learning, for he was born in another time."

Rabindranath Tagore

FURTHER READING

1. Allen M, Kambouri-Danos M. Substantive conceptual development in preschool science: Contemporary issues and future directions. Early child development and care.
2. Bruer JT. The myth of the first three years: A new understanding of early brain development and lifelong learning. New York: Free press. 1999. p. 235.
3. Damon W, Lerner RM. "Theories of human development: Contemporary perspectives." in Handbook of child psychology. Volume I: Theoretical models of human development, 5th Edition; 1998.
4. Lightfoot C, Cole M, Cole SR. The development of children, 3rd Edition.
5. Piaget J. "Piaget's theory" in Handbook of Child Psychology. Volume I: History, Theory and Methods, 4th Edition. New York: John Wiley; 1983. pp. 41-102.
6. Reynolds CR, Fletcher-Jensen E. Handbook of Clinical Child Neuropsychology, 3rd Edition; 2009.
7. Rosati AG, Wobber V, Hughes K, Santos LR. Comparative developmental psychology: How is human cognitive development unique? Evol Psychol. 2014;12(2):448-73.

Chapter 4

Developmental Concerns in Pediatric Practice

YK Amdekar

INTRODUCTION

There is a difference between family physician, pediatrician, and pediatric specialist. Family physician treats disease while pediatric specialist treats a disease that he thinks child has. Both function as "disease managers". But pediatrician is expected to treat the child in whom disease exists. It means pediatrician should be "health provider" and not just a "disease manager".

CONCEPT OF HEALTH

Health refers to physical (growth), mental (development), and social (behavior) well-being. Parents are generally concerned about growth or at least weight that is checked periodically and behavior is considered as parental responsibility. However, fact remains that growth faltering or behavior aberration if diagnosed late, may often be correctable but it is not so with development. This is because development is connected to functional maturation of brain that nearly achieves its potential by the end of 2 years. Hence, any developmental delay if not picked up early enough may leave behind permanent disability. Thus, developmental monitoring specially in first 2 years of child's life is an important part of pediatric practice. Of course, learning disability may surface subsequently but is often picked-up by parents or teachers.

GROUND REALITY

Present scenario of pediatric practice is far from the ideal and not even close to minimum-expected standards. Majority pediatricians are busy focusing on disease only without seeing the "child". Time spent per patient is so little that it is not enough to do justice to the disease itself, forget anything else about health. This results in failure to pick-up early deviation from normal development and such problems are addressed only after parents notice them, it is often too late. Lack of time is the excuse though it is lack of motivation to do the best. It is sad to diagnose autism spectrum disorder at the age of 3 years when parents are concerned about language delay or abnormal behavior. It is shameful that this very child was seen several times by a pediatrician who was not motivated to look beyond the disease. This child will move in the society as a proof of pediatrician's fault but everyone will blame destiny. I wonder whether pediatrician would take a note of his failure and commit for a change in future, may be, it escapes his attention as he is too busy.

PEDIATRICIANS MUST "DEVELOP"

Development constitutes change for the better. It is a process of transformation and in pediatric practice, it amounts to improvement to extend rational approach to health of children under their care. One of the specific objectives is to monitor child's development to pick-up early deviation, if any, and plan timely action. It is possible if pediatricians develop an approach to improve their power of observation and obtain relevant information from parents. With repeated practice, it does not take much time. Anyway taking time is worth it as it leads to excellence in practice that refers to joy—joy of fulfillment to yourself and spreading joy to children and their parents.

POWER OF OBSERVATION

It is the key to developmental screening in all domains and in all age groups. Child's every visit to a pediatrician offers such an opportunity, be it for routine immunization or any illness. During first 2 years, visits are more frequent and provides the perfect opportunity for monitoring development of child during the most vulnerable period. Note behavior of the child as he enters and observe from a distance while talking to parents. Observe child's response when you look at him, smile or talk to or when offered an age-appropriate object such as toy, picture, or book. Observe while carrying out physical examination and finally see his response when you say "bye-bye" or "namaste". Special attention is necessary for "at risk" children as in case of extreme prematurity, birth injury or dysmorphic features, and family history of delayed development.

AGE-APPROPRIATE BEHAVIOR

Behavior refers to the way child reacts to particular situation. Family dynamics and parenting skills decide child's behavior pattern and so within limits, variations are seen in normal children. Abnormal behavior may be the first sign of developmental delay. Stranger anxiety and enjoying attention at 6–10 months, negative emotions such as refusal or tantrums at 12–18 months, extreme behavior of stubbornness and anger at 2 years, play the major activity with sharing at 3–4 years and more independent and protective around 4–5 years are the patterns of expected behavior in normal children.

MINIMUM DEVELOPMENTAL SCREENING

Even a busy pediatrician is expected to observe few important milestones in every child as it may serve reasonable purpose of quick effective screening. At the age of 3 months, infant must achieve head control to some extent, social smile, recognizing mother, cooing, and finger to mouth coordination. This rules out major handicap as a result of antenatal or perinatal events. At the age of 12 months, child should be able to at least sit without support, respond to his name, and point at familiar objects, understands "no", plays a "pick-a-boo", holds a cup, and explores things around by banging or throwing. At 15 months, he is able to scribble in imitation and follows one-step command. At the age of 18 months, child should have developed expressive verbal language and is interested in pretend play, also makes tower of three blocks. At 2 years, can go up and down, imitates stroke by pencil, follows two-step instruction and has increasing vocabulary. It is ideal to use pen and paper (at 3 years a circle, 3.5 years cross, 4 years square, and 5 years a triangle), blocks (tower of increasing number of blocks and further different patterns such as bridge), draw a man test and naming colors and numbers beyond 4 years.

SUSPECT DEVELOPMENTAL ABNORMALITY

At around 1 year of age, if a child has no stranger anxiety, unaware of surrounding, difficult to stay in one place (though he may sit for longer time in front of TV), purposeless hyperactivity, lack of receptive language, no eye to eye contact, aggressive or undue separation anxiety, and short attention span, it is ideal time to seek expert opinion. At primary school age, if child is disorganized, has trouble with time and completing given tasks, defiant and disobeying attitude, or indulges in physical fighting or lying, it indicates need for referral. At school age, learning disability is suspected, if child has disproportionate poor performance as compared to his potential, inconsistent poor handwriting, reading difficulty, or problems with mathematical numbers.

CONCLUSION

It is pediatrician's responsibility to monitor development in growing children. "Develop" an attitude to become a "developed" pediatrician. Every pediatrician is capable of it, only if he is motivated to get rid of his own potential-performance discrepancy. Then he will enjoy his work and it will have positive impact on his life. Once you get started, habit will sustain it.

Chapter 5

Developmental Surveillance and Screening

Leena Deshpande

"Just Do IT!"

NIKE

Regular physical activity is the key to good mental and physical health. Similarly regular and effective developmental surveillance and screening program can lead to good developmental outcome in children.

INTRODUCTION

It is estimated that around 12–15% of children suffer from some developmental disorder. The benefits of identifying developmental disorders in these children as early as possible are well documented.

The prenatal period and the first 3 years after birth are together considered the single most transformative period in the entire life span for brain development. Neural circuits grow from simple to highly complex. Number of synapses increases rapidly and process of pruning occurs, where neural connections which are useful are strengthened and the ones not being used are lost. This process is highly dependent on environmental stimulation.

Early identification allows treatment to start during this most crucial time in the child's life when intervention can have the greatest impact on brain development. This has the potential to change the developmental trajectory of a child who is "at risk" for neurodevelopmental disabilities. This early identification is possible through effective implementation of a regular developmental surveillance and screening program in everyday office practice.

DEVELOPMENTAL SURVEILLANCE

Developmental surveillance is an informal but structured monitoring of a child's development and interpreting it in the light of the child's medical, social, and environmental factors. It is a flexible continuous process aimed at identifying children who may have developmental problems and is performed at every clinic visit of the child when he/she is well.

It includes:
- Identifying "at risk" children, by reviewing the child's medical history (e.g., prematurity and perinatal complications), family history (genetic, developmental, and mental health disorders), and social history (poverty and domestic violence) which may place the child at an increased risk of developmental problems.
- Reviewing developmental milestones by asking the parents relevant questions and attending to their concerns, if any.
- Developmental observation of motor skills, communication skills, and social engagement to look for slow or abnormal patterns of development.
- Relevant neurological examination.
- Documenting the findings with identification of any delays, dissociation, deviancy, or regression of milestones.

DEVELOPMENTAL SCREENING

Developmental screening is the use of a brief tool at specific ages of the child to identify children who are at risk of developmental disorder. A good screening test should be standardized, reliable, with acceptable sensitivity and specificity. It should be readily available at a low cost and can be administered fairly quickly (<15 minutes). There are various screening tests available, some can be completed by the parents while others are administered by the clinician. Each one covers different age groups.

Some of the common screening tests used are:
- *General screening*: These evaluate multiple areas of development and are commonly used:
  - Parent report: Ages and Stages Questionnaire (ASQ) and Parents' Evaluation of Developmental Status (PEDS)
  - Clinician administered: Bayley's Infant Neurodevelopmental Screen (BINDS), Denver Developmental Screening Test (DDST), Baroda Developmental Screening Test (BDST), Trivandrum Developmental Screening Chart (TDSC)
- *Domain-specific:* These evaluate one area of development:
  - Language Evaluation Scale Trivandrum (LEST)
  - The Early Motor Pattern Profile (EMPP)
- *Disorder-specific:* Helps to identify a specific developmental disorder:
  - Modified Checklist for Autism in Toddlers (M-CHAT-R/F)
  - Social Communication Questionnaire (SCQ).

The ages for screening are selected on the basis of times in the child's life when key developmental problems can be identified, e.g., gross and fine motor skills and early social skills at 9 months, early language, and emerging social skills at 18 months (when autism spectrum disorder can be detected) and expressive and receptive language development at 30 months of age.

It is vital to remember that screening tests are not diagnostic, rather it is a process by which child's development in one or more domains may be identified as atypical as compared with children of same age.

Screening tests help parents (irrespective of the parents' educational or socioeconomic status) to observe their child's development and behavior, making them understand the development expected at a particular age. It also helps the clinician to start a discussion with parents regarding potential delay in their child's development, if any.

Step-wise Approach

The current recommendations (by American Academy of Pediatricians) advocate developmental surveillance at each well baby visit. If no concerns are identified at the surveillance and the child is developing typically, the clinician apart from documenting this should also discuss age appropriate specific developmental stimulation activities for the child. If however, there are concerns identified during developmental surveillance, the child should undergo a standardized Developmental Screening Test (or referred directly for in-depth developmental evaluation, if significant concerns) to verify the concerns.

In addition to routine developmental surveillance, each child should undergo Developmental Screening Test at 9 months, 18 months, and 30 months of age. Autism screening is recommended at 18 months and 24 months of age. Screening at 4–5 years may also be useful for school readiness.

When screening confirms developmental concerns, next step is:
- Referral to appropriate professional for a complete developmental evaluation to diagnose a specific developmental disorder
- Medical evaluation to determine etiology of the developmental disorder
- Referral for therapeutic intervention to local early intervention program
- Parental counseling and ongoing support.

BEHAVIORAL SURVEILLANCE AND SCREENING

The focus of Developmental Surveillance and Screening program is in early infancy and preschool age children, behavioral surveillance requires extension into later childhood. Combining Developmental and Behavioral Surveillance is useful as often developmental delays may manifest through atypical behavioral patterns. Behavioral surveillance should include eliciting parental concerns of compliance, tantrums, activity levels, attention, and aggression. Any unusual patterns of behaviors such as repetitive speech, hand flapping, excess obsession with objects, self-injurious behavior, unusual visual gaze, etc., may be observed.

Behavioral screening: Standardized tools are available and are recommended over informal clinical judgment. Key ages for behavioral screening should be:
- 30 months
- Prior to school entry (4–5 years)
- 8 year visit
- Adolescence

Various behavioral screening tools recommended are:
- Pediatric symptom checklist (PSC) is a 35 quest checklist 4–16 years, is useful as a screening tool to identify moderate to severe impairments in children's psychosocial functioning.
- Ages and Stages Questionnaire-Social emotional (SE): 3–60 months
- Strengths and difficulties questionnaire: 3–17 years
- Vanderbilt Parent Rating Scale (VPRS): 6 years and older
- Child behavior checklist (CBCL).

If behavioral concerns are confirmed by the screening test, further evaluation by trained professional in developmental and behavioral pediatrics should be done.

Practical Tip

In the Indian scenario, developmental surveillance may work effectively if linked to the immunization ages. The child is seen for immunization at least 7–8 times in the first 2 years of life. This is the time when the child is well and parents are relaxed. The ages at which the child is given various immunization are good for looking at key developmental milestones.

There are many effective Developmental Screening Tests available. It is important that the clinician gets expertise in any one test and ensure regular use of the same in his everyday office practice.

This will help to have a sustainable developmental surveillance and screening program to detect developmental and behavioral problems early.

FURTHER READING

1. Pierce K, Courchesne E, Bacon E. To screen or not to screen for ASD universally is Not the Question: Why the Task Force Got it Wrong. J Pediatr. 2016;176:182-94.
2. Voigt RG, Macias MM, Myers SM. Developmental and Behavioral Pediatrics. Developmental and behavioral surveillance and screening within the medical home. Am Acad Pediatr. 2011;69-92.
3. William Carey, Allen Crocker et al. Developmental screening and assessment: Infants, toddlers, and preschoolers. Developmental-Behavioral Pediatrics. 4th Edition, 2009; 785-88.

Chapter 6

Approach to Global Developmental Delay

Leena Srivastava

"Many things we need can wait. The Child cannot...

Right now is the time his bones are being formed, his brain and his senses are being developed.

To him we cannot answer "Tomorrow". His name is "Today".
Adapted from the original by Gabriela Mistral

INTRODUCTION

Developmental delay is a term for the child who has a significant delay in the acquisition of milestones or skills, in one or more domains of development (i.e., gross motor, fine motor, speech/language, cognitive, personal/social, or activities of daily living). A significant delay has been operationally defined as discrepancy of 25% or more from the expected rate, or two standard deviations lower than the norm for the age. Global developmental delay (GDD) is defined as a delay in two or more developmental domains. GDD affects 1–3% of the population of children under 5 years of age. In India, the prevalence of developmental delay in children under 2 years of age is reported between 1.5–2.5%.

Unfortunately, the term "delay" is wrongly interpreted by many professionals and families alike that the child will eventually "catch up", thus delaying timely referrals. A recent international consensus conference has thus proposed early developmental impairment (EDI) as a more appropriate diagnostic term.

In addition to delays in development, other terms that we should recognize are deviations, dissociations, and regression in development.

The term "deviance" is used when a child develops milestones or skills outside of the typical sequence. An example can be seen in conditions such as cerebral palsy, in which the infant rolls over early even before neck holding in many instances due to increased extensor tone.

Developmental dissociation is the term used for a child who has widely differing rates of development in different developmental domains. For example, children with autism may have typical gross motor development but significantly delayed language development; thus language development is dissociated from gross motor development.

Developmental regression is the term used for a child who loses previously acquired skills or milestones and is a cause of concern as it is often associated with serious neurological and inherited metabolic disorders.

ETIOLOGY OF GLOBAL DEVELOPMENTAL DELAY (TABLE 1)

Table 1: Etiology of global developmental delays (GDDs).

Genetic or chromosomal syndromes	Down syndrome, fragile X syndrome, Rett syndrome, Prader-Willi syndrome, Angelman syndromes, Williams syndrome, neurocutaneous syndromes, i.e., neurofibromatosis type I, tuberous sclerosis, etc.
Metabolic disorders	Storage diseases, Phenylketonuria (PKU), urea cycle disorders, biotinidase deficiency etc.
Acquired causes:	
Prenatal or perinatal causes	• Exposure to teratogens or toxins (tobacco, alcohol, and illicit drugs) • Congenital infections • Intrapartum asphyxia and birth trauma • Intracranial hemorrhage • Prematurity • Congenital hypothyroidism
Postnatal causes	• Infection (meningitis and encephalitis) • Cranial trauma • Environmental causes, i.e., poor nutrition, family stress, child abuse or neglect, severe poverty, chronic iron deficiency anemia, vitamin B12 deficiency, and lead poisoning

CLINICAL APPROACH

History of presenting concerns (age and reason for the concern) along with:
- Detailed developmental history with documentation of milestone attainment. The child's current level of development in each domain should be noted (Note: The chronological age requires to be corrected for prematurity till 2 years of age)
- History of developmental deviancy, dissociation, and regression
- History and observation about social interaction and play skills (use of appropriate toys, crayons, and blocks, etc. may be used)
- Feeding and sleep patterns

- Behavioral history (with reference to maladaptive and self-injurious behaviors)
- History of seizures.

Family history with a three generation pedigree and history of consanguinity, miscarriages, or neonatal deaths.

Antenatal history of maternal diabetes, pregnancy-induced hypertension (PIH), bleeding, smoking, drug or alcohol use, TORCH infections, maternal phenylketonuria, etc.

Birth history with specific details of chorioamnionitis, duration of labor, mode of delivery, any complications, gestation, birth weight, APGARs, and need for any neonatal special care.

General Examination

- Height, weight, and head circumference should be charted on growth charts for short or tall stature, microcephaly, macrocephaly, and obesity.
- Pallor and knuckle hyperpigmentation should be looked for.
- Neurocutaneous stigmata-hypopigmented patches, cafe au lait spots, etc.
- Dysmorphic features
- Stigmata of congenital infections
- Spine.

Systemic Examination

- Organomegaly
- Detailed neurological examination with fundus examination.

Diagnosis is largely based on presenting concerns and features, detailed history, thorough clinical examination, and targeted individualized investigations for the etiological work-up.

Etiological Work-up

Vision and hearing assessment in all children to rule out sensory impairments.

Treatable conditions such as iron deficiency anemia, B12 deficiency, hypothyroidism, and lead levels (in risk for environmental exposure) should be looked for.

- *Iron deficiency anemia*: History of prematurity, low birth weight, improper weaning, cows milk intake, worm infestation, pica; pallor, platynychia, koilonychia; microcytic hypochromic anemia with low serum ferritin.
- *B12 deficiency:* History of exclusively breastfed infants with vegan mother; pallor, hyperpigmented knuckles, ankles, toes; tremors; megaloblastic anemia with neutropenia, thrombocytopenia; high serum lactate dehydrogenase (LDH), and low vitamin B12.
- *Congenital hypothyroidism*: Absence of neonatal screening or no/insufficient treatment with history of large baby at birth, prolonged neonatal physiological jaundice, constipation, hoarse cry, coarse features,

short stature; low free T4, high/normal thyroid-stimulating hormone (TSH), and absent/dysplastic/ectopic thyroid on scan.
- Biotinidase deficiency is a treatable disorder and may present as GDD/regression mostly with seizures, light hair, and sometimes with no other signs or symptoms.

Detailed formal developmental assessments by a developmental pediatrician and the team will help outline the domains involved and to guide the intervention plan goals.
- Bayleys Scale of Infant Development (BSID) assessing motor, mental, and behavior domains or Development Assessment Scale for Indian Infants (DASII) with motor and mental scale up to 30 months of age can be used for the development quotient (DQ).
- Intelligence quotient (IQ) for older children >3 years with age appropriate tests like Binet Kamat Test/Stanford Binet test/Wechsler preschool and primary scale of intelligence-Revised (WPPSI) Kaufman assessment battery for children (K-ABC)/Weschlers Intelligence Scale for Children (WISC).
- Colored progressive matrices for nonverbal performance-based testing.
- Vineland Social Maturity Scale or Vineland Adaptive Behaviour Scale for adaptive functioning should be used in addition to the formal IQ tests.
- Speech and language evaluation with assessment using REELS (Receptive and Emergent Language Scale), 3-dimensional Language Acquisition Test (3D LAT), linguistic profile test, and pragmatic assessment as indicated.
- Screening (MCHAT-R) or assessments for autism using INCLEN-INDT-ASD.
- Additional behavioral assessments with the use of tools like child behavior checklist (CBCL), if indicated as part of the profile.

POINTS TO REMEMBER
- A detailed history and careful examination are the most important components of the assessment of the child with GDD. One-third of etiological diagnoses are made on the basis of history and examination findings alone.
- Targeted investigations based on the positive findings and clinical suspicion of the final diagnosis.

TARGETED ETIOLOGICAL WORK-UP FOR GLOBAL DEVELOPMENTAL DELAY

Genetic Evaluation
Congenital malformation and dysmorphism are features suggestive of some genetic condition. Sensory impairments, unusual behavior patterns, and a

family history of a particular condition may indicate a syndrome diagnosis and prompt referral for a genetic work-up.

If clinical suspicion rests on a specific syndrome as an etiology for the GDD, laboratory tests to confirm, or rule out the syndrome should be performed.

- Chromosome analysis for Down syndrome
- Fluorescence in situ hybridization (FISH) testing when specific genetic disorders are suspected, such as Prader-Willi/Angelman syndrome, Williams syndrome, 22q11 deletion, etc.
- Females with moderate/severe cognitive impairment MECP2 for Rett's syndrome.
- Fragile X for boys with unexplained cognitive impairment or suggestive features
- Chromosomal microarray, next generation sequencing (NGS), whole genome sequencing, exome sequencing, or "next generation" genome sequencing is useful for unknown cause.

Neuroimaging: Variable detection rate mostly depending on selection criteria and imaging method used. The yield is increased by the presence of findings like abnormal head size or focal neurological signs. Magnetic resonance imaging (MRI) is preferable to computed tomography (CT) for the evaluation of children with GDD.

One study reported a yield of 13.9% from imaging performed on a screening basis, compared to 41.2% if carried out due to a clinical indication. A recent review reported that although abnormal MRI findings were found in approximately 30% of patients with developmental delay, these led to an etiology or syndrome diagnosis in fewer than 4% of cases.

Metabolic testing: The yield is 1% or less. Consider metabolic testing especially if newborn metabolic screening has not been carried out. Focus should be on identification of treatable causes due to the high potential for improved outcomes in cases with timely diagnosis. Features that warrant consideration are:

- Prior family history of a similarly affected sibling/death and parental consanguinity
- Documented developmental regression and episodic decompensation
- Failure to thrive and multiple organ system dysfunction
- Indicative dysmorphology and coarse features: Glycosaminoglycans (GAG) for mucopolysaccharidosis
- Suggestive ophthalmologic and retinal abnormalities
- Neuroimaging findings of basal ganglia involvement in the absence of any significant intrapartum asphyxia or unexplained white matter abnormality.

MANAGEMENT

- Specific management, parental counseling regarding realistic expectations, prognostication, counseling for future pregnancies with follow-up plan will be determined by the etiology found.
- Early intervention should be targeted toward maximizing the child's developmental potential.
- Multidisciplinary intervention plan with goals based on the detailed developmental profile should be outlined with the inclusion of physiotherapy, occupational therapy, speech and language therapy, and daily living activities along with cognitive stimulation play activities for home stimulation.
- Guidelines for regular follow up to monitor progress and review of the goals with documentation of the same are recommended.

APPROACH TO A CHILD WITH GLOBAL DEVELOPMENTAL DELAY (FLOWCHART 1)

Flowchart 1: Approach to a case of global developmental delay.

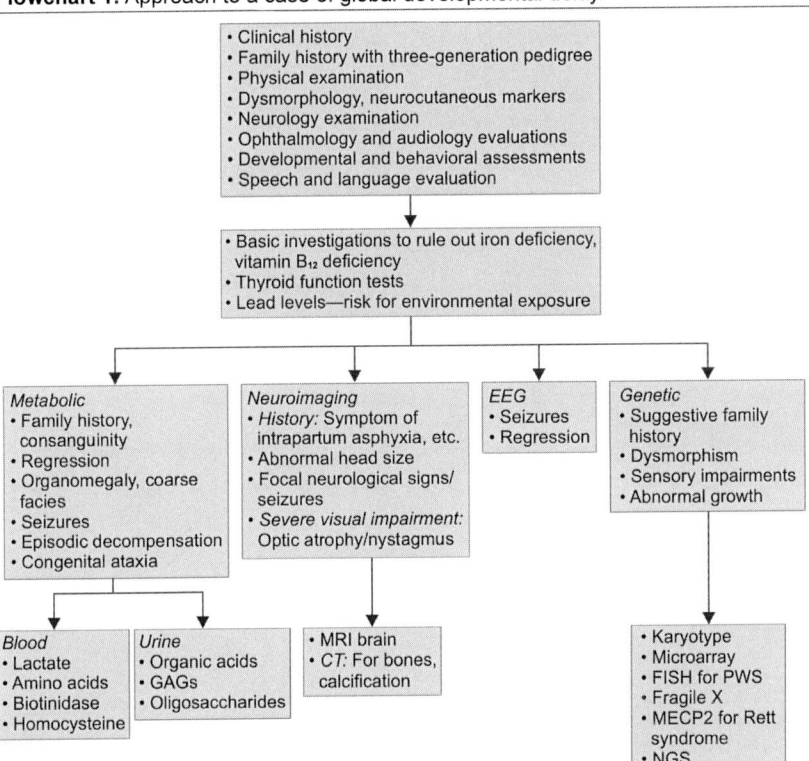

(CT: computed tomography; EEG: electroencephalography; FISH: fluorescence in situ hybridization; GAGs: glycosaminoglycans; MRI: magnetic resonance imaging; NGS: next generation sequencing; PWS: Prader-Willi syndrome)

FURTHER READING

1. McDonald LAB, Rennie AC. Investigating developmental delay/impairment. Paediatr Child Health. 2011;443-7.
2. Shevell M, Ashwal S, Donley D, Flint J, Gingold M, Hirtz D, et al. Practice parameter: Evaluation of the child with global developmental delay. Neurology. 2003;60(3):367-80.
3. Shevell M. Global developmental delay and mental retardation or intellectual disability: Conceptualization, evaluation, and etiology. Pediatr Clin North Am. 2008;55(5):1071-84.
4. Voigt RG, Macias MM, Myers SM. Section on Developmental and Behavioral Pediatrics, Cognitive Development. Am Acad Pediatr. 2010-2011. pp. 172-96.

Chapter 7

Developmentally Supportive Care

Naveen Jain

INTRODUCTION

Development supportive care (DSC) is a clinical care model that looks beyond survival of sick babies in intensive care unit. DSC aims at reducing stress and pain of babies in neonatal intensive care unit (NICU); this has consequences on immediate physiology—apnea, feed intolerance, sleep, etc., and long-term behavior and disability.

The sick/preterm baby's brain is extremely vulnerable. It is dependent on sensory inputs. Abnormal inputs from care processes that are not baby friendly can result in development and psychological problems.

Sick babies spend many days in NICUs separated from their parents. Parents are "allowed to visit" their own baby for only during visiting hours. DSC model understands that the baby is an individual and the baby's family is a critical component of baby's world. DSC addresses care processes beyond medications and procedures (feeding, position, sleep time, touch, pain control, NICU light and sound, etc.) that the baby experiences and that influence the baby's developing brain.

The NICU environment is very different from the in-utero world of the baby. The NICU has very bright lights and is noisy most of the "day and night" with alarms and activities of the unit. Loud conversations of busy doctors and nurses add to the stress.

The preterm baby spends many days in postures not conducive for development, the fact that the baby's postures have an impact on development of tone of the baby seldom crosses the minds, except when in DSC workshops.

Many painful procedures are part of the NICU care, like checking blood sugars; varying sensitivity exist on decreasing painful procedures and nonpharmacological/pharmacological analgesia.

Kangaroo care (KC), non-nutritive sucking, and massage are well known good practices, but often take back seat, as everybody is busy with X-rays, blood gases, fluids, and antibiotics decisions. Most NICUs fear accidental displacement of endotracheal tubes, central lines, or nasal prongs, if handled.

Family-centered developmentally supportive care has still not impressed the "evidence-based" medicine model of care; it is amazing that it requires a randomized trial to prove that a gentle mothers touch, a quite environment, allowing baby to sleep, etc., are good for a baby.

Most often the process of care giving that simply requires just the presence of parents. DSC has often been made to appear complicated—special nurses to understand the baby and multiple charts to decide if baby is in the right state or position. This has led to evaluating the worth of investing in resources and interfering with critical care to support physiology of a sick baby.

The guiding principles may be borrowed from many programs that have researched and evaluated the developmentally supportive care model.

MANAGEMENT—DEVELOPMENT SUPPORTIVE CARE IN NEONATAL INTENSIVE CARE UNIT

This chapter will evaluate various domains/care giving processes that are evidently beneficial to a sick baby in NICU that will decrease the stress of baby and the family.

Family-centered Care

Parents and the family must not be separated from the sick baby. Family-centered NICUs allow parents/family unlimited access to the baby. Some request parents to wait when invasive procedures are performed, sometimes restrict parent involvement if baby is unstable and critically ill. A few units restrict parent entry at unit handover time. Parents must be informed periodically and completely about baby's health care plans and must be a part of decision-making. Their cultural (religious) values, perception of disease, and health care must be respected. Efforts must be made to help the parents cope with stressful situations; avoid ambiguous messages, educate about care plans in advance, and involve counselors as necessary.

Parents must participate in care of the sick baby. They must hold the baby's hands, tuck the baby and provide comfort, perform KC, gently stroke, and massage the baby. Under supervision, units have involved parents in orogastric feeding, change of diapers, and many other care processes like taking weight of the baby. Early discharge from hospital and better transition from NICU to home resulted. Occasionally parents were overwhelmed and reported physical and mental exhaustion.

The way forward is couplet care or single-family room concept. The sick baby would be nurtured with the mother and the family living with the baby in the same room throughout the period of hospitalization. The room would be customized as per family traditions and culture. Baby would be mostly nursed by parents under medical supervision.

Neonatal Intensive Care Unit Environment—Light and Noise

Neonatal intensive care unit light should be dimmed, except when skilled procedures are performed. Day night cycling is expected to help baby's behavior maturation. Alarms should be muted once addressed, their volumes be reduced. Avoid loud conversations.

Many good developmentally supportive units have improved the designs of NICU by using sound absorbing floors and walls.

Care beyond Technology and Pharmacotherapy

Pain management and Procedural Support— Recognizing Stress Cues

Painful procedures must be minimized; example clubbing of blood tests that are not urgent can decrease painful pricks, e.g., lancet pricks are less painful than needle pricks. Tucking the baby, talking to the baby, and holding hands have all shown to decrease pain. Breast milk and sucrose decrease pain of procedures.

Topical anesthetics, paracetamol, and opioid analgesia may be required when more painful procedures are planned.

One must recognize infant behaviors that suggest stress like rapid breathing, change in skin color, stop sign of hand, etc.

Positioning

Placing the baby "frog legged" for prolonged periods in NICU results in external rotation at shoulder and hips. Gravity acting on forearms and legs (not present in utero) results in unequal lengthening of flexors and extensors and causes tone abnormalities.

Babies must be nursed with head in midline, hands brought to midline, toward the mouth. Legs and arms must be flexed, supported by boundaries. The baby must be contained in a nest like in-utero.

Practice tummy time, i.e., keeping baby prone for some time when baby is alert.

Cue-based Feeding

Most NICU feed babies by the clock, example 2-3 hourly. The baby may be sleeping when the nurse starts giving an orogastric feed. It is recommended to wait for baby cues that baby is waking up from sleep to decide the right time to feed. Nurses and parents are often concerned that feeds may be missed or delayed and hence, parental involvement is critical to implement cue-based feeding.

Even procedures considered routine like diaper change and cleaning of baby can cause unpleasant experiences to baby and must be planned based on babies' state of wakefulness.

Skin to Skin (Kangaroo) Care

Kangaroo care has been the most understood developmentally supportive care in the last decade. Scientific evaluation has demonstrated better sleep, saturations, heart rates, weight gain, exclusive breastfeeding rates, decrease in infections, and early hospital discharge.

Although long durations of KC are recommended, translation to practice requires counseling and education of family members. Hospitals should be able to provide support for the family to stay long hours, provide comfortable chairs, and privacy to perform KC.

Massage

Massage reduces behavioral and physiological response to pain and reduces cortisol levels. Better weight gain is demonstrated. Bonding to mother improves. Maturation of electroencephalogram (EEG) was shown to be better and development scores were also better in a study. Most studies enrolled stable preterm or term babies and performed massage for 15–20 min/day.

IMPLEMENTATION OF DEVELOPMENT SUPPORTIVE CARE

Development supportive health care practices implementation requires:
- Written policies on DSC
- Training of doctors, nurses, occupational therapists, and speech language therapists
- Parent participation
- Integration of DSC with clinical care (rather than a parallel service run by a specialist nurse or physiotherapist)
- Engineering changes of NICU structure.

FURTHER READING

1. Álvarez MJ, Fernández D, Gómez-Salgado J, Rodríguez-González D, Rosón M, Lapeña S. The effects of massage therapy in hospitalized preterm neonates: A systematic review. Int J Nurs Stud. 2017;69:119-36.
2. Boundy EO, Dastjerdi R, Spiegelman D, Fawzi WW, Missmer SA, Lieberman E, et al. Kangaroo mother care and neonatal outcomes: A meta-analysis. Pediatrics. 2016;137(1):e20152238.
3. Chan GJ, Valsangkar B, Kajeepeta S, Boundy EO, Wall S. What is kangaroo mother care? Systematic review of the literature. J Glob Health. 2016;6(1):010701.

4. Charafeddine L, Masri S, Ibrahim P, Badin D, Cheayto S, Tamim H. Targeted educational program improves infant positioning practice in the NICU. Int J Qual Health Care. 2018;30(8):642-8.
5. da Motta G de CP, da Cunha MLC. Prevention and non-pharmacological management of pain in newborns. Rev Bras Enferm. 2015;68(1):123-7.
6. Esser M, Dore S, Fitzgerald F, Kelley K, Kuller J, Ludwig S, et al. Applying developmentally supportive principles to diapering in the NICU: What we know. Neonatal Netw. 2018;37(3):149-54.
7. Fry TJ, Marfurt S, Wengier S. Systematic review of quality improvement initiatives-related to cue-based feeding in preterm infants. Nurs Womens Health. 2018;22(5):401-10.
8. Masri S, Ibrahim P, Badin D, Khalil S, Charafeddine L. Structured educational intervention leads to better infant positioning in the NICU. Neonatal Netw. 2018;37(2):70-7.
9. Pados BF, McGlothen-Bell K. Benefits of infant massage for infants and parents in the NICU. Nurs Womens Health. 2019;23(3):265-71.
10. Schiavenato M, Holsti L. Defining procedural distress in the NICU and what can be done about it. Neonatal Netw. 2017;36(1):12-7.
11. Westrup B. Family-centered developmentally supportive care: The Swedish example. Arch Pédiatrie. 2015;22(10):1086-91.

Chapter 8

Follow-up of the High-risk Newborn

Rhishikesh Thakre

INTRODUCTION

Neonatal intensive-care unit (NICU) graduates due to underlying illness, interventions, biological, and environmental factors are vulnerable and susceptible to injury to the growing brain. This insult may affect their physical growth, cognition, vision, hearing, speech, or behavior leading to handicaps of varying severity manifesting any time during infancy, childhood, adolescent, or adulthood. A systematic evaluation program is needed to identify delay, deviation, or dissociation which helps plan early intervention **(Table 1)**.

RISK STRATIFICATION FOR NEURODEVELOPMENTAL SCREENING (TABLE 2)

Follow-up Team

The core team includes pediatrician, developmental psychologist, physiotherapist, audiologist, ophthalmologist, social worker, and health nurse. Further specialist may be required based on patient problems.

Table 1: Comparisons of facilities: Pediatric clinic vs developmental clinic.

	Pediatric clinic	*Developmental clinic*
Parental concerns	Yes	Yes
Physical growth	Yes	No
Nutritional assessment	Yes	No
Development	Screening	Formal assessment
Vaccination	Yes	No
Medical care	Yes	No
Early intervention	No	Yes
Rehabilitation services	No	Yes

Table 2: Care provider based on risk stratification.		
At risk	Neonatal factors	Care
Mild	>37 w, >2.5 kg, HIE stage I, transient hypoglycemia, suspect sepsis, jaundice with phototherapy, preterm, and Grade I/II IVH	Pediatrician
Moderate	33–36 w, 1500–2500 g, HIE stage II, sepsis, jaundice with exchange transfusion, >Grade II IVH, prolonged encephalopathy, uncomplicated course on ventilation, hypoglycemia > 3d, and need for some resuscitation	Neonatologist/ developmental pediatrician
Severe	<1500 g, <33 weeks, multiorgan injury, HIE stage III, >7d ventilation, meningitis, kernicterus, abnormal neurologic exam at discharge, PVL or hydrocephalus, low Apgars at 5 min, and symptomatic hypoglycemia	Developmental center

(HIE: hypoxic ischemic encephalopathy; IVH: intraventricular hemorrhage; PVL: periventricular leukomalacia)

Components of High-risk Clinic

- Comprehensive, holistic, systematic, and humane assessment
- Assessment of growth and nutrition
- Neuromotor/sensory evaluation
- Responding to parental concerns
- Anticipatory guidance
- Early intervention

Timing of Examination

Developmental assessment is one of the fundamental evaluations in pediatric practice. At every opportunity, an attempt must be made to screen all infants and children, irrespective of their presenting complaints for developmental status. One of the best times to examine the infant is between feeds. The infant is assessed in a quiet room, when he or she is not hungry, sleepy, irritable, or sick.

CORRECTION FOR PREMATURITY

One needs to correct for prematurity till the age of 24 months while assessing development. Corrected age is the sum of chronologic age in weeks minus the difference between gestational age at birth and 40 weeks' gestation. The chronologic age is not taken into consideration while assessing milestones.

Table 3: Assessing development.

	Developmental screening	Developmental assessment
Candidates	For all	For "high risk", who fail screening
Incharge	Pediatrician	Developmental trained or psychologist
Purpose	Screen all for "delay"	Identify and quantify delay
Test	TDSC (Trivandrum Developmental Screening chart), Baroda Developmental Screening Test, and Denver Developmental Screening Test (DDST)	DASI (Development Assessment Scale for Indian Infants)

Table 4: Developmental quotient and its implications.

DQ	Implications
>85	Considered as within normal limits
<70	In two or more streams are considered as global developmental delay
<70	In any stream warrants serious consideration of the cause and early intervention
<50	Always implies an organic etiology

(DQ: developmental quotient)

ASSESSING DEVELOPMENT (TABLE 3)

The domains for developmental assessment are physical (motor and fine motor), cognitive (thinking, learning, and problem solving), communicative (listening, talking, and understanding), and social or emotional (playing, feeling secure and happy, feeding, sleeping habits, bladder/bowel habits, ability to play, and adapt to regulations).

Following developmental assessment developmental quotient (DQ) is calculated **(Table 4)**.

DQ = Developmental age/Chronological age × 100

ASSESSING TONE

Tone is assessed on inspecting the posture, feeling the muscle for stiffness or flabbiness, shaking the extremity to note the floppiness or stiffness, observing the range of motions, and comparing for symmetry and resistance to passive movement. Amiel Tison method is used early detection of tone abnormalities during first year of life **(Table 5)**.

Table 5: Ariel Tison method.				
Age (Months)	Adductor angle	Popliteal angle	Dorsiflexion angle	Scarf sign
0–3	40–80	80–100	60–70	Elbow does not cross the midline
4–6	70–110	90–120	60–70	Elbow crosses midline
7–9	110–140	110–160	60–70	Elbow goes beyond axillary line
10–12	140–160	150–170	60–70	

Note:
- A limitation of angles indicate hypertonia and wide angles indicate hypotonia.
- Does not replace developmental scales as mental development is not assessed.
- Predictive value at 3 months for normal development at 12 months is >93%.

Assessing Vision and Hearing

Screening for retinopathy of prematurity (ROP) is performed using indirect ophthalmoscopy. It is done on all high-risk newborns at 4 weeks—chronological age (<2000 g or <34 weeks gestation). The test is repeated if abnormal or till retinal vasculature is complete. Hearing screen is performed by otoacoustic emission (OAE) and confirmed by brainstem evoked response audiometric (BERA). In infants and children impedance audiometry, free field audiometry or behavioral audiometry is used.

Investigations

Not all infants need investigations. Neuroimaging [magnetic resonance imaging (MRI) preferred over computed tomography (CT) scan brain] is recommended as part of the diagnostic evaluation of the child with global developmental delay. Electroencephalogram (EEG) is done with seizure disorder or suspected epileptic syndrome. Metabolic testing and/or genetic testing may be pursued in the context of historical (parental consanguinity, family history, developmental regression, and episodic decompensation) or physical examination findings. All infants with global developmental delay should be screened for autism spectrum disorders.

Documentation

- Identifying risk factors
- Documenting and maintaining developmental history
- Eliciting parents' concern regarding the child's development
- Make accurate observations of the child
- Maintaining accurate record of findings
- Identifying strengths and weaknesses of child.

Table 6: Interpreting observations.

Test/Observation	Optimal response	Interpretation
Head circumference	Appropriate for age	Adequate brain growth
Cranial sutures	Edge to edge	No CNS depression
Fix, follow, and response to object	Present	
Social interaction	Present	
Sucking reflex	Efficient	
Raised to sit and reverse	Active flexor muscles	Upper motor control integrity
Passive axial tone	More flexion than extension	
Passive tone in limbs	Symmetrical and appropriate for gestation	
Fingers and thumb	Independent movements and abduction of thumbs	
Autonomic control during assessment	Stable color, heart rate, and respiration	Abnormality suggests autonomic instability
Primitive reflexes	Persistence beyond age	Significant brain insult

(CNS: central nervous system)

Box 1: Follow-up of high-risk newborn by pediatrician.
- Correction for gestational immaturity at birth should be done till 24 months of age for all preterms.
- Use corrected age for weaning and milestone screening.
- Use postnatal age for vaccination.
- Use Fentons/Wright's chart or intergrowth chart for preterm infants till term equivalent.
- Use WHO (2005) growth charts for term.
- Follow-up every 2 weekly until a weight of 3 kg. Then follow as per schedule below.

EARLY INTERVENTION

Early intervention is systematic stimulation programme for at risk infant to guide achieve normal developmental milestones. Early, intense, and sustained intervention produce the greatest and most sustained benefits **(Tables 6 and 7)**. For children with DQ of 75 and less, in any area then a center-based program is advised. For a child with a DQ between 76 and 85, a home program is given with regular review and follow-up **(Box 1)**.

Follow-up of the High-risk Newborn

Table 7: Age-based follow-up assessment of high-risk infants.

Components	1.5 m	2.5 m	3.5 m	6 m	9 m	12 m	18 m	24 m
Parental concerns	At every visit							
Medical problems	At every visit							
Vaccination	As per IAP schedule (2018–19)							
Anthropometry*	At every visit (Wt~, HC*, TL) use WHO growth charts (for boys/girls and separate)							
Nutrition:								
Diet	Exclusive breastfeeding			Weaning plus breast-feeding		Home diet		
Vitamin D	400 IU, daily							
Iron (per kg/day)	For preterm only (2–6 mg)			For term (2 mg)	For preterm		-	Yearly
Cal/PO$_4$ (2:1) Per kg/day	For preterm only (100 mg)			For term	-	-	-	Yearly
Formula: Shift to term formula at 2 kg weight:								
Neurologic exam	At every visit (Amil Tison method)							
Development test**	Screening at each visit	Formal testing		Screening at each visit		Behavioral assessment (MCHAT)	-	Formal testing
Eye evaluation	ROP Screening at 1 month age (All < 2 kg)		Formal Screening at 1 month age		For vision, squint, and optic atrophy	-	-	For vision, squint, and optic atrophy

Contd...

Contd...

Components	1.5 m	2.5 m	3.5 m	6 m	9 m	12 m	18 m	24 m
Hearing	OAE at discharge. BERA for testing or confirmation at 3 m. Screen clinically at each visit							
CT or MRI brain	As clinically indicated							
USG brain	At 36–40 weeks corrected age							
Language	-	-	-	-	LEST	-	LEST	-
Counseling	At every visit							
Biochemical screen	-	-	-	-	Hb and urine		Hb	Hb, urine, and BP

Note: *Danger signs: Weight gain < 20 g/day, Length growth < 0.5 cm/week, Head circumference < 0.5 cm/week
**Screening tests = History + TDSC (Trivandrum Development Screening Chart) OR DOC (Development Observation Card). Formal testing—DASII (Developmental Assessment Scale for Indian Infants)
LEST = Language evaluation scale Trivandrum; Behavioral assessment = CBCL (Achenbach Child Behavior Checklist), Pediatric Symptom Checklist. *Formal cognitive development, IQ is tested by 3 years of age.*

FURTHER READING

1. Lipner HS, Huron RF. Developmental and interprofessional care of the preterm infant: Neonatal Intensive Care Unit through high-risk infant follow-up. Pediatr Clin North Am. 2018;65(1):135-41.
2. Orton JL, Olsen JE, Ong K, Lester R, Spittle AJ. NICU Graduates: The role of the allied health team in follow-up. Pediatr Ann. 2018;47(4):e165-71.

Chapter 9

Genetics and Neurodevelopmental Disorders

Rashid Merchant, Snehal Mallakmir, Ami Shah

INTRODUCTION

Scientific discovery of trisomy 21 in Down syndrome opened the doors to detect chromosomal abnormalities as a cause of intellectual disability in the late 60s. Ever since, a wide variability of clinical presentations has stimulated the research into chromosomal and single gene causes to the finest level, giving us an insight into its applications to therapeutic management. Evolution of the knowledge of biochemical genetics, clinical cytogenetics, molecular genetics, and dysmorphology has paved the way for delineation of medical genetics as a specialty in medicine.

"Genome" is the term applied to the total complement of deoxyribonucleic acid (DNA). DNA molecules are functionally organized into approximately 20,000 genes. Alteration in the structure of single or multiple genes gives rise to genetic disorders called monogenic or polygenic disorders, respectively. Some disorders are multifactorial and are caused due to interaction of genes and other factors like environment. Genes are organized into microscopically visible structures called chromosomes. Alteration in the number of chromosomes (aneuploidy) and the structure of chromosomes (deletion, duplication, translocation, etc.) leads to disorders like Down syndrome (extra copy of chromosome 21) and Cri du chat syndrome (deletion in short arm of chromosome 5). Karyotype detects microscopically visible abnormalities in chromosomes (Down syndrome and Fragile X) while newer techniques such as microarray can detect submicroscopic microdeletions (William syndrome and Prader-Willi syndrome) or duplications (22q11.2 duplication syndrome).

In a clinically-diagnosed population, chromosomal aneuploidies may be detected by high resolution karyotype in up to 5%, and submicroscopic microdeletions and duplications recognized with chromosomal microarray in up to 10% of patients with autism spectrum disorders. About 20-25% patients may have single gene abnormalities like fragile X disorder (*FMR1* gene), Rett syndrome (*MECP2* gene), and *PTEN* gene mutations (in patients with macrocephaly and autism) and other genes; e.g., tuberous sclerosis

(*TSC1* and *TSC2* genes), neurofibromatosis (*NF1* gene), Angelman syndrome (*UBE3A* gene) identified by newer gene sequencing technologies.

In children with developmental disorders, screening for inborn errors of metabolic (IEM) diseases is very important since these are treatable (biotinidase deficiency) and if detected early can be prevented (amino acid disorders and hyperammonemia).

Mutations in single genes usually follow Mendelian patterns of inheritance such as autosomal dominant (AD), autosomal recessive (AR), or X-linked as shown in **Figures 1, 2,** and **3**.

Application of genetics into clinical practice in developmental disorders is important for precise diagnosis, prognosis, and management, as well as prevention of recurrence in the family.

Epigenetics refers to modification of gene activities without causing actual change in sequence of DNA. It may be caused due to change in chromatin-modifying enzymes, alterations in the function of histone modifiers, and methyl-DNA binding proteins. This is very important in cases with intellectual disability.

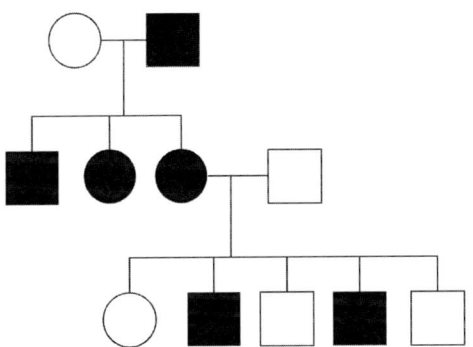

Fig. 1: Autosomal dominant inheritance pattern.

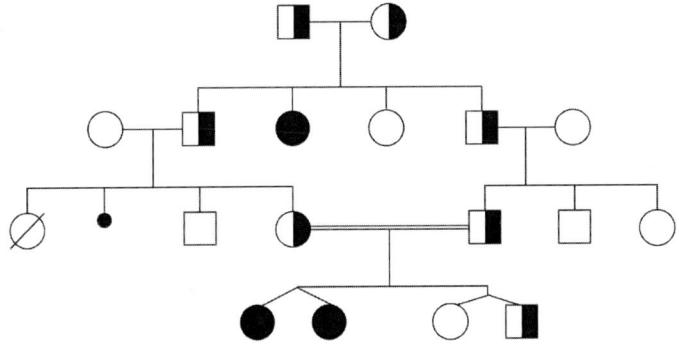

Fig. 2: Autosomal recessive inheritance pattern.

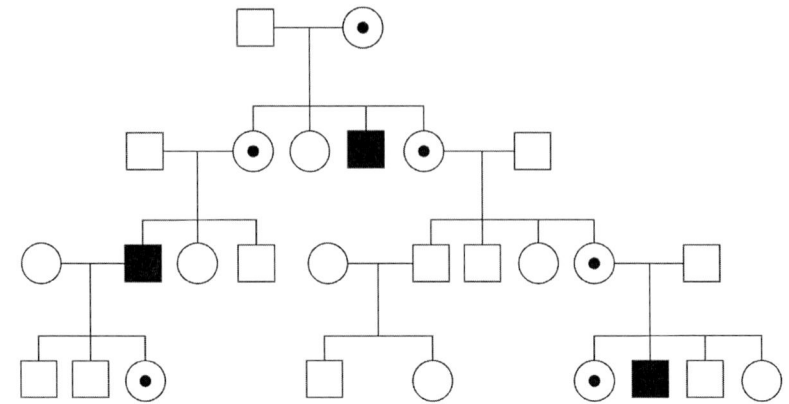
Fig. 3: X-linked inheritance pattern.

Increasing clinical interest of primary pediatricians with greater reporting and sample collection and analysis will go a long way in creating significant local Indian data which is likely to aid better genetic diagnoses in the near future.

CLINICAL FEATURES

Clinical history and construction of three degree pedigree chart to get detailed family history are of foremost importance. This often helps to:
1. Exclude pre or perinatal medical and environmental influences such as birth, injury, maternal disease, infections, drugs, nutrition.
2. Give an idea of the mode of inheritance in familial cases, whether X-linked, AR, or dominant.
3. Explain the risk of recurrence in each next pregnancy.

A family pedigree shown in **Figure 1** depicts AD inheritance. One of the parents may carry the mutated gene and it is transmitted to the next generation. However, many AD conditions like NF exhibit variable expression. It means different family members carrying the same mutation may show different degrees of clinical involvement ranging from asymptomatic, mild to severe (only café au lait spot or dermatological involvement to severe neurological involvement).

Pedigree in **Figure 2** shows AR inheritance like mucopolysaccharidosis (MPS) or many IEM (fatty acid oxidation disorders). The parents are usually asymptomatic carriers and presence of both mutated alleles in an affected child is needed to cause severe deficiency of the gene product like metabolic enzyme or structural protein.

In X-linked conditions like fragile X syndrome as shown in **Figure 3**, the carrier mother may or may not show manifestations but disease is severe in affected children. Fragile X, in addition, shows feature of anticipation which means the severity of disease mutations increases in next generations.

History of previous investigations like normal karyotype or metabolic screening helps to exclude overlapping clinical phenotypes. Record of monitoring of growth and developmental parameters over a period of time points to associated endocrine abnormalities like thyroid deficiency (present in many chromosomal syndromes like Down syndrome and Turner syndrome) and growth hormone deficiency (in Russell–Silver, Noonan syndrome, etc.).

Careful clinical examination should be done for presence of dysmorphism, e.g., upslanting eyes in Down syndrome, hypertelorism in Noonan syndrome as well as major or minor systemic abnormalities such as cardiac defects, scoliosis, renal anomalies along with careful search for neurocutaneous markers such as café-au-lait spots, hypopigmented macules, and hemangiomas.

Examination of parents and siblings as well as other family members suspected or diagnosed to have genetic disorders is important. The parents may show presence of café au lait spots as in NF. In Noonan syndrome, one of the parent carrying the mutation may show facial dysmorphic features similar to the child and/or cardiac involvement like hypertrophic cardiomyopathy. Mutations in completely different genes may end up causing the same clinical phenotype, as happens in Noonan syndrome which is caused by mutations in any one of the following genes—*PTPN11* (AD inheritance), *KRAS* (AD inheritance), *LZTR1* (AR inheritance), etc.

One should never miss looking for systemic problems associated with dysmorphology. Easily recognizable syndromes such as trisomy 21, Turner syndrome, and William syndrome are associated with cardiac, neurological, or renal anomalies. It is important to note that typical facial dysmorphism may not be apparent in early infancy or milder phenotype may be seen. Presence of characteristic systemic abnormalities in cases with mild or atypical dysmorphism may suggest a close follow-up for evolution of further clinical spectrum or facial features (e.g., supravalvular aortic stenosis in William syndrome).

Many inborn metabolic disorders give rise to specific clinical symptoms and signs like neurological complications (dyskinesia in glutaric aciduria, behavioral abnormalities in MPS III, and seizures in tuberous sclerosis), organomegaly in storage diseases, skeletal abnormalities in MPS, or may present with metabolic derangements like acidosis.

It is important to remember that many children with developmental disorders may not have any clues such as facial dysmorphisms, metabolic, or clinically apparent systemic abnormalities.

MANAGEMENT

While one decides about an evaluation plan, it is necessary to maintain a balance between rapidly expanding list of tests, reporting of causative genetic abnormalities, careful clinical correlation, and possible final conclusion, along with the issues of cost, expected yield, and parental understanding of applications of tests and result. Hence, the evaluation plan should be customized to individual case scenario after confirmation of the diagnosis of developmental disorder by a trained developmental team using objective criteria, tools, and cognitive tests.

Visual and auditory screening are necessary in all patients. Electroencephalogram (EEG) in cases of seizures and magnetic resonance imaging of brain in known genetic syndromes with central nervous system anomalies is important. Similar careful search is done for other systemic problems such as cardiac, renal malformations, or skeletal abnormalities. Routine metabolic screening for MPS, organic acids, serum lactate, amino acids, ammonia, and acylcarnitine profile is done as per the clinical suspicion.

High-resolution chromosomal karyotype is done in recognizable syndromes like Down syndrome and Turner syndrome. Fragile X studies in males with developmental delay and *MECP2* gene studies in females with suspected Rett syndrome is appropriate. Specific tests such as fluorescent in situ hybridization (FISH) or multiplex ligation-dependent probe amplification (MLPA) may be done when clinical diagnosis is specific to that disorder (e.g., William syndrome with 7q11.23 deletion, Prader–Willi syndrome with 15q11-q13 deletion); however, limitations of the tests should be discussed with parents, as these tests may not detect all patients with the disease and further tests such as microarray or gene sequencing may be needed in few patients for further confirmation of diagnosis. Comparative genomic hybridization (chromosomal microarray) is recognized as the first tier testing in intellectual disabilities. In syndromes with single gene etiologies like Noonan or Cornelia de Lange syndrome, disease-specific gene panels by next generation sequencing technique are available.

Whole exome or genome analysis is a recent important useful tool to screen for single gene pathogenic variations in unidentified etiologies; however, identification of variants of unknown significance (VUS) and benign variants may pose interpretation challenges. Investigation of the child and both parents simultaneously significantly helps to explain pathogenicity of identified variation; this may also be indicated, along with evaluation of the fetus if the mother presents with a subsequent pregnancy.

Management is also focused on pretest and post-test counseling of parents and counseling after final diagnosis. Prognosis and management by multidisciplinary team need to be discussed for better outcome in every child. Many genetic disorders need care by specialists for systemic problems, particularly in cardiac, orthopedic, and neurological complications as well as specific nutrition and rehabilitative measures.

The genetics of neurodevelopmental disorders are complex and includes a wide spectrum. But the significant positive change in the yield of diagnosis with evolving tests as well as accessibility in India is improving management and outcome of these children.

FURTHER READING

1. Kapoor D, Mukherjee SB. Global developmental delay and intellectual disability in Indian children—Where do we stand? Indian Pediatr. 2018;55(12):1083-5.
2. Michelson DJ, Shevell MI, Sherr EH, Moeschler JB, Gropman AL, Ashwal S. Evidence Report: Genetic and Metabolic Testing on Children with Global Developmental Delay: Report of the Quality Standards Subcommittee of the American Academy of Neurology and the Practice Committee of the Child Neurology Society. Neurology. 2011:77(17):1629-35.
3. Narayanan DL, Girisha KM. Genomic testing for diagnosis of genetic disorders in children: Chromosomal microarray and next-generation sequencing. Indian Pediatr. 2020;57(6):549-54.
4. Puri RD, Tuteja M, Verma IC. Genetic approach to diagnosis of intellectual disability. Indian J Pediatr. 2016;83(10):1141-9.
5. van Bokhoven H. Genetic and epigenetic networks in intellectual disabilities. Annu Rev Genet. 2011;45:81-104.
6. Schaefer GB, Mendelsohn NJ. Clinical genetics evaluation in identifying the etiology of autism spectrum disorders. Genet Med. 2008;10(4):301-5.

Chapter 10

Intellectual Disability

Samir H Dalwai, Aradhana Rohil

"Only 50 years ago persons with intellectual disabilities were scorned, isolated, and neglected. Today, they are able to attend school, become employed, and assimilate into their local community."

Nelson Mandela

INTRODUCTION

Intellectual disability (ID) is a commonly acknowledged developmental disorder. It has replaced the notorious term "mental retardation".

Cognitive and intellectual advancement with age and greater control over the environment by learning to adapt (i.e., acquiring new skills to achieve new functions) is the developmental hallmark of humans.

Intellectual disability is a neurodevelopmental disorder that has impairment in both, the cognitive (intellectual) ability and adaptive function of the individual in the environment. ID begins in childhood (before 18 years of age) and affects approximately 1% of the population. It manifests as failure of the child to progressively achieve skills to receive, analyze, and process information to function adequately and age-appropriately in one's environment. These skills impact learning, reasoning, problem solving, abstract thinking, and judgment. It is soon evident that the child is "lagging behind" peers and even younger siblings in participation in multiple settings like home, community, school, and requires support.

Children with ID may exhibit dysmorphic and other physical features due to genetic disorders that may be recognizable as a syndrome; this is termed as syndromic ID. These may be diagnosed in infancy. Most severely affected children are recognized earlier, some even before 2 years of age. Children who have mild ID may be missed until school age; mild delays are more common than severe.

Global developmental delay (GDD) refers to children under 5 years of age who fail to meet expected developmental milestones in multiple domains with significant impairments in functioning. As they grow older, many but

Intellectual Disability 55

not all children with GDD meet criteria for ID. ID is usually provided as a diagnosis at 5 years of age after comprehensive standardized testing; the term GDD may be used provisionally until then.

CLINICAL DIAGNOSIS

Children present with language delay, and detectable adaptive delay, like age-inappropriate behavior or play and self-help skills, learning difficulties, lagging behind a younger sibling, or may be identified during routine pediatric examination. Generally, the social and communication development is equivalent with the child's level of cognitive functioning. It is pertinent to note that gross motor functions may not be affected to the same extent.

Conditions commonly associated with ID worsen the prognosis but when treated can significantly improve the clinical situation **(Table 1)**.

Elaborate history and examination may help identify the etiology and associated conditions, as well as the subdomains and degree of impairments.

Key points in history:
- Three-generation family pedigree chart (neurodevelopmental and genetic disorders, poor obstetric history, neonatal deaths, and consanguinity)
- Prenatal, perinatal, and postnatal problems, medications, infections, congenital abnormalities, substance abuse in pregnancy, or other environmental exposures
- Detailed developmental, behavioral, medical, family, social, educational history, and quality of life
- History of associated conditions **(Table 1)**.

Table 1: Conditions commonly associated with intellectual disability (ID).

Medical conditions	Neurodevelopmental disorders
Vision impairment (e.g., strabismus, cataract, and refractive errors)	Genetic disorders (trisomy 21, fragile X syndrome, and Klinefelter syndrome)
Hearing loss	Autism and ADHD
Sleep disorders	Learning disabilities
Constipation	Cerebral palsy
Dental caries	Seizures
Obesity	Feeding and eating disorders pica
Endocrine abnormalities (e.g., hypothyroidism and short stature)	Depression and anxiety and post-traumatic stress disorder (PTSD)
Gastroesophageal reflux disease	Injury, neglect, physical and sexual abuse
Lead poisoning	Self-injurious behaviors
Congenital heart disease (e.g., AV canal defect in Down syndrome)	Movement disorders

(ADHD: attention deficit hyperactivity disorder; AV: atrioventricular)

Key points in examination:
- Anthropometry (height, weight, and head circumference)—syndromic ID and growth disorders
- Dysmorphic features—genetic or syndromic etiology
- Cutaneous findings—café-au-lait macules (neurofibromatosis), ash-leaf spots (tuberous sclerosis), and bruises or other signs (neglect and physical abuse)
- Complete neurologic, neurodevelopmental assessment, including behavioral phenotype (attention and impulsivity), social skills, and communication
- Sensory screening—ophthalmologic examination and audiometry.

Investigations:
- Thyroid testing is recommended for infants and children presenting with ID in countries without newborn screening programs.
- *Genetic testing:* G-banded karyotyping for Down syndrome; fragile X testing is recommended in all children with unexplained ID or autism.
- Neuroimaging and neurophysiology are indicated in the presence of specific neurological signs or seizures.

Assessments:
Screening tests for development (ages and stages questionnaire—third edition) and behavior (ages and stages—social and emotional, second edition) are recommended for early recognition.

When a screening test suggests delay, comprehensive developmental evaluation is warranted. A diagnosis of ID requires impaired intellectual and adaptive functioning in at least one of three domains **(Table 2)** and includes standardized assessments **(Table 3)**.

Points to remember:
- An Intelligence Quotient (IQ) Score that is two standard deviations or more below the mean (<70) indicates significant intellectual impairment, but not a diagnosis of ID.
- Although ID severity is no longer classified according to an IQ Score, IQ measures of intellectual impairment may be considered as in **Table 4**.
- In the absence of adaptive impairment, even if the child's IQ is <70, a diagnosis of ID cannot be given. Other factors or conditions can sometimes

Table 2: Domains of impaired adaptive functioning.

Conceptual	Social	Practical
Literacy and mathematics: language, reading, writing, number, and money concepts	Interpersonal and social communication, and social problem-solving	Activities of daily living or personal care: eating, dressing, mobility, toileting, and managing money
Reasoning	Following rules	Following schedules
Memory	Gullibility, avoiding bullying—victimization	Health care and safety

Table 3: Standardized tests for diagnostic assessment of intellectual disability (ID).

Age	Cognitive and adaptive testing	Adaptive testing
Below 2 years	Bayley Scales of Infant and Toddler Development, third edition (BSID-III) (2005) Griffiths Scales of Child Development, third edition (Griffiths III) (2015)	The Vineland Adaptive Behavior Scale, third edition (Vineland-III) (2016) The adaptive behavior assessment system, third edition (ABAS-III) (2015)
	Intellectual testing	
2–5 years	Wechsler Preschool and Primary Scale of Intelligence, fourth edition (WPPSI-IV) (2012)	The Vineland Adaptive Behavior Scale, third edition (Vineland-III) (2016)
Above 5 years	Wechsler Intelligence Scales for Children, fifth edition (WISC-V) (2014)	

Table 4: Traditional classification of Intelligence Quotient Scores [intellectual impairment, not intellectual disability (ID)].

Mild	Between 50–55 and 70	Moderate	Between 35–40 and 50–55
Severe	Between 20–25 and 35–40	Profound	<20–25

contribute to poor performance (hearing and vision impairment, and attention problems).
- The severity of ID is defined according to the level of adaptive impairment and the level of support needed and not as per IQ test scores.

MANAGEMENT

Management of ID requires:
- Early diagnosis
- Intervention
- Appropriate support

The goals are to:
- Prevent or minimize further deterioration
- To lessen the effects of disability and improve functioning and
- To promote optimal functioning in all areas at home, school, and in the community.

For maximal benefit, interventions should begin as early as possible but must be appropriate and holistic. Both, early and appropriate, are equally important.

Since ID encompasses a wide range of functioning and attention to disability, needs, and strengths, the developmental pediatrician (DP) and the pediatrician should address all aspects as per the needs of the child and family as well as individual patient characteristics. Interventions should be individualized and sustained to achieve ongoing results. As intervention involves multiple disciplines, it is important to plan and organize these as part of an overall intervention program in a collaborative, interdisciplinary, and dynamic manner by the DP.

Depending on the child's program, the DP may include aspects of speech and language therapy, occupational therapy, physical therapy, vision and hearing referrals, behavioral intervention, family counseling, educational assistance, and group interventions. Desirable behaviors should be positively reinforced, and restraining or punitive aversive approaches should be avoided. Goals that achieve inclusion, independent functioning, and life skills learning are important. It is observed that rather than namesake referrals, a well-organized program with individualized goals for each professional with dynamic monitoring by the Pediatrician and DP results in better outcomes for the child and family.

Pharmacologically treatable causes of ID (inborn error of metabolism and congenital hypothyroidism) and psychopharmacological therapy for mental health disorders should be promptly initiated. Medications should be used only as part of a clear, comprehensive program with specific goals of target behaviors; monitoring is essential for limiting use to the minimum dose and duration, and to prevent undesirable effects.

Early "labelling" does not accurately predict intelligence in the long-term and may result in stigmatization. Ultimate outcome depends on multiple factors such as the cause and severity of ID, the presence and severity of other-associated conditions, environmental and social factors, and appropriate individualized services. With early and appropriate supportive services, some mildly-affected children progress by 5 years of age such that they do not meet diagnostic criteria for ID.

Various governments and school boards offer provisions to children with ID.

The Pediatrician has an important role to play in early detection, appropriate dynamic intervention, and the advocacy for children with ID and to ensure their rights as well as to stand up to prevent their abuse and neglect and to ensure that they are truly included in all sections of the community.

FURTHER READING

1. American Psychiatric Association. Intellectual Disability (Intellectual Developmental Disorder). In: Diagnostic and Statistical Manual of Mental Disorders, 5th edition, American Psychiatric Association.
2. American Association on Intellectual and Developmental Disabilities (AAIDD). [online] Available from http://aaidd.org/intellectual-disability/definition (Last accessed December, 2021).
3. Council on Children with Disabilities, Section on Developmental Behavioral Pediatrics, Bright Futures Steering Committee, Medical Home Initiatives for Children with Special Needs Project Advisory Committee. Identifying infants and young children with developmental disorders in the medical home: An algorithm for developmental surveillance and screening. Pediatrics. 2006;118(1):405-20.

Chapter 11

Multiple Disabilities

Leena Deshpande

"I am only one, but still, I am one. I cannot do everything, but still, I can do something; and because I cannot do everything, I will not refuse to do something that I can do."

Helen Keller

Helen Keller, who is one of the most famous disabled persons in the world overcame her struggle of being deaf and blind and dedicated her life to helping others. Based on her struggle with multiple disabilities, a popular Bollywood movie 'Black' depicts a child's life journey living with visual and hearing impairment. This movie has brought forth the many difficulties people with multiple disabilities face in daily life.

INTRODUCTION

Multiple disabilities is a general and broad term describing a child affected with more than one disability. Different combinations of disabilities are possible; it could be a combination of a physical and cognitive deficit, cognitive and behavioral disability, physical and sensory impairment, or a combination of any of these difficulties. In America, according to their Individuals with Disabilities Education Act (IDEA), deaf-blindness has a separate classification, however, in India it is included under the category of multiple disability.

Apart from the developmental and behavioral management in children with multiple disabilities, the care for the medical needs can also be challenging and complex as they require health-related services in addition to that required by typically developing children.

In India, as per the Census 2011 of the total disabled children in the age group of 0–19 years, 9% have multiple disabilities.

Multiple disabilities are seen in children with genetic syndromes, cerebral palsy, central nervous system malformations, metabolic disorders, chromosomal abnormalities, intrauterine infections, neurological disorders like spina bifida, and other-related conditions.

CLINICAL FEATURES

The clinical features depend on the disability the child has and its etiology. The main symptoms seen are difficulties with mobility, poor communication ability, and the need for assistance in daily activities. The combined effect of multiple disability can be more than the combination of two individual disabilities.

An example of multiple disability seen in office practice is a child with quadriparetic cerebral palsy with microcephaly who also has visual impairment, epilepsy, and cognitive impairment.

Hypoglycemic injury at birth may also cause multiple disabilities and the child may suffer from corticovisual impairment, features of autism spectrum disorder, and intractable seizures.

Syndromes like CHARGE as well as intrauterine infections like rubella will affect multiple systems.

Associated problems can be complex and multiple. Feeding problems, seizures, respiratory issues, failure to thrive, neurogenic bladder and bowel, orthopedic problems like hip dislocation and scoliosis, and endocrine issues like delayed or precocious puberty, along with combination of hearing or visual deficit are common.

Comorbid behavioral and psychological conditions such as anxiety, depression, aggressive behavior, and self-injurious behaviors are seen commonly as the child grows older.

Educational challenges are common and finding a school suitable to a child's intelligence level and commensurate with the multiple challenges can be quite difficult.

MANAGEMENT

The role of a pediatrician is crucial, both as a support to the family and as a care coordinator. It requires great dedication and compassion. Awareness regarding various comorbid conditions will help counseling the family.

The main goal is to foster independence as much as possible and help the child develop to the best of his potential.

Points to note:
- It is important to identify the types of disabilities the child has and their individual severities. Understanding how they affect the child's mobility and balance, his communication ability and learning potential is crucial to guide the family. Most children will need some level of support throughout life and the amount of support needed will depend on the disabilities involved and their severity.
- Coordination between the different pediatric medical and surgical specialists involved in the child's care can be best done by a developmental pediatrician and/or the primary pediatrician of the family.

- Depending on the problem areas, the developmental pediatrician will make an intervention program allotting goals to a multidisciplinary team including physiotherapist, occupational therapist, speech and language therapist, psychologist, special educator, and dietician.
- Awareness regarding available technology which can help the child's mobility and communication will optimize the child's progress.
- Recurrent respiratory infections due to multiple factors like gastroesophageal reflux and poor immunity worsen the general health. Advice regarding prevention of infections, e.g., influenza and routine vaccines may be needed. Poor weight gain and failure to thrive are common.
- Issues like feeding disorders, sleep problems, constipation, and seizures will cause daily difficulties and proactive, prompt, and appropriate guidance will help parents manage the child calmly and effectively.
- Children with multiple disabilities clock more frequent visits to the hospital and hospitalization rates are higher and longer.
- Etiological diagnosis will help in prognostication, proactive anticipatory guidance, and genetic counseling.
- The multiple problems of the child tend to be overwhelming for the family and empathy, ongoing support from the pediatrician helps them come to terms with the long-term morbidity.
- Many families get desperate and want to try alternative and complementary treatment modalities. Guiding them gently regarding evidence-based treatment, being nonjudgmental and helping them make informed choices is necessary.

"However difficult life may seem, there is always something you can do and succeed at. Concentrate on things your disability does not prevent you doing well and do not regret the things it interferes with. Do not be disabled in spirit as well."

Stephen Hawking

FURTHER READING

1. National Institute for Empowerment of Persons with Multiple Disabilities. https://niepmd.tn.nic.in.
2. William Carey, Allen Crocker, Ellen Roy Elias et al. Children with multiple disabilities and special heath care needs. Developmental -Behavioral Pediatrics. 4th edition, 2009.

Chapter 12

Down Syndrome

A Somasundaram

"I'm not a 'Down's. I am a person with Down syndrome—Down syndrome is just something I have, not who I am."

Anonymous

INTRODUCTION

Trisomy for the human chromosome 21 causes what is known as Down syndrome (DS) in about one of every 800 live births. It is a complex condition which results in multiple lifelong health problems, including varying degrees of intellectual disability (ID) and delays in speech, memory, and learning. Individuals with DS show a wide range of effects in many organ systems, some of which are congenital and some progressive. These include cardiac malformations, gastrointestinal anomalies, craniofacial and skeletal anomalies, and contrasting cancer phenotypes which include an increased frequency of childhood leukemia and reduced prevalence of many types of cancer in adults. There is broad variability in both the occurrence (penetrance) and severity (expressivity) of these phenotypes across the DS population. In recent years, increased research, education, health care, and intervention programs have all contributed to people with DS now working and leading longer and healthier lives.

All individuals with DS have some degree of ID making this the most frequent genetic cause of ID with intelligence quotients (IQs) that can range from mild to severe; the mean IQ in DS is ~50.

NEUROBIOLOGY OF DOWN SYNDROME

Despite being one of the first genetic diseases identified, only recently have we begun to understand how trisomy 21 may impact cognitive function. Cognitive disabilities in DS appear to result mainly from two pathological processes: neurogenesis impairment and Alzheimer-like degeneration. In DS, suboptimal network brain architecture and altered synaptic communication arising from neurodevelopmental impairment are key determinants of cognitive defects. Hypocellularity and hypoplasia start at early developmental stages and likely depend upon impaired proliferation of neuronal precursors, resulting in reduction of numbers of neurons and synaptic contacts. The impairment of neuronal precursor proliferation extends to adult neurogenesis and may affect learning and memory. Neurodegenerative mechanisms also contribute to cognitive impairment. Early-onset Alzheimer disease occurs with extremely high incidence in DS patients and is causally-related to overexpression of beta-amyloid precursor protein (beta APP), which is one of the triplicated genes in DS.

DEVELOPMENTAL MILESTONES

Children with DS will achieve the same milestones as other children, albeit at a delayed development. In monitoring the development of a child with DS, it is more useful to look at the sequence of milestones achieved, rather than the age at which the milestone is reached **(Table 1)**.

Table 1: Comparison of developmental milestones in a Down syndrome and a normal child.

Milestone	Range for children with Down syndrome	Typical range
Gross motor		
Sits alone	6–30 months	5–9 months
Crawls	8–22 months	6–12 months
Stands	1–3.25 years	8–17 months
Walks alone	1–4 years	9–18 months
Language		
First word	1–4 years	1–3 years
Two-word phrases	2–7.5 years	15–32 months
Social/Self-help		
Responsive smile	1.5–5 months	1–3 months
Finger feeds	10–24 months	7–14 months
Drinks from cup unassisted	12–32 months	9–17 months
Uses spoon	13–39 months	12–20 months
Bowel control	2–7 years	16–42 months
Dresses self-unassisted	3.5–8.5 years	3.25–5 years

RELATIVE STRENGTHS

Social Development

The social functioning of babies and children with DS is relatively less delayed than other areas of development. Babies with DS look at faces and smile only a week or two later than other children and they are usually sociable infants. Infants with DS enjoy communicating and make good use of nonverbal skills including babbling and gesture in social situations.

Most children and adults with DS continue to develop good social skills and appropriate social behavior, though a significant minority may develop difficult behaviors, particularly those with the greatest delays in speech and language development.

Learning with Visual Supports

Research suggests that people with DS learn better when they can see things illustrated. This finding has been demonstrated across a number of areas of development including the acquisition of language, motor skills, and literacy. This suggests that teaching will be more effective when information is presented with the support of pictures, gestures, or objects.

Word Reading

Many children with DS can develop reading abilities in advance of what might be expected for their cognitive and language levels. Reading makes an important contribution to vocabulary and language development for all children and this may be a particular benefit for children with DS, given their specific language delays.

CHARACTERISTIC DIFFICULTIES

Motor Development

Motor skills develop at a slower rate for children with DS than for those without. These delays in motor development reduce the infants' opportunities for exploring and learning about the world around them and therefore further affect cognitive development. Poor oral motor control may impact the development of language skills.

Expressive Language, Grammar, and Speech Clarity

Children with DS show specific delays in learning to use spoken language relative to their nonverbal understanding. Almost every child will have expressive language that is delayed relative to their language comprehension.

The children experience two types of expressive difficulty—delay in mastering sentence structures and grammar, and specific difficulties in developing clear speech production.

Several issues can affect speech and language development for children with DS:
- Cognitive development
- Hearing problems in some children
- Decreased muscle tone, strength, and coordination in mouth and throat

The gap between the children's understanding and their ability to express themselves is a cause of much frustration and can sometimes lead to behaviour problems. It can also result in the children's cognitive abilities being underestimated. Language delay also leads to cognitive delay as much human learning is through language and language is internalized for thinking, remembering, and self-organization.

Number Skills

Most children with DS struggle with basic number skills and their number skills are typically some 2 years behind their reading skills. There is a need for more research into the reasons for this. Currently, the best available advice is to draw on what is known about the children's learning strengths and to use maths teaching systems that make full use of visual supports to teach number concepts.

Verbal Short-term Memory

Short-term memory is the immediate memory system which holds information "in mind" for short periods of time and supports all learning and cognitive activity. It has separate components specialized for processing visual or verbal information.

The ability of children with DS to hold and process verbal information is not as good as their ability to hold and process visual information. These verbal short-term memory problems make it more difficult to learn new words and sentences. They also make it more difficult to process spoken language and this can adversely affect learning in the classroom.

Studies suggest that the processing and recall of spoken information is improved when it is supported by relevant picture material. This information has led to educators stressing the importance of using visual supports including pictures, signs, and print when teaching children with DS as this approach makes full use of their stronger visual memory skills.

BEHAVIORAL ISSUES

At least half of all children and adults with DS face a major mental health concern during their life span. Children and adults with multiple medical problems experience an even higher rate of mental health problems.

The pattern of mental health problems in DS vary depending on the age and developmental characteristics of the child or adult with DS as follows.

Young and early school age children with limitations in language and communication skills, cognition, and nonverbal problem solving abilities present with increased vulnerabilities in terms of:
- Disruptive, impulsive, inattentive, hyperactive, and oppositional behaviors (raising concerns of coexisting oppositional disorder and ADHD)
- Anxious, stuck, ruminative, inflexible behaviors (raising concerns of coexisting generalized anxiety and obsessive-compulsive disorders)
- Deficits in social relatedness, self-immersed, and repetitive stereotypical behaviors (raising concerns of coexisting autism or pervasive developmental disorder)
- Chronic sleep difficulties, daytime sleepiness, fatigue, and mood-related problems (raising concerns of coexisting sleep disorders and sleep apnea).

Older school age children and adolescents, as well as young adults with DS with better language and communication and cognitive skills presenting with increased vulnerability to:
- Depression, social withdrawal, diminished interests, and coping skills
- Generalized anxiety
- Obsessive compulsive behaviors
- Regression with decline in loss of cognitive and social skills
- Chronic sleep difficulties, daytime sleepiness, fatigue, and mood-related problems (raising concerns of coexisting sleep disorders and sleep apnea).

Older adults present with increased vulnerability to:
- Generalized anxiety
- Depression, social withdrawal, loss of interest, and diminished self-care
- Regression with decline in cognitive and social skills
- Dementia.

All these changes in behavior often seem to occur as a reaction to (or triggered by) a psychosocial or environmental stressor, e.g., illness in, separation from, or loss of a key attachment figure.

OBSESSIVE COMPULSIVE SYMPTOMS

Increased level of restlessness and worry may lead the child or adult to behave in a very rigid manner, even resulting in a state of being "stuck", as is often reported by caregivers where the child or adult needs to follow familiar routines in these situations. They also engage in repetitive, compulsive as well as ritualistic behaviors that raise the question of obsessive-compulsive disorder. The child or adult under these circumstances tends often to be unhappy, fearful, and the two states generalized anxiety and obsessive-compulsive behaviors may often coexist. The disruptive, oppositional, and inattentive child with DS often does not tend to be unhappy, but rather quite silly, happy, and excited. The problems are quite challenging for parents or caregivers to navigate, as the child/adult with DS with generalized anxiety or obsessive-compulsive profile has a tendency to be stuck, frozen, and require great degree of negative attention that, in turn, is reinforced and continues in a vicious cycle.

Sleep

Children and adults with DS commonly experience a range of sleep-related difficulties either as primary sleep disorder or associated with mental health problems (e.g., generalized anxiety and mood disturbances). Irrespective of the etiology, sleep difficulties impair the ability of a child or adult with DS to maintain alertness and attention during the day, as well as maintain better control, e.g., frustration tolerance. Chronic sleep difficulties in children and adults with DS need to be evaluated thoroughly by interdisciplinary team in order to rule out any contributory medical conditions.

Children and adults with DS, in particular, are at increased risk for development of obstructive sleep apnea with mild to moderate cessation of breathing during sleep that leads to reduction of oxygen saturation in the blood. Although the diagnosis of sleep apnea is suspected on the basis of history that often includes evidence for periods of daytime sleepiness, fatigue, it is necessary to conduct further tests to confirm this diagnosis by means of referral for a sleep study at a sleep disorder laboratory often available in major medical centers.

Prevalence of Autism Spectrum Disorder Symptomatology

Autism spectrum disorder (ASD) has previously been thought to be rare in individuals with DS but recent research suggests that ASD characteristics might occur in 5–35% of individuals with DS. Individuals with DS + ASD showed more stereotyped behaviour, repetitive language, over activity, and self-injury than those with DS only. Individuals with DS + ASD were less withdrawn from their surroundings than individuals with ASD only.

Hearing Impairment

The anatomical ear structure of children with DS has characteristics that may predispose them to hearing deficits. They are more prone to conductive hearing loss secondary to cerumen impaction and middle ear pathologies, including, among others, middle ear effusion, acute otitis media, and eardrum perforations. They can experience permanent (conductive, sensorineural, and mixed hearing losses were identified in significant numbers) and transient hearing loss secondary to a middle ear disease.

MANAGEMENT

For children with DS, the definition of a "behavior problem" varies but certain guidelines can be helpful in determining if a behavior has become significant.
- Does the behavior interfere with development and learning?
- Are the behaviors disruptive to the family, school, or workplace?
- Is the behavior harmful to the child or adult with DS or to others?
- Is the behavior different from what might be typically displayed by someone of comparable developmental age?

The first step in evaluating a child or adult with DS who presents with a behavior concern is to determine if there are any acute or chronic medical problems related to the identified behavior. The following is a list of the more common medical problems that may be associated with behavior changes.
- Vision or hearing deficits
- Thyroid function
- Celiac disease
- Sleep apnea
- Anemia
- Gastroesophageal reflux
- Constipation
- Depression
- Anxiety

Evaluation by the primary care physician is an important component of the initial work-up for behavior problems in children or adults with DS.

Finally, caveats or steps to consider in addressing any of the above potential medical concerns in the context of treatment of "behavioral problems" include the following:
- *Step 1:* Emotional/behavioral problems in children and adults with DS occur commonly and are not always due to an underlying medical condition. Nevertheless, these medical conditions associated in children and adults with DS need to be ruled out as part of a comprehensive assessment approach.
- *Step 2:* Medical conditions, even if they may not cause the emotional/behavioral issues, may nevertheless exacerbate them or make the child or adult with DS resistant to treatment of the emotional/behavioral problem.
- *Step 3:* Correction of a medical condition, e.g., hypothyroidism, may not remove the underlying emotional/behavioral issues. The opposite is also true; e.g., a child or adult with hypothyroidism plus depression is unlikely to respond to treatment of depression with antidepressant medication alone unless the hypothyroidism is corrected. Because emotional/behavioral and physical issues are intertwined, the two need to be treated concurrently.

FURTHER READING

1. Baburamani AA, Patkee PA, Arichi T, Rutherford MA. New approaches to studying early brain development in Down syndrome. Dev Med Child Neurol. 2019;61(8):867-79.
2. Contestabile A, Benfenati F, Gasparini L. Communication breaks-down: From neurodevelopment defects to cognitive disabilities in Down syndrome. Prog Neurobiol. 2010;91(1):1-22.
3. Cooling G. Hearing loss in children with Down syndrome, Nightengale, Emily AuD. The Hearing Journal. 2018;71(2):10-12.
4. Moss J, Richards C, Nelson L, Oliver C. Prevalence of autism spectrum disorder symptomatology and related behavioural characteristics in individuals with Down syndrome. Autism. 2013;17(4):390-404.
5. Vicari S, Pontillo M, Armando M. Neurodevelopmental and psychiatric issues in Down's syndrome: assessment and intervention. Psychiatr Genet. 2013;23(3):95-107.

Chapter 13

Turner Syndrome

Shambhavi Seth

TURNER SYNDROME

Turner syndrome is a chromosomal disorder which affects only females. The normal female karyotype comprises of two X chromosomes but in Turner syndrome one X chromosome is deficient or structurally altered. Hence, it is also known as **45, X,** or **45, X0.**

INTRODUCTION

The incidence of Turner syndrome worldwide is 1:2000–1:5000 females at birth but the incidence is said to be more in female fetuses which do not survive. Up to 95–99% of Turner syndrome conceptions are thought to end in miscarriages or still births.

Almost 50% of individuals with Turner syndrome have monosomy that is single X chromosome (**Fig. 1**). This occurs due to nondisjunction at the time of cell division which leads to missing chromosome in reproductive cells. When one of these cells forms the genetic makeup, it will present as single X chromosome. In most of the cases of monosomy, the functional X chromosome comes from mother.

Other condition in which Turner can present is as mosaic Turner syndrome (**Fig. 2**), in which females may have missing X chromosome in some but not in all the cells. Both monosomy and mosaic Turner syndrome are not inherited which means that a family having one child with Turner may not have increased risk in subsequent pregnancies. Only in rare circumstances where there is a balanced translocation of X chromosome in a parent, or where the mother has 45X mosaicism restricted to her germ cells, there may be an exception.

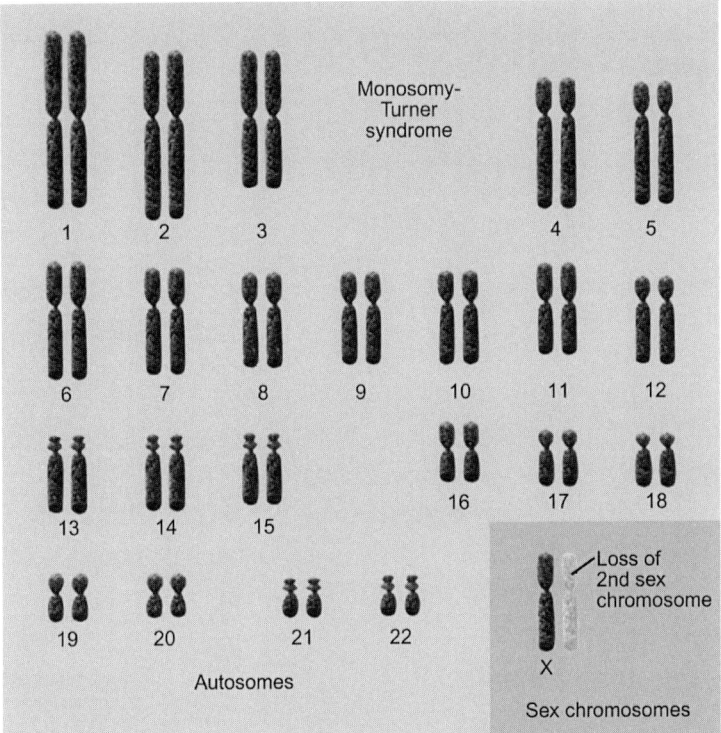

Fig. 1: Monosomy—Turner syndrome.
Source: National Library of Medicine. Turner Syndrome. Bethesda, United States. [online] Available from https://ghr.nlm.nih.gov/ condition/turner-syndrome (Last accessed December, 2021).

CLINICAL FEATURES

Before birth: Prenatal ultrasound may show edema or fluid collection on the back of the neck or other abnormal fluid collections, heart abnormalities, and abnormal kidneys.

Newborns: Clinical presentation may vary from small for gestation age, webbing of neck, protruding ears, and lymphedema of hands and feet to a normal phenotype.

Infancy: Broad chest with widely spaced nipples, low hairline at the back of the head, receding or small lower jaw, high narrow palate, cubitus valgus, congenital hip dislocation, patella dislocation, fingernails, and toenails that are narrow and turned upward, short fingers and toes.

Congenital heart defects may be present in 40% of cases. Most common heart defects being bicuspid aortic valves, coarctation of aorta, aortic stenosis, and mitral valve prolapse.

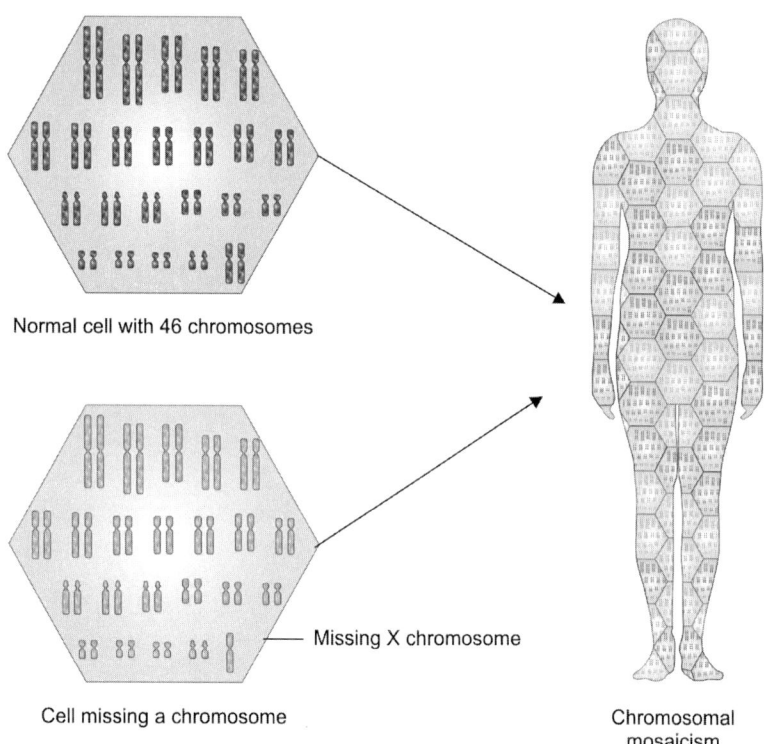

Fig. 2: Mosaic Turner syndrome.
Source: National Library of Medicine. Turner syndrome. Bethesda, United States. [online] Available from https://ghr.nlm.nih.gov/ condition/turner-syndrome (Last accessed December, 2021).

Structural renal anomalies are also fairly common (60% cases). Mostly present as horseshoe kidney, an abnormal urine-collecting system, and poor blood flow to the kidneys.

Older children and adults: Most common features are short stature and ovarian insufficiency. There is underlying gonadal dysgenesis which leads to primary amenorrhea, lack of secondary sexual characters, and infertility.

Effect on development: Most patients tend to be of normal intelligence but up to 6% have underlying intellectual disability. They are also at increased risk for learning disabilities (up to 70% cases). The verbal skills are better preserved compared to nonverbal skills—particularly arithmetic, visuospatial skills, and processing speed. Social awkwardness and increased risk of behavioral problems like attention deficit hyperactivity disorder is there.

Other features: Hypothyroidism may be seen in 15–20% cases. Women with Turner syndrome are at a moderately increased risk of developing type 1 diabetes in childhood and a substantially increased risk of developing type 2 diabetes by adult years. Strabismus, cataracts, recurrent otitis media, sensorineural hearing loss, inflammatory bowel disease, and increased incidence of celiac disease may be present.

MANAGEMENT

Chromosomal karyotyping is the test of choice for diagnosis of Turner syndrome and can be done at any age. Prenatally amniocentesis or chorionic villus sampling for diagnosis during pregnancy can be done.

There is no definitive cure for Turner syndrome but therapies are targeted to improve quality of life and alleviation of clinical symptoms.

The primary treatment for all cases includes hormone therapies:
- Growth hormone therapy is recommended to increase the final height and can be started in early childhood. Oxandrolone is a hormone that helps to increase height by increasing the body's production of protein and improving bone mineral density and may be recommended in addition to growth hormone.
- Estrogen therapy is given to induce puberty. Often, estrogen therapy is started around age 11 or 12 years. Estrogen helps to promote breast development and improve the uterine volume. Estrogen replacement therapy usually continues throughout life, until the average age of menopause is reached.
- Fertility treatments are required for conception. Females with Turner syndrome have relatively high-risk pregnancies in most cases.

Since Turner syndrome can result in various developmental problems and medical complications, a team of specialists is required for holistic management.

FURTHER READING

1. Beit-Aharon C. Standing Tall with Turner Syndrome. Lulu Press. 2013.
2. Donaldson MDC, Gault EJ, Tan KW, Dunger DB. Optimising management in Turner syndrome: From infancy to adult transfer". Arch Dis Child. 2006;91(6):513-20.
3. Danielsson K. Turner Syndrome (Monosomy X) and Pregnancy Loss. 2009.
4. Gravholt CH, Andersen NH, Conway GS, Dekkers OM, Geffner ME, Klein KO, et al. Clinical practice guidelines for the care of girls and women with Turner syndrome: Proceedings from the 2016 Cincinnati International Turner Syndrome Meeting. Eur J Endocrinol. 2017;177(3):G1-70.
5. Kliegman R. Nelson Textbook of Pediatrics: First South Asia edition, Volume 3. Elsevier.
6. National Library of Medicine. Turner Syndrome. Bethesda, United States. [online] Available from https://ghr.nlm.nih.gov/ condition/turner-syndrome (Last accessed December, 2021).

Chapter 14

Noonan Syndrome

Kawaljit Singh Multani

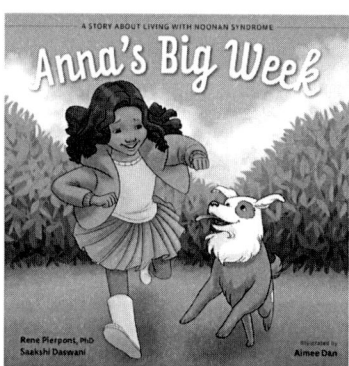

"Anna's Big Week" by Rene Pierpont and Saakshi Daswani tells the story of a spunky 9-year-old girl who has been diagnosed with Noonan syndrome and describes week long events at her home, school, and hospital visits.

INTRODUCTION

In two separate reports, one in 1883 by Kobylinski and the other in 1902 by Funke, two separate patients were described with webbed neck and short stature. This led to interest in a phenotype dubbed as the "male Turner syndrome". Ullrich described similar features in an 8-year-old girl in 1930. In 1968, a pediatric cardiologist Jacqueline Noonan described a series of 19 patients in the American Journal of Diseases of Children titled "Hypertelorism with Turner phenotype" who had short stature associated with significant facial, cardiac, and chest wall abnormalities. Dr Noonan was the first to highlight that this condition occurred in both males and females, along with congenital heart disease in many cases and familial occurrence in certain cases. The eponym "Noonan Syndrome (NS)" was adopted in recognition of her work in 1971 at the symposium of cardiovascular defects.

Noonan syndrome is an autosomal dominant disorder, which is seen equally in males and females. With the advancements in the field of genetics, NS is now a part of the group of disorders termed RASopathies, occurring in 1 in 1,000–1 in 2,500 live births, caused by defective Ras/mitogen-activated protein kinase (MAPK) signaling pathway. Mutations in genes encoding for the proteins or regulators of the Ras/MAPK signaling pathway have profound effects on development of the fetus which results in defects in developmental processes of multiple organs in varying degrees causing a wide spectrum of phenotypical features.

CLINICAL FEATURES

- Dysmorphic facial features such as hypertelorism, ptosis, low set ears, webbed neck, and low posterior hairline are characteristic.
- More than 80% cases may have congenital heart disease in the form of pulmonary valve stenosis, hypertrophic cardiomyopathy, and atrial septal defects.
- *Developmental delay*: Gross motor and fine motor delays are seen in 50-75% of cases most of which persist in childhood and adolescence.
- Most cases with NS have intelligence quotient (IQ) in the average range, 6-23% of cases have IQ < 70 and slow processing speed and nonverbal reasoning.
- Feeding problems like poor suck/swallow, gagging, gastroesophageal (GE) reflux, recurrent vomiting, food refusal, and intestinal dysmotility are seen early in life.
- Delayed speech and poor language development are seen in 40-65% of cases and are more common in males.
- *Behavior issues*: Higher rates of attention deficit hyperactivity disorder (ADHD) and autistic spectrum disorder (ASD), social immaturity, and reduced peer interaction.
- *Musculoskeletal disorders*: Chest deformities and scoliosis
- *Endocrine disorders:* Short stature, growth hormone (GH) deficiency, hypothyroidism, and delayed puberty.
- Cryptorchidism (unilateral/bilateral)
- Renal disorders, e.g., dilated renal pelvis, horse shoe kidney, polycystic kidney disease, renal hypoplasia, and unilateral renal ectopia/agenesis
- Neurological disorders, e.g., seizures, hydrocephalous, and Chiari I malformation
- Skin disorders, e.g., keratosis pilaris and ulerythema
- Coagulation defects and lymphatic dysplasias.

DIAGNOSIS AND GENETICS

Noonan syndrome should be suspected in all children with characteristic facial features, short stature, and congenital heart disease. Most cases are sporadic **(Fig. 1)**. The risk of NS developing in the sibling of an affected person is 50% if one parent is affected, but is <1% if none of the parent(s) is affected. Mutation testing will confirm a diagnosis of NS in 70-75% of cases (PTPN11, SOS1, RAF1, R1T1, and KRAS) which has implications for management and

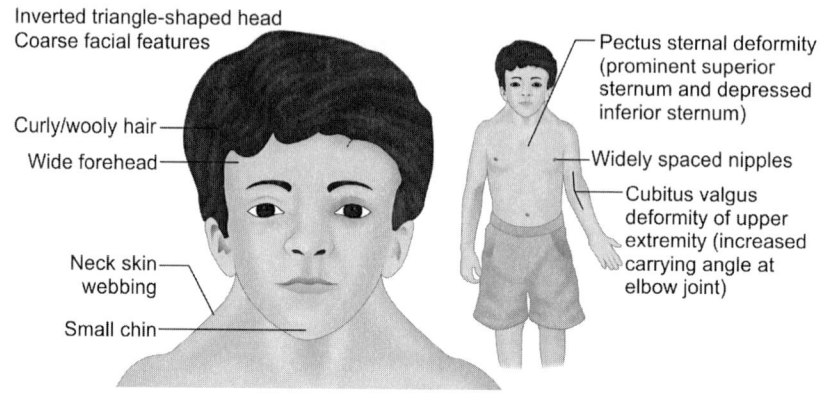

Fig. 1: Facial features in Noonan syndrome.

genetic counseling. Individuals with PTPN11 and SOS1 have little or no cognitive impairment. Preimplantation genetic diagnosis in familial cases with known mutations can be offered.

DIFFERENTIAL DIAGNOSIS

Cardiofaciocutaneous syndrome: Characterized by cardiac abnormalities, distinctive craniofacial appearance, and cutaneous abnormalities.

Costello syndrome: Characterized by growth problems, developmental delay or intellectual disability, coarse facial features, curly or sparse fine hair, soft skin with deep palmar and plantar creases, papillomata of the face and perianal region, diffuse hypotonia, joint laxity, and cardiac disease.

LEOPARD syndrome: An acronym for the cardinal features of lentigines, electrocardiogram (ECG) conduction abnormalities, ocular hypertelorism, pulmonary stenosis, abnormal genitalia, retardation of growth, and sensorineural deafness.

MANAGEMENT

Multidisciplinary team approach is required for evaluation and follow-up of cases with NS **(Table 1)**. Age-based Noonan growth charts and treatment guidelines are available **(Figs. 2A and B)**. Cardiovascular anomalies are managed as per general population guidelines. Recently, trametinib [a mitogen-activated extracellular signal-regulated kinase (MEK) inhibitor] has been used in treatment of cardiac conditions of NS and has been found to reverse hypertrophic cardiomyopathy and valvular obstruction in patients with RIT1-associated NS. Endocrinologist, nephrologist, hematologist,

Noonan Syndrome

Table 1: Routine screening guidelines for children with Noonan syndrome at different ages.

	Prenatal	Birth–3 months	3 months–1 year	1–5 years	5–15 years
Counseling regarding prenatal diagnosis*					
Physical exam for evidence of Noonan syndrome with particular attention to cardiac examination, cryptorchidism, skin examination, and GIT (feeding problems)					
ECHO by pediatric cardiologist					
Mutation testing to confirm diagnosis					
Newborn hearing screening and follow-up					
Growth and development assessment			Monitor OFC, length and weight 3 monthly; use Noonan specific growth charts. Assess development at each visit and refer early for developmental delay		
Thyroid screening (if not done as part of newborn screen)			Baseline assessment at the time of diagnosis		
CNS evaluation			Low threshold for investigation of neurological symptoms like headache, etc.; refer for MRI early		
Ophthalmology assessment			Baseline assessment at the time of diagnosis		
Renal ultrasound			Baseline assessment at the time of diagnosis		
Coagulation screening			Prior to any major surgery OR once in childhood		
Skin problems and lymphedema			Avoid skin dryness and hot baths		
Behavioral issues					
Learning difficulties**					

Note: *In case of an earlier affected child; **At school entry
(CNS: central nervous system; GIT: gastrointestinal tract; MRI: magnetic resonance imaging)

ophthalmologist, otolaryngologist, neurologist, behavior therapist, and speech therapist form the part of team based on the clinical features of the case.

NOONAN SYNDROME GIRLS
2–20 years
Stature and growth velocity for age*
Name:
DOB:
ID:
Mother's stature:
Father's stature:
Mean parental height:
Date
Age
Weight
Stature
BMI[b]
Tanner[c]
bTo calculate BMI: Weight (kg) ÷ stature (cm) ÷ stature (cm) x 10,000
or weight (lb) ÷ stature (in) ÷ stature (in) x 703
cTanner stages of pubic hair (P1,P2,P3,P4,P5) and breast development (B1,B2,B3,B4,B5)
Age (years)
STATURE
Entire female population
97%
50%
3%
%
SD
97 1.88
90 1.28
75 0.67
50 0.00
25 -0.67
10 -1.28
3 -1.88
cm
in
cm/y
GROWTH VELOCITY
Late maturer (=2SD)
Growth velocity for age in normal population

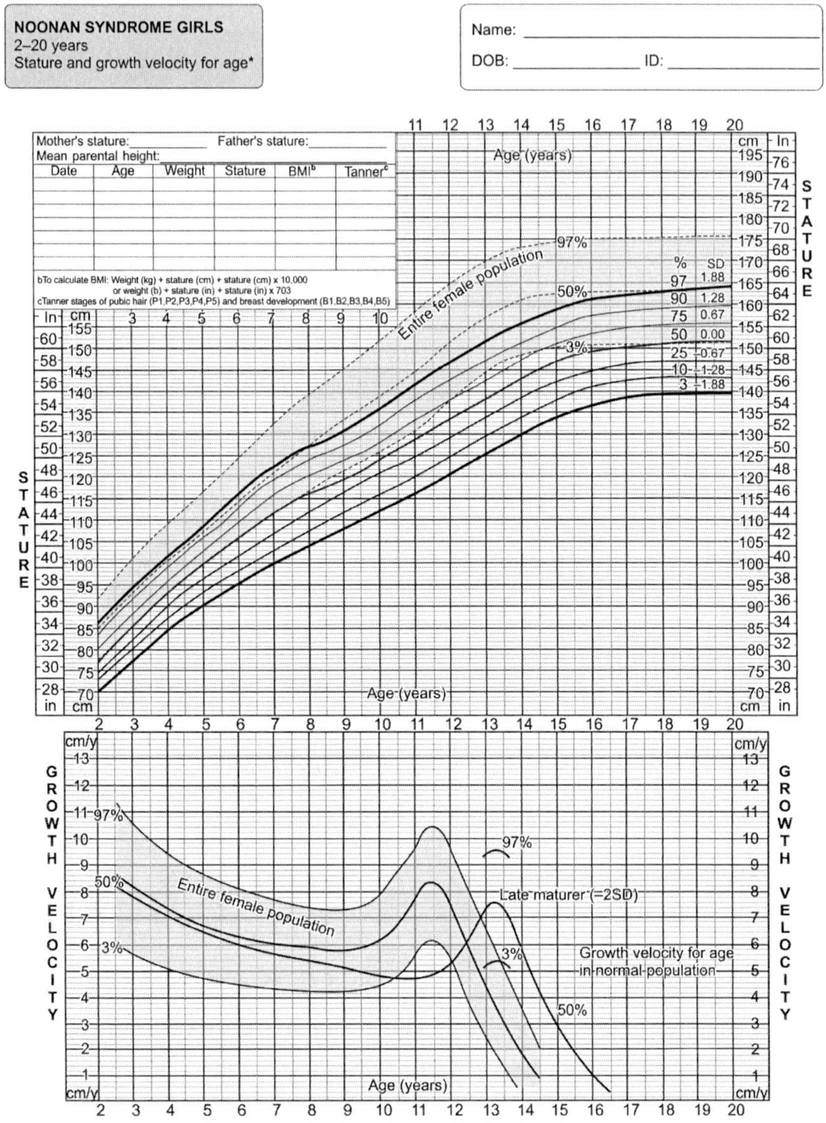

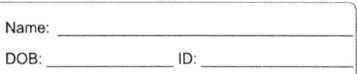

Fig. 2A

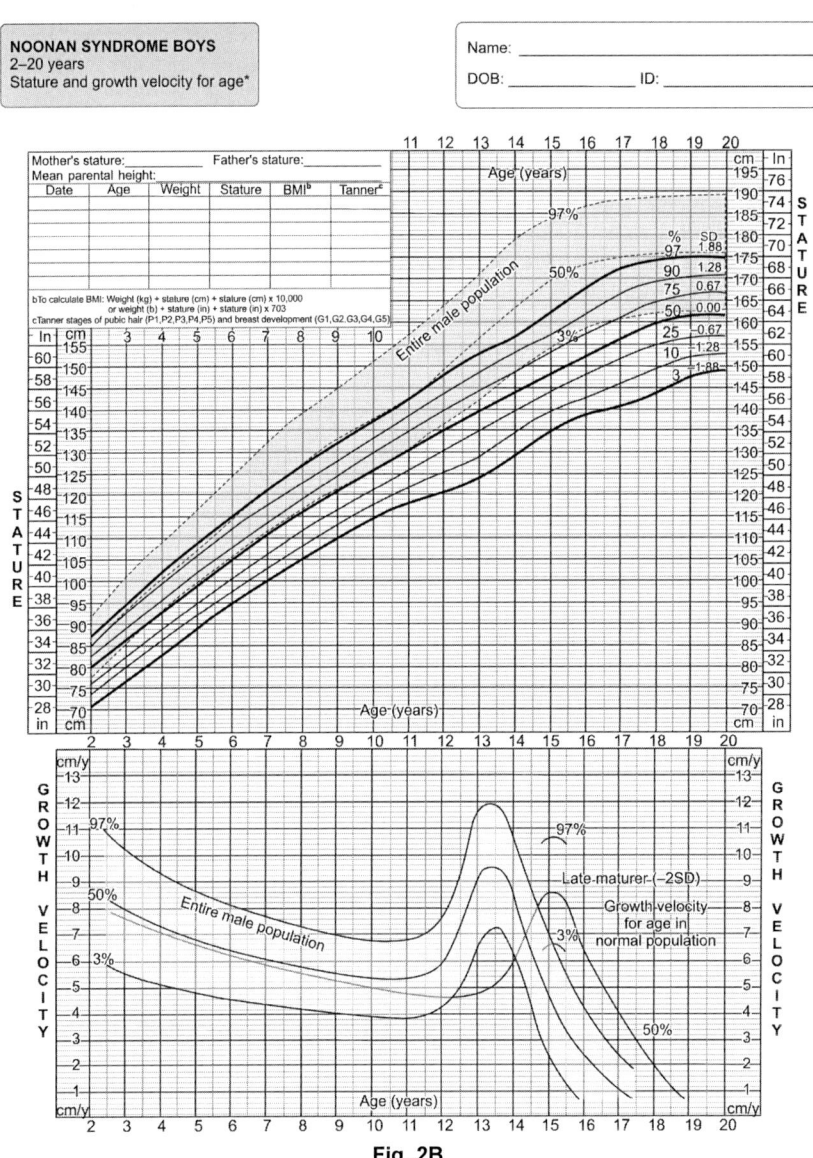

Fig. 2B
Figs. 2A and B: Growth charts for Noonan syndrome.
Source: http://www2.dyscerne.org

FURTHER READING

1. Bhambhani V, Muenke M. Noonan syndrome. Am Fam Physician. 2014;89(1): 37-43.
2. Kim YE, Baek ST. Neurodevelopmental aspects of RASopathies. Mol Cells. 2019;42(6):441-7.
3. Meštrović T. Noonan Syndrome History. [online] Available from https://www.news-medical.net/health/Noonan-Syndrome-History.aspx (Last accessed December, 2021).
4. Noonan Syndrome Guideline Development Group. (2011). Management of Noonan syndrome: A clinical guideline. [online] Available from http://www2.dyscerne.org (Last accessed December, 2021).
5. Pierpont EI. Neuropsychological functioning in individuals with Noonan syndrome: A systematic literature review with educational and treatment recommendations. J Pediatr Neuropsychol. 2016;2:14-33.
6. Roelofs RL, Janssen N, Wingbermühle E, Kessels RP, Egger JI. Intellectual development in Noonan syndrome: A longitudinal study. Brain Behav. 2016;6(7):e00479.

Chapter 15

Fragile X Syndrome

MA Florita, B Yambao-Dela Cruz, Kaye M Napalinga, Randi J Hagerman

INTRODUCTION

Fragile X syndrome (FXS) is a genetic condition that is the most common inherited cause of intellectual disability and the most common monogenic cause of autism spectrum disorders (ASD).

The mean prevalence of FXS was estimated at 1 in 5,000–7,000 for males and 1 in 8,000–11,000 for females although the prevalence can vary in different parts of the world. It is inherited as an X-linked dominant trait. Males carrying the full mutation (FM) [>200 CGG repeats in the front end of the gene *FMR1* (fragile X mental retardation 1)] are always affected and females carrying the FM are less affected (~30–50%). The prevalence of the premutation (PM) ranges from ~1 in 250 to 1 in 813 males and ~1 in 110 to 1 in 270 females.

CLINICAL FEATURES

The FXS phenotype is caused by inactivation of the *FMR1* gene. Manifestations are variable and depend on differences in FMRP (Fragile X mental retardation protein) production caused by *FMR1* inactivation. Several factors affect the level of FMRP. These include: sex, background genetic effects, environmental influences, and molecular variations (the level of methylation or the presence of mosaicism of repeat size or methylation). Physical, medical, and neuropsychiatric manifestations comprise the FXS phenotype.

The clinical presentation of FXS begins in infancy, but becomes more specific and prominent as the individual gets older. Infants with FXS initially present with hypotonia, poor suck, reflux, and frequent regurgitation. Delays in language development, hyperactivity, anxiety, sensory overload, sleep disturbances, and recurrent otitis media become manifest in the first 2 years of life. This is followed by impulsivity, aggression, autism symptoms, poor eye contact, tantrums, anxiety, and seizures (in 16%) in early childhood.

The classic physical features of FXS that include prominent ears, a long face, flat feet, hyperextensible finger joints, double-jointed thumbs, and soft skin are usually seen in childhood. Macroorchidism develops at puberty. Other features include hernias, joint dislocations, and flat feet with pronation.

Behavioral symptoms in adolescence include increasing aggression, persistent anxiety, impulsivity, hyperactivity, inattention, and perseveration. In adulthood, there is episodic dyscontrol, persistence of poor attention, anxiety, and perseveration. In aging, patients with FXS can present with symptoms of Parkinsonism and cognitive decline. The clinical presentation is also different for males and females, with females having less severe manifestations than males.

The clinical presentation of the *FMR1* PM differs from the FM. These include: (1) fragile X-associated neuropsychiatric disorders (FXAND) that can affect 50% of carriers and includes anxiety, depression, attention-deficit/hyperactivity disorder (ADHD), insomnia, chronic fatigue, chronic pain, or social deficits or ASD; (2) fragile X-associated tremor/ataxia syndrome (FXTAS), a neurodegenerative disorder that can start in the 60s and affects 40% of male carriers and 16% of female carriers, and (3) fragile X-associated primary ovarian insufficiency meaning ovarian dysfunction or menopause before age 40 (FXPOI).

MANAGEMENT

A physician or health care provider should order *FMR1* deoxyribonucleic acid (DNA) testing in any child that presents with a substantial developmental delay, intellectual disability, or ASD without a known reason. For each child diagnosed with FXS, they have other family members with PM or FM alleles. In addition, we recommend testing the siblings of individuals with FXS, cascade testing (i.e., *FMR1* DNA testing of other extended family members) once a proband is diagnosed.

Management is multidisciplinary. Early diagnosis and intervention is recommended and children diagnosed with FXS benefit from early intervention that includes speech and language therapy, physical therapy, behavioral therapy, occupational therapy with a sensory integration approach and special education programs.

Pharmacologic interventions include the conventional psychotropic medications commonly used for treatment of individuals with FXS such as stimulants, selective serotonin reuptake inhibitors (SSRIs) and in some cases, atypical antipsychotics. Stimulants are usually beneficial for the treatment of ADHD symptoms in children with FXS who are ≥5 years of age. For individuals with severe hyperactivity who are <5 years of age, the use of an α-adrenergic agonist, such as guanfacine or clonidine, can be helpful. Anxiety is also common and a low dose of sertraline can be of help in children with FXS who are 2 years and older. For children with FXS who demonstrate aggression or severe anxiety that is not improved with an SSRI, use of an atypical antipsychotic, such as aripiprazole or risperidone, can also be useful.

Associated medical conditions are common among individuals with FXS. Conductive hearing loss due to recurrent otitis media is common which can be managed with antibiotic treatment or early ventilation tube (pressure-equalization tube) placement. Hearing monitoring should be done successively. Adenoidectomy and or tonsillectomy maybe carried out when there is chronic infection of the adenoids or obstructive sleep apnea. Accordingly, monitoring and managing obstructive sleep apnea and other sleep problems are of particular importance in individuals with FXS, as they are linked to decrements in daytime performance and behavior. Sleep problems may also be ameliorated with melatonin and if this does not work then low dose clonidine can help with sleep. Visual screening is recommended within the first 3–4 years of life to address vision problems such as strabismus. Seizures are seen in 16% of children with FXS and should be identified by electroencephalography and proceeded with a neurology referral and treatment with an anticonvulsant. Other complications of FXS include gastro-esophageal reflux wherein antacids may be used for treatment to prevent pain, esophagitis, and resulting behavioral decompensation. Some individuals with FXS benefit from orthotics or shoe inserts for the management of foot pronation and flat feet, and this can help with motor development in younger patients and to avoid leg pain and reduce gait problems when older. Lifestyle modification is also highly recommended encouraging patients to follow a healthy diet, including food restriction when necessary because of obesity, and partaking in exercise programs to minimize the health problems associated with weight gain.

Targeted treatments include the following medications; metformin, a common type 2 diabetes medication, is beneficial for language and eating behavior in children and adults with FXS. Controlled trials of metformin are currently taking place to see if cognitive improvements occur with metformin treatment. Another medication cannabidiol (CBD) has been very helpful in a topical preparation for children with FXS in open label studies and a controlled trial is currently taking place internationally. In addition, low dose sertraline has been helpful for development and behavior in young children with FXS.

ACKNOWLEDGMENTS

This work was supported in part by the NICHD grant HD036071, the Azrieli Foundation and the NICHD funded MIND Institute Intellectual and Developmental Disabilities Research Center (grant U54 HD079125) and the National Center for Advancing Translational Sciences and National Institutes of Health (grant UL1 TR001860).

FURTHER READING

1. Hagerman RJ, Berry-Kravis E, Hazlett HC, Bailey DB Jr, Moine H, Kooy RF, et al. Fragile X Syndrome. Nat Rev Dis Primers. 2017;3:17065.
2. Hagerman RJ, Hagerman PJ. Fragile X Syndrome: Diagnosis Treatment and Research, 3rd edition. Baltimore, Maryland: The John Hopkins University Press; 2002. pp. 3-22.
3. Hunter J, Rivero-Arias O, Angelov A, Kim E, Fotheringham I, Leal J. Epidemiology of fragile X syndrome: A systematic review and meta-analysis. Am J Med Genet A. 2014;164A(7):1648-58.
4. Willemsen R, Kooy RF. Fragile X Syndrome from Genetics to Targeted Treatment. University of Antwerp, Antwerp, Belgium: Elsevier. 2017.

Chapter 16

Klinefelter Syndrome

Kawaljit Singh Multani

"Children are not things to be molded, but are people to be unfolded."
Jess Lair

INTRODUCTION

"Klinefelter syndrome" (KS) is the most common genetic cause of male infertility and has an estimated frequency of 1 in 500–1 in 1,000 males. Harry Klinefelter, Fuller Albright, and EC Reifenstein reported a series of nine men with gynecomastia, small testes, and azoospermia in 1942 which was named as Klinefelter–Reifenstein–Albright syndrome. Later in 1959, it was demonstrated by Patricia Jacobs and John Anderson that such cases have an additional X chromosome resulting in a 47, XXY karyotype. This additional X chromosome results in disruption of many aspects of fetal development which results in characteristic phenotype of KS.

Most of the cases (80–90%) have the karyotype (47,XXY) while the rest (10–20%) either have mosaic pattern (47,XXY/46,XY), or additional X chromosomes (48,XXXY or 48,XXYY) or structurally abnormal X chromosomes (47,XiXqY). The condition is not inherited and the additional X chromosome results from nondisjunction of sex chromosomes during meiosis I in the gonads and is inherited from the father in 50% and the mother in 50% of the cases. The risk is increased with increased maternal age as chromosomal abnormalities tends to increase with age.

CLINICAL DIAGNOSIS

Most of the children born with KS are normal at birth and the initial few years. Few cases have cleft palate, clinodactyly, cardiac abnormalities, inguinal hernia, cryptorchidism, hypospadias, or micropenis and these are more frequently seen in cases with higher degree of chromosomal abnormalities. Children with KS are taller than others and have muscle weakness which becomes more pronounced with age. Motor delays (developmental coordination disorder), speech delays (poor expressive speech), and learning disabilities [reading problems and specific learning disability (SLD)] are also found in patients with KS. They also tend to have emotional issues, anxiety, depression, limited problem-solving skills, and poor social skills. 10% of the cases can have autism spectrum disorder (ASD).

More than 75% of the cases are diagnosed after puberty. At puberty, boys (>50% of cases) develop gynecomastia, have small testes (<4 mL testicular volume) and less facial and bodily hair. Eunuchoid body structure (tall, slim with long legs and arms, and arm span exceeding height by ≥5 cms) with gynecomastia and androgen insufficiency is the hallmark of a case of KS. In a large case series of 44 patients, it was seen that two-thirds of the cases were diagnosed after 18 years of age and dysmorphism, developmental delays, cardiac abnormalities, intellectual disabilities, and behavioral issues [depression and attention deficit hyperactivity disorder (ADHD)] were commonly seen in pediatric population as compared to adults. Due to the additional X chromosomes, these males are prone to autoimmune disorders, thromboembolic phenomenon and osteoporosis. Almost half of the cases develop a metabolic syndrome (increased belly fat, hypertension, elevated lipids, and type II diabetes mellitus). Persons with KS have a 20-50 folds increase in risk of breast cancer as compared to normal population.

Differential diagnosis of KS includes Fragile X syndrome, Kallman syndrome, and Marfan syndrome. Diagnosis of KS should be suspected in all male children with delayed puberty, tall stature, small testes, and gynecomastia. Diagnosis can be confirmed by karyotyping. They have low testosterone levels and elevated follicle-stimulating hormone/luteinizing hormone (FSH/LH) levels with FSH levels being much higher as compared to LH. Serum testosterone levels continue to fall with age. Semen examination may reveal azoospermia or low sperm count with poor motility. Fibrosis of seminiferous tubules is seen in testicular histology.

MANAGEMENT

As the condition is genetic, the management is mainly supportive once the diagnosis has been made. A developmental intervention program in cases with motor delay as well as specific case-based interventions can be of use in school going children who have school/socialization issues and dyspraxias.

Hormonal replacement therapy with testosterone can be used for improving masculinity (increase in muscle mass and hair growth) as well as reduce the chances of osteoporosis. Intramuscular injections of testosterone can be given every 3 weeks; initial doses are kept low and as puberty advances the dose is increased **(Fig. 1)**. Depot preparations of testosterone (once in 3 months) are also available. Gynecomastia may persist despite treatment

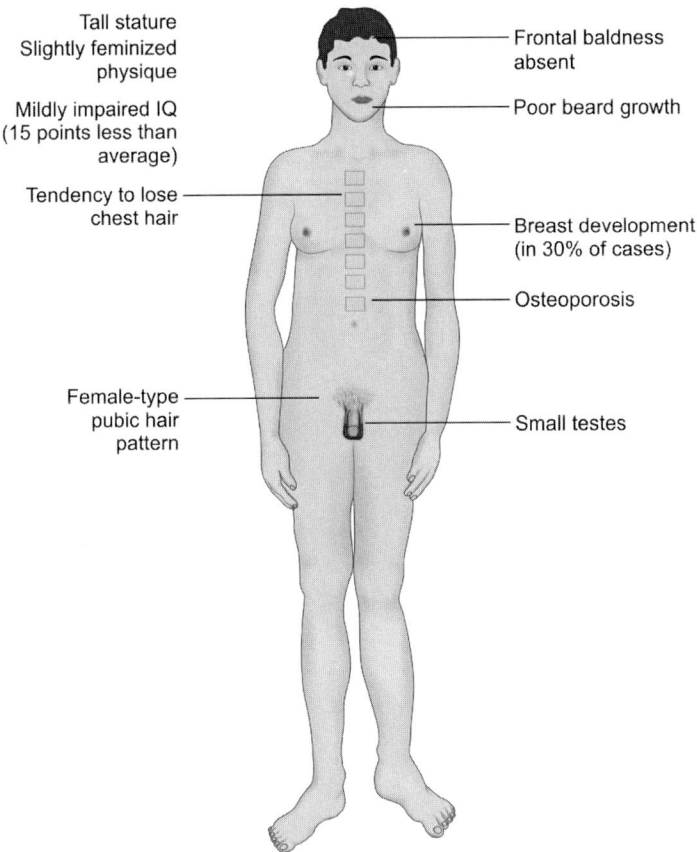

Fig. 1: Features of Klinefelter's syndrome.

with testosterone and require surgical resection. About 3.1% of all males with infertility have KS. With the availability of intracytoplasmic sperm injection (ICSI) and testicular sperm extraction (TSE), it is now possible for men with KS to father children.

FURTHER READING

1. Alcan N, Poyrazoglu S, Bas F, Bundak R, Darendeliler F. Klinefelter syndrome in childhood: Variability in clinical and molecular findings. J Clin Res Pediatr Endocrinol. 2018;10(2):100-7.
2. Asirvatham AR, Pavithran PV, Pankaj A, Bhavani N, Menon U, Menon A, et al. Klinefelter syndrome: Clinical spectrum based on 44 consecutive cases from a South Indian Tertiary Care Center. Indian J Endocrinol Metab. 2019;23(2): 263-6.
3. Bearelly P, Oates R. Recent advances in managing and understanding Klinefelter syndrome. F1000Res. 2019;8 (F1000Faculty Rev).

4. Klinefelter HF, Reifenstein EC, Albright F. Syndrome characterized by gynecomastia, aspermatogenesis without A-Leydigsm and increased excretion of FSH. J Clin Endocrinol Metab. 1942;2(11);615-27.
5. Nieschlag E, Ferlin A, Gravholt CH, Gromoll J, Köhler B, Lejeune H, et al. The Klinefelter syndrome: Current management and research challenges. Andrology. 2016;4(3):545-9.
6. Peynirci H, Erturk E. Klinefelter syndrome—Review. Turk Jem. 2013;17:63-7.

Chapter 17

Prader–Labhart–Willi Syndrome

Manju George Elenjickal, Neethu Mary Mathew

INTRODUCTION

Prader-Willi syndrome (PWS) is a complex multisystem genetic disorder that shows great variability, with changing clinical features during the lifespan. It is a relatively common congenital disorder with an incidence of about 1 in 10,000 live births. The syndrome is caused by the loss of expression of several paternally acquired genes encoded on the proximal long arm of chromosome 15 (15q11.2–q13). It was first described by Prader, Labhardt, and Willi in 1956 in nine children with the tetrad of small stature, mental retardation, obesity, and small hands and feet. The complex phenotype is most probably caused by a hypothalamic dysfunction that is responsible for hormonal dysfunctions and for absence of the sense of satiety. Thus, the child develops hyperphagia during infancy which can lead to obesity and its complications. Many children with PWS display a range of behavioral problems that become more noticeable and interfere with the quality of life as they grow older. The chief characteristics of PWS include:
- Pre and postnatal muscular hypotonia
- Obesity due to insatiable hunger and overeating
- Low intelligence
- Small hands and feet
- Dysmorphic facies
- Hypogonadism.

CLINICAL FEATURES

Because of its multigenetic pathology, clinical features vary from patient to patient and across the lifespan.

Prenatally decreased fetal activity, breech delivery, low birth-weight, and length are seen. Newborns exhibit marked axial hypotonia, associated with lethargy, decreased movement, weak crying, poor reflexes and poor sucking, leading to failure to thrive. Dysmorphic features like narrow bifrontal diameter, dolichocephaly, almond-shaped eyes, downturned angles of the mouth with abundant and thick saliva, and small hands and feet are less distinct at birth but can become more apparent with age. Hypogonadism is a typical finding. In males, small penis and hypoplastic scrotum which is poorly rugated and pigmented are noted; in females, genital hypoplasia often goes unnoticed—the clitoris and the labia, especially the labia minora, are generally small from birth.

By preschool age, the child develops a food obsession, which leads to becoming overweight. Their eating habits are complex and multifactorial. Children with PWS usually have a mild to moderate level of intellectual disability, usually associated with cognitive difficulty, poor motor development, reduced speech clarity, and difficulty in processing higher language concepts are seen. Temper tantrums especially related to food denial, obsessive-compulsive, or repetitive-restricted behaviors are seen.

During adolescence, hyperphagia (3-6 times more than the normal caloric intake) and behavioral problems become more pronounced. This can lead to obstructive sleep apnea, cardiorespiratory insufficiency, thrombophlebitis, and chronic leg edema which is the major causes of morbidity and mortality.

Hypogonadism leads to delayed puberty and in all cases infertility. Women may have to undergo treatment to attain menarche. Even though hypogonadism is the general rule in PWS, 15-20% of patients may show features of premature adrenarche or precocious puberty.

The quality of life of adults with PWS is largely limited by the degree of obesity, the presence of its complications, and behavioral problems.

DIAGNOSIS

Features, such as neonatal hypotonia and feeding problems in infancy, during the first years of life, excessive eating, and global developmental delay during early childhood are useful to select patients for referral for genetic analysis.

The PWS region is found in a 5-6 Mb genomic region on the proximal long arm of chromosome 15 (15q11.2-q13). Paternal microdeletion (75-80%), maternal uniparental disomy (UPD) (20-25%), and imprinting defect (ID) (1-3%) are the three main molecular mechanisms result in PWS. Other defects such as balanced and unbalanced translocations, which, together with ID, are responsible for the majority of familial cases.

MANAGEMENT

Early diagnosis of PWS is important for effective long-term management and a multidisciplinary approach is fundamental to improve quality of life, prevent complications, and prolong life expectancy.

Patient management has to be individualized as per the clinical presentation. A multidisciplinary team of neonatologist, pediatrician, developmental pediatrician, endocrinologist, orthopedic surgeon, urologist, psychologist, psychiatrist, and physiotherapist has to deal with all of the patient's medical and psychological problems.

Nutritional intervention includes feeding support as well as dietary control. Feeding support can be provided using special nipples or tubes for poor muscle tone and a high-calorie formula to gain adequate weight gain.

The onset of overeating starts between the age group of 2–4 years; hence, strict supervision will help minimize obesity and rapid weight gain. Parents should focus on a balanced, low-calorie diet, and regular exercise for these children.

The Developmental Pediatrician intervention for physical therapy to target hypotonia and psychological support for behavioral problems to promote quality of life of these children is indicated in adolescence and adulthood period. Psychological support is essential for parents and children equally. Similarly, the Developmental Pediatrician needs to factor in a range of interventions to improve speech and language skills, everyday skills, age appropriate behaviors, social skills, and interpersonal skills.

Researchers suggest a regular 30 minutes physical activity for children and adolescents with PWS.

Endocrinological advice for human growth hormone treatment and sex hormone replacement therapy is solicited when the child reaches the normal age of puberty to reduce the risk of developing osteoporosis. Surgery may have a role to correct undescended testicles.

FURTHER READING

1. Bittel DC, Butler MG. Prader-Willi syndrome: Clinical genetics, cytogenetics and molecular biology. Expert Rev Mol Med. 2005;7(14):1-20.
2. Crinó A, Schiaffini R, Ciampalini P, S Spera, L Beccaria, F Benzi, et al. Hypogonadism and pubertal development in Prader-Willi syndrome. Eur J Pediatr. 2003;162(5):327-33.
3. Elena G, Bruna C, Benedetta M, Stefania DC, Giuseppe C. The Prader-Willi-Syndrome: Clinical Aspects. J Obes. 2012;2012:1-13.
4. Gunay-Aygun M, Schwartz S, Heeger S, O'Riordan MA, Cassidy SB. The changing purpose of Prader-Willi syndrome clinical diagnostic criteria and proposed revised criteria. Pediatrics. 2001;108.
5. Holland AJ, Treasure J, Coskeran P, Dallow J, Milton N, Hillhouse E. Measurement of excessive appetite and metabolic changes in Prader-Willi syndrome. Int J Obes Relat Metab Disord. 1993;17(9):527-32.

Chapter 18

Angelman Syndrome

Shabina Ahmed

INTRODUCTION

Angelman syndrome (AS) is a neurodevelopmental disorder presenting with delay in developmental milestones with speech delay or absence of speech and may be associated with severe learning difficulties and autism.

Angelman syndrome is caused by a variety of genetic abnormalities involving the 15q11–q13 region of maternal chromosome 15, which leads to deficient UBE3A gene expression. This gene product has a role in ubiquitin-mediated proteolysis, which is essential in central nervous system development through alteration of synaptic connectivity.

Normal development requires a genetic contribution of this region, namely, 15q11–q13 region of maternal chromosome 15, from both male and female parents. The dependence on parental origin of this region gives rise to distinct functions and this is known as gene imprinting. If the deficiency is expressed maternally, it leads to AS and if derived paternally, it leads to Prader-Willi syndrome. AS is most commonly caused due to absence of the maternal contribution on the imprinted region of chromosome 15q11–q13. A similar paternal deletion of the 15q11–q13 region gives rise to the Prader-Willi syndrome.

The genetic abnormalities include maternal deletions—70% of patients have denovo deletion. 2% have paternal uniparental disomy while 2–3% have imprinting mutations and point mutations.

CLINICAL FEATURES

- Characterized by subtle dysmorphic facial features, e.g., wide smiling mouth, prominent chin, deep set eyes, and intermittent thrusting of tongue.
- Characteristic behavioral profile of a happy sociable disposition, easily provoked laughter, often laugh in inappropriate situations.

They are often seen mouthing objects or fingers and have irregular sleep patterns.
- Some may have motor difficulties like broad-based ataxic gait, jerky motor movements, flapping of hands, and variable tone in limbs.
  Some of the above features led to the term "Happy Puppet Syndrome".

Additional Comorbid Features

- Epilepsy is seen in 90% of children with AS. The electroencephalogram (EEG) has a distinctive pattern—typically rhythmic, triphasic delta waves of high amplitude, and maximally over frontal regions. This EEG pattern gives a clue to AS. Atypical seizures and myoclonic seizures are most prevalent in the early years and may decline as a child grows, but may reappear in adulthood.
- Varying degrees of learning difficulties in reading and writing with cognitive delay may be seen.
- Some may be associated with social communication deviation resulting in symptomatology of autism.
- There may be microcephaly and slowing of head growth in the first year of life.
- Other comorbidities including hyperactivity, anxiety, and aggressive behavior may present over time.

Differential Diagnosis

There is significant phenotype overlap with Rett syndrome. However, Rett syndrome has a unique hand wringing behavior and chromosomal studies show mutation of MECP2 location on Xq28.

MANAGEMENT

A holistic approach to the diagnosis and long-term clinical care of individuals with AS is important.

Management of epilepsy is difficult. It might be improved by better understanding of pathophysiology. Current hypothesis involves inhibitory transmission due to impaired regulation of GABA receptors, related to functional absence of UBE3A, and abnormal hippocampal CaMK11 activity. Most effective antiepileptic drugs are valproate, clonazepam, or phenytoin.

Dietary therapy, low glycemic index treatment (LGIT) containing high fat, and limited carbohydrate have also proved effective in some cases.

Children with AS need specialized individualized intervention services as part of a customized dynamic intervention program to address their unique cognitive and behavioral issues.

FURTHER READING

1. Bird LM. Angelman syndrome: Review of clinical and molecular aspects. Appl Clin Genet. 2014;7:93-104.
2. Kishino T, Lalande M, Wagstaff J. UBE3A/E6-AP mutations cause Angelman syndrome. Nat Genet. 1997;15(1):70-3.
3. Laan LA, Renier WO, Arts WF, Buntinx IM, von der Burgt IJ, Stroink H, et al. Evolution of epilepsy and EEG finding in Angelman syndrome. Epilepsia. 1997;38(2):195-9.
4. Laan LA, V Haeringen A, Brouwer OF. Angelman syndrome: A review of clinical and genetic aspects. Clin Neurol Neurosurg. 1999;101(3):161-70.
5. Nicholls RD. Genomic imprinting and uniparental disomy in Angelman and Prader-Willi syndrome: A review. Am J Med Genet. 1993;46(1):16-25.
6. Nurmi EL, Bradford Y, Chen Y, Hall J, Arnone B, Gardiner MB, et al. Linkage disequilibrium at the Angelman syndrome gene UBE3A in autism families. Genomics. 2001;77(1-2):105-13.
7. Pelc K, Boyd SG, Cheron G, Dan B. Epilepsy in Angelman syndrome. Seizure. 2008;17(3):211-7.
8. Thibert RL, Larson AM, Hsieh DT, Raby AR, Thiele EA. Neurologic manifestations of Angelman syndrome. Pediatr Neurol. 2013;48(4):271-9.
9. Williams CA, Beaudet AL, Clayton-Smith J, Knoll JH, Kyllerman M, Laan LA, et. al. Angelman syndrome 2005: Updated consensus for diagnostic criteria. Am J Med Genet A. 2006;140(5):413-8.

Chapter 19

Williams Syndrome

Jyoti Bhatia

INTRODUCTION

Williams syndrome (WS) was first described by Dr John CP Williams in 1961 for children with supravalvular aortic stenosis, mental retardation and characteristic facial features. It was later described by Beuren in 1962 hence, the name William-Beuren syndrome.

It is an uncommon genetic disorder caused by microdeletion of 26–28 genes on the long arm of chromosome 7. It is a multisystem disorder affecting approximately 1 in 7,500 live births. Boys and girls are equally affected.

CLINICAL FEATURES

In addition to the neurodevelopmental problems, children with WS have a distinct facial morphology, cardiac problems, growth failure, connective tissue, and endocrine abnormalities.

The elfin-like facial appearance along with some systemic manifestations provide the clue to the presence of this disorder. Almost all affected children show these facial features—face is narrow, eyes have a stellate iris with periorbital puffiness, nose is short with an upturned bulbous tip, mouth is wide with full lips and a long philtrum, and chin is small and tapering. This facies with a broad smile owing to their unique personality makes it easy for a clinician to pick-up these children in the clinic **(Fig. 1)**.

Infants with WS are generally small for gestational age and have a slower growth rate. They may be hypotonic in the first year of life with significant feeding issues. Idiopathic hypercalcemia, if present, further aggravates the medical and growth issues.

The cardiovascular and endocrine abnormalities cause significant morbidity and mortality. There is a generalized narrowing of medium and large arteries leading to stenosis. The supravalvular aortic area and the pulmonary arteries are most commonly affected. Other cardiac issues include septal

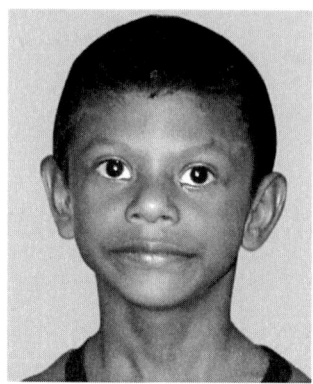

Fig. 1: Facial dysmorphism in a child with Williams syndrome. *Courtesy:* Dr. Kaushik Mandal.

defects, valve abnormalities, and hypertension. Endocrine abnormalities include episodes of hypercalcemia especially in infancy, hypothyroidism, impaired glucose tolerance, and higher risk of diabetes mellitus.

Neurodevelopmental profile: There is a global developmental delay in early years of life. Hyperextensible joints and hypotonia exaggerate the delay in motor milestones and most children walk by around 2 years. Fine motor difficulties are common. Older children have mild to moderate intellectual disability [intelligence quotient (IQ) averages 50-60].

Children with WS have a unique cognitive profile. Though their language acquisition is delayed, it shows good progress with age and older children are talkative with good vocabulary. Language skills are better than overall cognition. There is, thus, a relative strength in language skills but a profound weakness in visuospatial and visuomotor skills. Incidence of strabismus and refractive errors is also high. Academically, they may perform well with word reading but reading comprehension is poor. Difficulty with writing, drawing, and mathematics is significant. Attention deficit hyperactivity disorder may coexist in a large proportion of these children.

The other unique feature is their highly sociable personality. Children with WS have a pleasant personality and are happy to interact. But they lack the social skills for appropriate interactions and building relationships. This personality profile has directed recent research toward understanding the genetic basis of human social behavior.

"It's not just warmth or openness that we value; these traits must be coupled with a more sophisticated sense of when to turn them on or off. People with WS never turn them off. They have the social drive but not the cognitive ability to use it effectively."

—**Jennifer Latson**
in "The Boy Who Loved Too Much: A True Story of Pathological Friendliness."

Despite being keen to develop social relationships, most of them are socially rejected and isolated. Emotional issues are common with a very high incidence of anxiety and specific phobias. Children may be irritable, worrisome, and fearful.

Other common problems seen in children with WS include hearing loss, hypersensitivity to sound, recurrent otitis media, sleep problems, joint laxity and contractures, urinary tract diverticula, and dental issues.

ASSESSMENTS AND INVESTIGATIONS

The diagnosis is suggested by the characteristic clinical features. It needs to be confirmed by testing for the deletion of the Williams-Beuren syndrome critical region (WBSCR) by fluorescence in situ hybridization (FISH) or chromosomal microarray (CMA).

Monitoring and investigations needed for systemic problems include regular serum calcium monitoring, thyroid function tests, renal and bladder ultrasound, and echocardiography. These children need regular growth and blood pressure monitoring.

All children should undergo complete vision assessment including assessment of visuospatial skills and a detailed hearing assessment. Detailed developmental assessment is done to assess the degree of delay in all developmental areas and identify functional strengths and weaknesses. Detailed speech and language assessment are important keeping in view that these children have a unique language profile. To identify challenges in academics, IQ assessment and screening for attention deficit hyperactivity disorder and specific learning difficulty should be routinely done. Mental and emotional health should be regularly reviewed in view of higher incidence of anxiety, depression, and emotional issues.

Williams syndrome is autosomal dominant but most cases are new deletions; parent to child transmission is uncommon. Testing of parents or siblings is not warranted if they have no clinical features. Prenatal testing should be offered if a parent has the deletion or to parents who already have a child with WS.

MANAGEMENT

Management of systemic issues has to be done through appropriate referrals. A multidisciplinary developmental intervention program guided by a developmental pediatrician is needed to optimize skill development. Functional level of the child at every age helps design the intervention program. This is achieved through appropriate goals laid down in all areas of development—gross motor, fine motor, language and cognition, and behavior from an early age and can be provided with the help of trained professionals.

As the child grows, he needs additional inputs in education and social-emotional skill training. Socially appropriate behaviors and understanding subtle social-communication cues need to be taught. ADHD and specific learning difficulties need to be addressed, if present. Anxiety management includes cognitive behavioral therapy and pharmacologic treatment. Self-calming techniques should be taught from an early age.

The Pediatrician's role is crucial in making an early diagnosis in suspected cases, counseling the families, and helping the Developmental Pediatrician design the appropriate intervention program for the specific requirements of managing this developmental disorder.

FURTHER READING

1. Committee on Genetics. American Academy of Pediatrics: Health care supervision for children with Williams syndrome. Pediatrics. 2001;107(5): 1192-204.
2. Morris CA. Williams Syndrome. In: Adam MP, Ardinger HH, Pagon RA, et al., (Eds). GeneReviews®. Seattle (WA): University of Washington, Seattle; 1993-2019.
3. Pober BR. Williams-Beuren syndrome. N Engl J Med. 2010;362(3):239-52.

Chapter 20

Neurofibromatosis

Z Bassi

Neurofibromatosis is a term that encompasses at least two distinct disorders, neurofibromatosis type 1 (NF1) and neurofibromatosis type 2 (NF2).

Both NF1 and NF2 are genetically determined disorders.

Neurofibromatosis type 2 (NF2) affects 1 in 35,000 people. It is characterized by acoustic neuromas usually bilateral (vestibular schwannomas), as well as other tumors of the peripheral and central nervous system, mononeuropathies, and cataracts. The features of NF2 are often not apparent in early childhood. NF2 has a lower incidence of cutaneous findings, higher incidence of central nervous system (CNS) tumors, and a worse prognosis than NF1 and less likely to present primarily to a Developmental pediatrician. NF2 will not be discussed in detail here.

INTRODUCTION

Neurofibromatosis type 1 (otherwise known as von Recklinghausens disease) is an autosomal dominantly-inherited neurocutaneous disorder affecting approximately 1 in 2,500 children. About half of the people with NF1 are de novo new mutations and have no family history.

Although the condition mainly affects the skin and nervous system, its effects are wide ranging and other organs can be involved. The severity and type of clinical problem varies between individuals even within families. Individuals with NF1 are at increased risk for the development of benign and malignant tumors.

Mosaic NF1 occurs occasionally as a result of a somatic mutation in the *NF1* gene, the proportion of the body affected depending on the time of mutation in embryonic development. If an early somatic mutation occurs, then the phenotype can be very similar to nonmosaic presentation and a later mutation can cause more localized and often unilateral in distribution.

The *NF1* gene was identified on chromosome 17q11.2 which codes for a tumor suppressor neurofibromin. NF1 is caused by a heterozygous loss of function mutation in this gene.

CLINICAL FEATURES

The diagnostic criteria in current clinical use are those developed by the National Institute of Health **(Box 1)**.

The clinical features of NF1 accumulate with age and most children with NF1 meet the National Institutes of Health (NIH) criteria by 8 years of age. Hence, a child may need to be followed up or monitored over time. Genetic testing may aid early diagnosis and may be used when diagnosis is in doubt, or where this may affect treatment (e.g., in optic pathway gliomas) or for genetic counseling.

All children with NF1 should have an annual review to monitor for key symptoms and complications in a number of systems. The common systemic presentation of NF1 are described here.

- *Skin:*
  - Café au Lait: These may be present at birth or early infancy and are seen in 99% of patients with NF1 by 3 years of age. These have a smooth outline, may increase in size and number over time and can fade with age. 1-2 Cal are found in 10% of the general population. Only cosmetic treatment may be offered, if indicated.
  - Freckling: Hyperpigmented macules 1-3 mm in diameter are found in 85% of children usually after the age of 3 years. These are typically found in the axilla and groin but can also be found at the base of the neck, upper eyelids, or over the trunk.
  - Xanthogranulomas: Yellowish orange nodules or papules about 1 cm in diameter are seen over the head, neck, trunk, and limbs. A link between these and juvenile chronic myelogenous leukemia (CML) has been suggested but routine screening is not warranted.
  - Glomus tumors: These present as purplish discoloration around the nail bed and the lesions are exquisitely tender. Pain is precipitated by

---

Box 1: Diagnostic criteria of neurofibromatosis type 1 (NF1) [National Institutes of Health (NIH) consensus statement 1988].

Clinical diagnosis can be made when a child has two or more of the following features:
- Six or more café au lait macules or hyperpigmented macules (>5 mm in diameter in prepubertal children and >15 mm in postpubertal)
- Two or more cutaneous/subcutaneous neurofibromas or one plexiform neurofibroma
- Axillary or groin freckling
- Optic pathway glioma
- Two or more Lisch nodules (iris hamartomas seen on slit lamp examination)
- Bony dysplasia (sphenoid wing dysplasia, bowing of long bone +/- pseudarthrosis)
- A first degree relative with NF1

cold or trauma. Magnetic resonance imaging (MRI) will help localize these and treatment is surgical removal.
- *Neurofibromas*:
  - Cutaneous: Develop in teens/early twenties and occasionally in early childhood, benign, removed for cosmetic reasons, or if causing discomfort, e.g., get caught in clothes.
  - Subcutaneous: Present in approximately 15% of patients. Evident on palpation of the skin and may cause pain and paresthesia, but malignant change is rare. Removal may result in neurological deficit and should be considered carefully with a specialist.
  - Plexiform: Present in about 30% of patients and associated with major physical problems in about 6% of patients. These grow along the length of a nerve and may involve multiple nerve fascicles and branches. The growth rate is unpredictable. Facial plexiform neurofibromas (1–2% of patients) causing facial disfigurement develop usually in the first few years.

There is about a 10% lifetime risk of malignant change in plexiform neurofibromas, most common in the second and third decade.
- *Eyes*:
  - Optic pathway gliomas present in 15–30% of children with NF1 but only a third become symptomatic. All children should have regular ophthalmology screening until the age of 8 years and annual vision testing thereafter.
  - Glaucoma usually seen in early childhood.
  - Congenital sphenoid dysplasia resulting in proptosis, exophthalmos/enophthalmos.
  - Plexiform neurofibroma involving eyelids.
- *Growth*:
  - Short stature (10–25th centile) is seen in a third of children with NF1.
  - Children with NF1 often have macrocephaly however, investigation is required, if rapid increase in head circumference is seen.
- *Cardiovascular:*
  - Congenital heart disease: Pulmonary stenosis is common. If a murmur is heard, the child should be referred for echocardiogram.
  - Hypertension: Blood pressure (BP) should be checked annually. Consider renal artery stenosis (in children and young adults or older individuals with refractory hypertension assess for abdominal bruit), coarctation, pheochromocytoma (if additional symptoms, e.g., paroxysmal palpitation and sweating), or early-onset essential hypertension and investigate accordingly.
- *Orthopedic*:
  - Bowing of long bones with/without pseudarthrosis usually presents in infancy but has been noted in older children in clinical practice.

- Scoliosis—idiopathic or dystrophic and can be associated with underlying plexiforms. Dystrophic scoliosis usually presents earlier and is associated with kyphosis. Referral for orthopedic assessment is required.
- Osteoporosis.
- *Nervous system*:
  - Malformations including aqueduct stenosis (this is one of the acute presentations of NF1) and tumors (optic pathway glioma/cerebral tumors presenting) presenting with signs/symptoms of increasing intracranial tension
  - Epilepsy particularly complex partial seizures
  - Pressure on peripheral nerves, spinal nerve roots, spinal cord, or neuropathy (symmetrical distal tingling/numbness or weakness)
  - Cerebrovascular/neurovascular conditions.
- *Cognitive and behavior:* Cognitive problems are common and these range from average to low intelligence quotient (IQ) or specific learning difficulty, developmental coordination difficulties, dyslexia, visual spatial, or attentional difficulties. There is an increased frequency of autism spectrum disorder (25–40%) and attention deficit hyperactivity disorder (40–50%).

Hence, children presenting to the Developmental Pediatrician for neurodevelopmental assessment [autism spectrum disorder (ASD)/attention-deficit hyperactivity disorder (ADHD)/learning disability (LD)] should have a detailed examination of their skin preferably with a woods light to exclude underlying NF1.

Psychological problems can present in adolescents due to cosmetic issues and symptoms of anxiety and depression should be assessed for.

INVESTIGATIONS

Routine imaging (X-rays, MRI scans, and echo) is not recommended. Investigations are based upon clinical findings and are used to assess for diagnostic uncertainty or emergent complications. The most common findings on brain MRIs are focal areas of signal intensity on T2-weighted images [focal abnormal signal intensity (FASI)]. They are most commonly seen from 8 to 16 years and tend to disappear in adulthood. They have no association with other CNS pathologies, nor is there clear correlation with learning problems.

Referral to a geneticist is recommended to consider genetic testing and for genetic counseling.

Urgent advice should be sought if:
- There is acute/progressive sensory, motor deficit, incoordination, or sphincter disturbance
- Headaches on waking associated with altered consciousness

- If the following develop in a plexiform or subcutaneous neurofibroma—persistent pain for more than a month or nocturnal pain or new neurological deficit or change in texture from soft to hard or rapid increase in size
- New onset of vision signs/symptoms.

MANAGEMENT

All children with NF1 should have, at the least, an annual review to monitor the multiorgan manifestations. More frequent assessments, referral to appropriate specialists, or therapy teams or investigations are required based on clinical presentation. Developmental Pediatricians are best placed to carry out annual reviews and follow-up of these children. The following should be assessed at every review:

- Detailed review of any new symptoms/clinical signs
- *Vision:* look for visual symptoms, squint, proptosis, visual acuity, color vision, and field of vision at appropriate developmental age and optic disc
- *Anthropometry:* Height/weight/head circumference and plot on reference charts
- Assessment of development, behavior, and progress at school
- *Pubertal development*: Tanners staging (delayed/precocious due to hypothalamic or pituitary lesions)
- *Blood pressure*: If high, should be checked three times in a month to verify and consider investigations
- Evaluation of the skin
- Evaluation of the spine and bones
- Neurological examination
- Cardiovascular examination
- Systemic examination, if any symptoms
- Evaluation of mood.

FURTHER READINGS

1. Dunning-Davies BM, Parker AP. Annual review of children with neurofibromatosis type 1. Arch Dis Child Educ Pract Ed. 2016;101(2):102-11.
2. Ferner RE, Huson SM, Thomas N, Moss C, Willshaw H, Evans DG, et al. Guidelines for the diagnosis and management of individuals with neurofibromatosis 1. J Med Genet. 2007;44(2):81-8.
3. Garg S, Green J, Leadbitter K, Emsley R, Lehtonen A, Evans DG, et al. Neurofibromatosis type 1 and autism spectrum disorder. Pediatrics. 2013;132(6):e1642-8.
4. Garg S, Lehtonen A, Huson SM, Emsley R, Trump D, Evans DG, et al. Autism and other psychiatric comorbidity in neurofibromatosis type 1: Evidence from a population-based study. Dev Med Child Neurol. 2013;55(2):139-45.
5. Neurofibromatosis. Conference statement. National Institutes of Health Consensus Development Conference. Arch Neurol. 1988;45(5):575-8.

Chapter 21

Tuberous Sclerosis

Z Bassi

INTRODUCTION

Tuberous sclerosis complex (TSC) is a multisystem disorder affecting approximately 1:6000–1:10000 newborns. It is an autosomal dominantly-inherited condition but 60–70% of the cases are sporadic.

There are two genetic loci linked to disease: the *TSC1* gene on chromosome 9 and the *TSC2* gene on chromosome 16. TSC is an extremely variable disease that can affect virtually any organ in the body but usually involves the skin, brain, kidneys, lung, and heart.

CLINICAL FEATURES (BOX 1)

Some common systemic features of TSC with manifestations:

Skin

- Hypomelanotic macules are seen in about 90% of individuals with TSC, they typically appear at birth or infancy, and may be a presenting sign of TSC. Poliosis (circumscribed hypomelanosis of hair) is also included in this.
- Angiofibromas occur in about 75% of TSC patients with onset typically between ages 2 and 5 years. They are solid red or pink papules, bilaterally symmetrical over the nose, cheeks, and chin. Treatment—laser and topical rapamycin ointment.
- *Fibrous cephalic plaque*: The forehead plaque is observed in about 25% of TSC patients and are histologically similar to angiofibromas.
- Ungual fibromas are usually multiple. These can occur in the general population in response to trauma but are usually solitary. The frequency is about 20% overall.
- Shagreen patches commonly take the form of large plaques on the lower back that have a bumpy or orange-peel surface. These are observed in about 50% of individuals with TSC and typically have their onset in the first decade.

> **Box 1:** Diagnostic criteria: [2012 International Tuberous Sclerosis Complex (TSC) Consensus Conference].
>
> **Genetic diagnostic criteria**
> The identification of either a TSC1 or TSC2 pathogenic mutation in deoxyribonucleic acid (DNA) from normal tissue is sufficient to make a definite diagnosis of tuberous sclerosis complex. Note that 10–25% of TSC patients have no mutation identified, and a normal result does not exclude TSC, or have any effect on the use of clinical diagnostic criteria to diagnose TSC.
>
> **Clinical diagnostic criteria**
> *Major features:*
> - Hypomelanotic macules (≥3, at least 5-mm diameter)
> - Angiofibromas (≥3) or fibrous cephalic plaque
> - Ungual fibromas (≥2)
> - Shagreen patch
> - Multiple retinal hamartomas
> - Cortical dysplasias*
> - Subependymal nodules (SENs)
> - Subependymal giant cell astrocytoma
> - Cardiac rhabdomyoma
> - Lymphangioleiomyomatosis (LAM)†
> - Angiomyolipomas (≥2)†
>
> *Minor features:*
> - "Confetti" skin lesions
> - Dental enamel pits (>3)
> - Intraoral fibromas (≥2)
> - Retinal achromic patch
> - Multiple renal cysts
> - Nonrenal hamartomas
>
> *Definite diagnosis:* Two major features or one major feature with ≥2 minor features
> *Possible diagnosis:* Either one major feature or ≥2 minor features
>
> Notes: *Includes tubers and cerebral white matter radial migration lines.
> †A combination of the two major clinical features (LAM and angiomyolipomas) without other features does not meet criteria for a definite diagnosis.

- Confetti skin lesions are numerous 1–3-mm hypopigmented macules scattered over regions of the body such as the arms and legs. Their frequency varies from 3% in children to about 58% overall.

Mouth

- Dental enamel pits are much more common in TSC patients than the general population, with a study (Mlynarczyk et al.) reporting 100% of adult TSC patients (n = 50) as having pitting compared with 7% of 250 adult control subjects.
- Intraoral fibromas occur in about 20–50% of individuals with TSC, on the buccal or labial mucosa and even the tongue.

Eye

Multiple retinal hamartomas are observed in 30–50% of TSC. These lesions usually do not cause problems with vision.

Central Nervous System

- Cortical dysplasias in TSC are commonly associated with intractable epilepsy and learning difficulties. They are congenital abnormalities caused, at least in part, when a group of neurons fail to migrate to the proper area of the brain during development. The cortical tubers are observed in ~90% of TSC.
- Infants may present with infantile spasms in early life and can be the first manifestation of TSC. Vigabatrin is the first line for treatment of infantile spasms.
- *Subependymal nodules (SEN) and subependymal giant cell astrocytomas (SEGAs)*: SENs are benign growths in the lining of the lateral and third ventricles. They are seen in 80% of TSC patients. SEGAs have an incidence of 5–15% in TSC they are much more likely to arise during childhood or adolescence. They can cause serious neurologic compromise including obstructive hydrocephalus.

Renal

- Angiomyolipomas are benign tumors composed of vascular, smooth muscle, and adipose tissue. These are common in the kidney but can occur in other organs and seen in 80% of TSC patients.
- Multiple renal cysts.

Cardiovascular

- Cardiac rhabdomyomas are benign tumors of the heart. They are highly specific to TSC and often the first noted manifestation of disease sometimes noted antenatally. These often regress and need to be monitored. They can occasionally cause ventricular outflow tract obstruction.
- Cardiac arrhythmias, including atrial and ventricular arrhythmia and Wolff-Parkinson-White syndrome, may occur.

Pulmonary

Lymphangioleiomyomatosis (LAM) patients typically present with progressive dyspnea on exertion and recurrent pneumothoraces in the third to fourth decade of life.

Endocrine

- Adrenal angiomyolipoma can be present in a quarter of TSC patients

- Thyroid papillary adenoma have been reported in TSC patients
- There are case reports of angiomyolipomas or fibroadenomas in the pituitary gland, pancreas, or gonads.

Gastrointestinal
- Liver angiomyolipomas are reported in 10-25% of TSC patients
- Hamartomatous rectal polyps.

LEARNING AND BEHAVIOR

Tuberous sclerosis complex is associated with a range of behavioral and cognitive difficulties in individuals with and without intellectual disability. Behavioral problems include sleep disturbance, aggressive behaviors, phobias, self-injury, temper tantrums, depressed mood, and anxiety disorder. In particular, there is strong evidence of attention deficit hyperactivity disorder (ADHD) and autistic spectrum disorder (ASD) (up to 60-70%), and intellectual disability [intelligence quotient (IQ) < 70].

Due to the spectrum of presentation these children may present first to a developmental Pediatrician and hence, review for neurocutaneous markers is an essential part of management of children with learning or neurodevelopmental disorders.

MANAGEMENT

Complications of TSC can be life-threatening with significant impact on patients' quality of life. Regular surveillance and early management of complications improve outcomes.

Baseline Assessments/Investigations with Newly-diagnosed Children with Tuberous Sclerosis Complex

- Genetics referral
- Assessment of learning and development
- *Examination*: Skin, teeth, eyes, blood pressure (BP), and evaluation for TSC-associated neuropsychiatric disorder (TAND-via a checklist)
  - Electroencephalogram (EEG) if indicated—if abnormal 24 hour video EEG
  - Baseline electrocardiogram (ECG) in all ages
- Echocardiogram in pediatric patients, especially if younger than 3 years of age
- *Renal functions*: Magnetic resonance imaging (MRI) brain and abdomen
- Pulmonary function testing and high-resolution chest computed tomography (HRCT), if symptomatic or in older females.

Regular Surveillance for Children with Tuberous Sclerosis Complex

- Assessment of learning and development
- *Examination*: Skin, teeth, eyes, BP, and evaluation for TSC-associated neuropsychiatric disorder (TAND)—annually
- Electroencephalogram—determined by clinical need; video EEG when seizure occurrence is unclear or when unexplained behavioral or neurological changes occur
- Baseline ECG—every 3-5 years; more frequently, if symptomatic
- Echocardiogram—every 1-3 years if rhabdomyoma present in asymptomatic children; more frequently in symptomatic individuals
- Renal functions—annually
- Magnetic resonance imaging brain—every 1-3 years up to age 25 and then less frequently depending on symptoms
- Magnetic resonance imaging abdomen—every 1-3 years (some suggest annual USS)
- Pulmonary function tests—annually only if cysts detected on CT or if symptomatic (rare in children).

Treatment of Complications

Refer to appropriate specialists for management of medical complications identified on assessment and surveillance. Treatment is dependent on presentation and is a combination of medical and surgical intervention.

Everolimus [mammalian target of rapamycin (mTOR) inhibitor] is a condition-specific treatment that can be used in certain children who fulfill strict criteria under the guidance and monitoring of a specialist [e.g., for refractory epilepsy by neurologist, rapidly increasing acute myeloid leukemia (AML) by a renal physician].

FURTHER READING

1. Amin S, Kingswood JC, Bolton PF, Elmslie F, Gale DP, Harland C, et al. The UK guidelines for management and surveillance of Tuberous Sclerosis Complex. QJM. 2019;112(3):171-82.
2. Krueger DA, Northrup H; International Tuberous Sclerosis Complex Consensus Group. Tuberous Sclerosis Complex surveillance and management: Recommendations of the 2012 International Tuberous Sclerosis Complex Consensus Conference. Pediatr Neurol. 2013;49(4):255-65.
3. Northrup H, Krueger DA; International Tuberous Sclerosis Complex Consensus Group. Tuberous sclerosis complex diagnostic criteria update: Recommendations of the 2012 International Tuberous Sclerosis Complex Consensus Conference. Pediatr Neurol. 2013;49(4):243-54.

Chapter 22

Mucopolysaccharidoses: Developmental and Behavioral Outcomes

Shibani Kanungo, Neelkamal Soares

INTRODUCTION

Lysosomes are cellular organelles with their main role aiding in cellular debris digestion and recycling. This degradation of one substrate to another in this intracellular process of digestion utilizes multiple enzymes. The enzyme deficiencies within the lysosome result in accumulation of undegraded substrates. This storage process leads to the clinical spectrum depending on the site (organ system) of the accumulation and the specific substrate, and constitute a group of inborn errors of metabolism (IEM) disorders called the lysosomal storage disorders (LSD).

Mucopolysaccharides (MPS) or glycosaminoglycans (GAGs) are complex long sugar chain units in repeating fashion, hence called "polysaccharide", are essential component of connective tissues and are found in skin, cartilage, cornea, vascular walls, heart, brain, liver, and spleen. Dermatan sulfate, heparan sulfate, keratan sulfate, hyaluronic acid, and chondroitin sulfate are some of the known GAGs. These GAGs when bound to specific core proteins form the proteoglycans. The degradation of GAGs occur in the lysosomes utilizing several acid hydrolase enzymes. The deficiencies of these enzymes collectively result in the group of LSD disorders called MPS.

Historically, the first two MPS were described independently before 1920 by clinicians in Canada and Germany, but the biochemical basis for these conditions was understood only after the 1950s. Advances in molecular analysis technology helped us understand the genotype-phenotype of each MPS, while the partially-degraded GAG accumulations in body fluids diagnostic biochemical confirmation of these disorders. Though our understanding of lysosomal function and role in disease presentation is evolving, successful strides in treatment of few LSDs have helped improve health outcomes.

CLINICAL FEATURES AND DIAGNOSIS

Chronic and progressive multiorgan system involvement and wide spectrum of clinical presentations **(Table 1)** often delay a diagnosis of MPS. A high

Table 1: Mucopolysaccharidoses (MPS).*

Type of MPS	Enzyme deficiency	Accumulated product	Prominent systemic findings
I (Hurler/Schie)	α L-iduronidase	Dermatan sulfate and heparan sulfate	Coarse features, macrocephaly, hirsutism, corneal clouding, obstructive sleep apnea (OSA), progressive skeletal dysplasia, and arthropathy, hepatosplenomegaly, cardiomyopathy, and hernias
II (Hunter)	Iduronate 2-sulfatase	Dermatan sulfate and heparan sulfate	Coarse features (no corneal clouding), macroglossia, ankylosis of temporo-mandibular joint, hoarse voice, hearing loss, joint contractures, dysostosis multiplex. Cardiac valvular disease, hepatomegaly and/or splenomegaly, hernia, inelastic ivory-white papular ridges on skin
III (Sanfilippo)	Depending on subtypes: Heparan n-sulfatase, α-N-acetylglucosaminidase, α-glucosaminidase acetyltransferase, N-acetylglucosamine 6-sulfatase	Heparan sulfate	Mildly coarse facial features, ear, and respiratory infections, hirsutism, scoliosis, lumbar lordosis, hip dysplasia, and pain

Contd...

Contd...

Type of MPS	Enzyme deficiency	Accumulated product	Prominent systemic findings
IV (Morquio)	Galactose 6-sulfatase, N-acetylgalactosamine-6-sulfate sulfatase	Chondroitin 6-sulfate and keratan sulfate	Ligamentous laxity, kyphoscoliosis, hip pain, hip subluxation, atlantoaxial instability, hepatomegaly, OSA, cardiac hypertrophy, valvular regurgitation, coarse facial features, corneal clouding, cataracts, and hearing loss
VI (Maroteaux-Lamy)	N-acetylgalactosamine-4-sulfatase	Chondroitin 4-sulfate and dermatan sulfate	Pectus carinatum, joint contractures, scoliosis/kyphosis, cervical stenosis, severe pulmonary obstruction, cardiac valve regurgitation, hernias, hepatosplenomegaly, coarse facial features and hirsutism, OSA, hearing loss, corneal clouding, optic nerve damage
VII (Sly)	β-D-glucuronidase	Chondroitin 4-sulfate, chondroitin 6-sulfate, dermatan sulfate, and heparan sulfate	Coarse facial features, macrocephaly, macroglossia, hirsutism, chronic rhinorrhea, hearing impairment, corneal opacity, hepatosplenomegaly, hernia, AV malformation, and OSA Coronary valvular disease, cardiomyopathy, contractures, scoliosis, and kyphosis

Note: *MPS IX which is extremely rare, and MPS V and MPS VIII are not defined.
(AV: arteriovenous; OSA: obstructive sleep apnea)

index of clinical suspicion on even few of the constellation of findings such as coarse facial features, growth failure, skeletal deformities, learning difficulties, behavioral problem, and cognitive decline can help timely diagnosis. Though most MPS seem to be normal appearance at birth, GAG accumulation starts in utero and can present as hydrops fetalis or intrauterine death or with skeletal deformities at birth or with recurrent hernias and recurrent ear and respiratory infections in early childhood.

Urine GAGs analysis using electrophoresis or thin layer chromatography can identify the specific pattern of GAG excretion suggesting specific MPS disorder. And diagnostic confirmation includes enzyme activity assays in leukocytes or cultured fibroblast with molecular analysis of MPS specific genes. Inheritance of all MPS is autosomal recessive and consanguinity within a family increases the risk. The only exception is MPS II (Hunter's), which is X-linked and the differential diagnostic clinical pearl is lack of corneal involvement or vision problems (good eyesight is essential to hunt).

Successful early treatment and easy detection of enzyme activity in asymptomatic newborn have helped inclusion of MPS I in the newborn screening panel.

DEVELOPMENTAL AND BEHAVIORAL PERSPECTIVES OF MUCOPOLYSACCHARIDOSES

In determining developmental functioning and outcomes, it is important to understand the natural history of specific MPS as well as disease attenuation as a result of treatment and secondary comorbidities. A good understanding of cognitive and developmental testing tools, to determine when and on which age ranges to use, helps provide best interventions. Also, most tools are normed on children without MPS or other neurological or genetic conditions.

The general pattern for the MPS is the deteriorating/progressive forms present with developmental deterioration earlier in life. Often, seizures can worsen the progress. Meanwhile, attenuated forms present later (and often with milder presentations).

Mucopolysaccharidoses-IH (Hurler) presents with normal early psychomotor development, though progressive learning difficulties become notable by second year of life. A deceleration is followed by a gradual decline in skills with resulting severe intellectual disability. In the more attenuated form, MPS-IS (Schie) are intellectually normal though can present with learning disabilities. Clinical spectrum in between these two extreme forms [Hurler–Scheie syndrome, (MPS IH-S), present with variable intellectual dysfunction usually between 3 and 8 years of age.

Mucopolysaccharidoses-II also present with normal early development, generally followed by regression in early childhood and results in intellectual disability, though in attenuated form, normal intelligence can be present.

Mucopolysaccharidoses-IV generally present with normal developmental/intellectual functioning, though neurologic symptoms such as hearing loss and nerve compression might lead to poor developmental and behavioral outcomes.

Mucopolysaccharidoses-VI generally follow a pattern of normal development.

Mucopolysaccharidoses-VII in its severe form can have plateau followed by regression in language skills, though attenuated form can have normal intelligence and just learning disabilities.

Mucopolysaccharidoses-III have very mild clinical or dysmorphic features but mainly affects the central nervous system presenting with learning difficulty progressing to behavioral problems and cognitive delays later in childhood with delay in diagnosis. There are four subtypes of MPS III (A, B, C, and D); initial presentation usually at age <3 years includes speech delay, with recurrent ear infections, and failed hearing tests. Behavioral problems such as sleep issues, anxiety, ADHD-like features (hyperactivity and impulsivity), opposition/defiance, and behaviors that might be consistent with autism spectrum disorder can become severe and impair family functioning. In the attenuated forms, behavior problems can emerge later and are generally more manageable.

MANAGEMENT

Supportive educational and rehabilitative management are usually required for developmental and behavioral consequences of MPS. Educational interventions include specialized instruction for learning disabilities and cognitive impairment, while a developmental intervention program with appropriate speech, physical, and occupational therapy goals are needed for developmental delays and specific regressive developmental patterns. Specific treatment of seizures, hearing loss, and psychiatric conditions are also recommended with the latter being addressed by behavioral interventions and medications (as indicated).

All patients with MPS should be under care of a metabolic geneticist and undergo genetic counseling for MPS specific gene findings. Hematopoietic stem cell transplantation (HSCT) has been used in MPS patients (especially MPS-I) with some success in addressing systemic symptoms with prolongation of survival, but has not been found to have consistent impact on neurological outcomes, unless started earlier than 2 years of age. In general, HSCT at younger age (<2 years) in patients without significant cognitive impairment results in better developmental outcomes. Enzyme replacement therapy is effective treatment for systemic symptoms, but while attempts to deliver enzyme through intrathecal or directly into cerebral ventricles to improve neurological symptoms showed promising results in animal studies, clinical trials in humans are still ongoing. While gene therapy has promise, there are yet to be successful interventions using gene therapy in MPS. Best management approach includes multidisciplinary/subspecialty [developmental behavioral pediatrics, ear nose and throat (ENT), cardiology, neurology, psychology, and social work] collaboration to address each organ system manifestation with metabolic genetics clinic or consultant serving as the core speciality helps unique needs of these families with such rare disorders.

FURTHER READING

1. Scarpa M, Orchard PJ, Schulz A, Dickson PI, Haskins ME, Escolar ML, et al. Treatment of brain disease in the mucopolysaccharidoses. Mol Genet Metab. 2017;122(S):25-34.
2. Shapiro EG, Escolar ML, Delaney KA, Mitchell JJ. Assessments of neurocognitive and behavioral function in the mucopolysaccharidoses. Mol Genet Metab. 2017;122S:8-16.
3. Sun A. Lysosomal storage disease overview. Ann Transl Med. 2018;6(24):476.
4. Tomatsu S, Fujii T, Fukushi M, Oguma T, Shimada T, Maeda M, et al. Newborn screening and diagnosis of mucopolysaccharidoses. Mol Genet Metab. 2013;110(1-2):42-53.
5. Valstar MJ, Ruijter GJG, van Diggelen OP, Poorthuis BJ, Wijburg FA. Sanfilippo syndrome: A mini-review. J Inherit Metab Dis. 2008;31(2):240-52.
6. Wijburg FA, Wegrzyn G, Burton BK, Tylki-Szymańska A. Mucopolysaccharidosis type III (Sanfilippo syndrome) and misdiagnosis of idiopathic developmental delay, attention deficit/hyperactivity disorder or autism spectrum disorder. Acta Paediatr. 2013;102(5):462-70.

Chapter 23

Rett Syndrome

Leena Srivastava

*"The girl I see has gone slow,
In both her mental and motor shores,
Whilst the head does not well grow,
Her hand wringing has stopped her chores,
Seizures also appear as she lay,
Get the MECP2, I say!"*

Leena Srivastava

INTRODUCTION

Rett syndrome (RS) is an X-linked dominant neurodevelopmental disorder and not a progressive, degenerative disorder as once thought. RS predominantly affects females and is occasionally identified in males. It is characterized by normal early growth and development for the first 6 months followed by a regression of development, loss of purposeful use of the hands, repetitive hand movements, acquired microcephaly, problems with walking, seizures, and intellectual disability. The disorder was first described by an Austrian pediatrician, Dr Andreas Rett in 1966.

The incidence of classic forms is 1:10,000–1:15,000 whereas atypical forms are much rarer. About 70% children survive to age 35 years. It occurs sporadically in 99.5% cases and hereditary factors contribute in about 0.5%.

In 1999, the discovery of a genetic mutation [methyl-cytosine binding protein 2 (MECP2)] on the X chromosome (Xq28) provided significant insight into the cause of Rett syndrome.

Methyl-cytosine binding protein 2 (pronounced: meck-pee-too) codes for a protein that binds to methylated deoxyribonucleic acid (DNA) and regulates gene transcription. This mutation has now been found in >95% of those meeting criteria for typical RS and >50% meeting those for atypical RS.

Rett syndrome is most often misdiagnosed as autism, cerebral palsy, or neurodegenerative disorders. Diagnostic and statistical manual 4 (DSM4) classified it under pervasive developmental disorders. DSM5 groups it under autism spectrum disorder but as a separate neurogenetic disorder with a known genetic origin.

CLINICAL FEATURES AND DIAGNOSIS

Stages of Rett Syndrome

Stage I: Developmental stagnation (6–18 months): These are early signs and changes may be gradual and subtle, after normal development in the first 6 months.
- Hypotonia
- Unsteady immature ambulation problems in sitting, crawling, and walking
- Reduced hand function
- Delay in development of speech
- Reduced eye contact and lack of interest in surroundings.

Stage II: Stage of regression (1–4 years): Also called rapid destructive phase where the child starts losing some of her abilities.
- Slowing of head growth
- Loss of purposeful hand function with hand stereotypes like hand wringing, clasping, and washing
- Regression of communication
- Inconsistent social interaction with social withdrawal
- Problems in mobility and coordination—ataxic/apraxic gait, and tremors
- Seizures
- Episodes of irritability/screaming
- Sleep disturbances
- Hyperventilation/apnea
- Feeding difficulty.

Stage III: Plateau phase (5–7 years): Latent period with plateauing or relative improvement in the development, communication, and behavioral repertoire. Here, symptoms get no worse or their intensity lessens.
- Seizures and breathing problem
- Bruxism
- Deterioration of autonomic function
- Arrhythmias
- Osteopenia
- Growth failure

Stage IV: Late motor deterioration (5–25 years—up to decades):
- Scoliosis and spasticity

- Losing the ability to walk
- Communication and language do not worsen; repetitive hand movements may improve.

Atypical/variant presentations of Retts have also been described:
- Zappella variant with preserved speech variant, where some improvement of speech and motor may be seen. Head circumference is also often in the normal range.
- Rolando or the congenital variant may show developmental delay from the beginning with hypotonia.

POINTS TO REMEMBER
- Siblings can have differences in severity.
- In females, unusual X inactivation patterns with MECP2 mutations may be asymptomatic or have mild learning disability and will not be identified unless they transmit the mutation to a daughter who develops RS.
- Mostly believed that males with the disorder are not compatible with life and may result in miscarriages or stillbirths but males with severe encephalopathy have been described.
- The majority of deaths in RS are either sudden and unexpected, or secondary to cardiac arrhythmias or pneumonia.

Key Points to Look for in History and Examination
- Female child
- History of developmental regression around 6–18 months of age with apparent normal development earlier
- "Autism-like" features
- Decelerating head growth velocity especially in the latter half of the first year
- Hand wringing or such stereotypic hand movements with loss of functional hand use
- Seizures

Evaluation
- History with detailed developmental history.
- Examination with head circumference measurement and detailed neurological examination.
- Hearing and vision evaluation.
- Deoxyribonucleic acid analysis for mutations in MECP2. If negative for MECP2, mutations in *FOXG1* (the congenital variant) or *CDKL5* (the

early seizure variant). DNA analysis may also be offered to the mother for carrier state and prenatal testing for future pregnancies.
- If genetic work up is negative, other investigations to rule out neurometabolic and degenerative disorders such as magnetic resonance imaging (MRI) brain, serum amino acids, urine organic acids, chromosome microarray analysis, and others may be offered as appropriate. Electroencephalogram (EEG) in children with seizures.
- Detailed developmental evaluation with developmental quotient (DQ) and an adaptive functioning scale like Vineland Social Maturity Scale (VSMS) may be used to formulate goals for the intervention plan and monitor progress.

Diagnosis is mainly clinical. Mutations on the *MECP2* gene confirm the diagnosis. The fact that not all *MECP2* mutations will have RS and not all RS will have a *MECP2* mutation makes the clinical impression more reliable along with the genetic work up.

Differential Diagnosis

Depending on the age and stage of presentation, rule out hearing/visual disturbances, autism spectrum disorder, neurodegenerative or metabolic disorders such as neuronal ceroid lipofuscinosis, phenylketonuria, urea cycle defects, leukodystrophies, central nervous system (CNS) infections, cerebral palsy, spinocerebellar ataxias, epileptic syndromes like Lennox-Gastaut and conditions like Angelman syndrome.

MANAGEMENT

Psycho education and psychosocial support and genetic counseling with anticipatory guidance for the family form the back bone of management. An intervention plan for the developmental problems is mandated which should be multidisciplinary and goal based. This should include the domains of communication, motor, hand function, behavior along with management of the nutrition, control of seizures, sleep, and other issues such as respiratory problems and osteopenia.

Developmental interventions like communication goals for speech and language and/or alternative and augmentative communication (AAC) aids may be helpful with appropriate use of pictures or gadgets. Physiotherapy helps with goals for mobility, balance, coordination and posture, screening and management of scoliosis, hypotonia/spasticity with prevention of contractures, and control deformities. Scoliosis may be managed with braces to maintain truncal stability; occasionally spine surgery may be indicated. Occupational therapy focuses on goals for promoting hand function with feeding, dressing, and other goals for activities of daily living. Hand or elbow restraints may be used to control hand movements (especially, if self-injurious) or to aid function. Behavioral management is indicated as per the behavioral problems and applicability in individual cases.

Medical management focuses on:
- *Feeding/nutrition*: Detailed feeding evaluation with oral motor and oropharyngeal function and appropriate positioning and neck posture is advised. Additional factors like gastroesophageal reflux, constipation, and drooling management should be taken into consideration and nutritionally adequate diet of right consistencies and textures should be planned.
- *Seizures*: Antiepileptic drugs and ketogenic diet.
- Sleep disturbances are managed with sleep hygiene, behavioral approaches, and medications like melatonin.

Management of respiratory problems, monitoring for cardiac abnormalities with annual electrocardiography (ECG), and management of osteopenia with orthopedic care as indicated. Specific-targeted treatments for RS are still under ongoing clinical development.

FURTHER READING

1. Iris Etzion. Neurodevelopmental disabilities: Conceptual framework. Swaiman's Pediatric Neurology: Principles and Practice. 6th ed. Edinburgh: Elsevier Saunders; 2018: p. 413-17.
2. Neul JL, Kaufmann WE, Glaze DG, Christodoulou J, Clarke AJ, Bahi-Buisson N, et al. Rett syndrome: Revised diagnostic criteria and nomenclature. Ann Neurol. 2010;68(6):944-50.
3. National Institutes of Health. Rett Syndrome Fact Sheet. [online] Available from https://www.ninds.nih.gov/Disorders/Patient-Caregiver-Education/Fact-Sheets/Rett-Syndrome-Fact-Sheet (Last accessed December, 2021)
4. Rett syndrome. [online] Available from https://www.omim.org/entry/312750 (Last accessed December, 2021).

Chapter 24

Sleep Disorders

Leena Srivastava, Kawaljit Singh Multani

"Sleep, sleep, baby" said the tired mom
Dad on laptop yet working was the norm,
"No, I want to play!" screamed the boy
And jumping, he flung the toy!
Our daily routine, we are unable to keep
Please, Doc, guide us to help our child sleep!"

INTRODUCTION

Once considered a state of rest, research in the field of sleepover last few decades has changed the way we look at sleep. Sleep is now considered as important function as awake state which is essential for healthy development and body homeostasis and longevity across species. Sleep can be defined as a "prolonged state of behavioral quiescence which is reversible and has specific electroencephalogram (EEG) correlates." Although most animals sleep, large variations in sleep patterns are seen among different species. Sleep problems, though common in children, are considered a disorder when they occur at least three times in a week for more than 3 months and cause functional impairment in the child or family's life.

Sleep problems may be caused in children due to behavioral factors such as resistance to being put to bed, etc. to medical causes such as obstructive sleep apnea (OSA), etc. In infancy, differentiating behavioral from medical causes may be challenging and requires vigilance. Sleep problems in children can be a major cause of distress to the parents affecting a child's behavior and overall family functioning. Sleep problems are reported in 20–25% of all children in a well baby clinic visits. Certain conditions in children may be associated with a higher incidence of sleep problems, e.g., acute illnesses such as middle ear infections, chronic illnesses such as asthma, pain-related conditions, neurodevelopmental or psychiatric disorders, and medications such as steroids and stimulants.

PHYSIOLOGY OF SLEEP

Sleep in humans has been found to evolve with time from newborn period to adulthood and research indicates that sleep in early years of life greatly influences the development of the child and cognitive abilities later in life. The fetus spends most of its time in utero sleeping, interspersed with small periods of wakefulness. At the time of birth, the brain of a newborn is structurally complete on a macro level but it is still changing at a microscopic level (neuronal migration, synapse formations, myelination, and synapse sculpting), which is essential for the development of higher brain functions later in life, including language and cognitive thinking. This activity results in accumulation of waste products in the central nervous system (CNS) and hence, the newborn sleeps for prolonged periods which is needed to clear the waste products. Newborns do not have an established circadian rhythm and it takes 3-4 months to settle into a set pattern of sleep-wakefulness. A newborn has three types of sleep—quiet sleep [non-rapid eye movement (REM) sleep, active sleep (REM sleep/dream sleep), and indeterminate sleep]. In the first few weeks after birth, newborns have short sleep cycles lasting 50-70 minutes with REM sleep at onset and most time in sleep is REM sleep. By 6 months, REM sleep constitutes about 50% of total sleep and further reduces to 20% in adults. Melatonin (sleep hormone) is produced by the pineal gland in the brain which is crucial for the chronobiotic control (biologic clock) of circadian rhythm of sleep-wake cycle in the newborn. Melatonin production is suppressed by light and after birth, melatonin secretion increases over 3-6 months thereby establishing the sleep-wake pattern in the infant. Electrophysiologically, the sleep EEG of the newborn reaches adult pattern by 6 months. From 4 months to 1 year of life, the infant continues to take multiple day-time naps and the night sleep consolidates to adult-like pattern, though night wakings are common. Day-time naps generally stop by 5 years of age. The sleep pattern of an individual is influenced by genetic, behavioral, environmental, and social factors (parenting styles, cultural factors, etc.). With age, the average sleep time reduces with most sleep at night.

CLINICAL FEATURES

Since most neurodevelopmental disorders (NDDs) have underlying CNS malformations at either structural or cellular levels; it is easy to understand that they will be associated with problems of normal sleep evolution/development in the child. More than half of these children having sleep issues (50-95%) reported in various studies. Various mechanisms postulated to sleep disorders are neurochemical—abnormal melatonin, gamma-aminobutyric acid (GABA) and serotonin levels, poor and inconsistent sleep habits, and factors such as anxiety in older children. Another common theory proposed is the relationship between iron deficiency and periodic leg movements. Common causes of sleep disturbances in children with NDD include comorbid behavioral disorders, medical and neurological disorders, epilepsy, medications, lack of consistent limit setting or routines, limitation in comprehending verbal communication, etc. Sleep deprivation can lead to increasing maladaptive behaviors, aggravation of the features of the primary disorder while making the handling of these children more difficult for their caretakers thus affecting the quality of life of the whole family. Some NDDs such as Angelman syndrome and Rett syndrome have characteristic sleep disturbances as one of the diagnostic criteria.

Classification (as per Diagnostic and Statistical Manual 5 and International Classification of Sleep Disorders 3)

- Insomnia disorders—difficulty with the initiation or maintenance of sleep without caregiver intervention causing impairment in functioning areas occurring at least 3 nights a week, for >3 months despite adequate opportunity to sleep.
- Sleep-related breathing disorders—like OSA, central apnea, and sleep-related hypoventilation present with repeated movements of the limbs, neck, etc., during sleep. Common disorders in this group include snoring, restless leg syndrome, or sleep-related leg cramps.
- Central disorders of hypersomnolence (narcolepsy)—these children may show excess sleep time during the night and/or day and have difficulty in awakening after a nap.
- Circadian rhythm sleep-wake disorders (CRSWD)—significantly delayed sleep timing compared to the desired schedule of sleeping awakening. The presentation may be similar to insomnia or excessive daytime sleepiness (EDS).
- Sleep-related movement disorders (SRMD)
- Parasomnias—events with arousal events such as sleep walking or sleep terrors occurring in sleep.

Sleep problems in children may present with consequences such as sleepiness during the day, irritability and other behavioral problems, and poor academic performance **(Table 1)**. Based on the learned ability to fall asleep and maintain sleep, behavioral insomnia often presents as resistance to bedtime, delayed sleep-onset, night awakenings, or a mix of all significant enough to need parental intervention. Most behavioral problems are either related to sleep onset associations or to inadequate limit settings. Sleep onset associations can be rocking, patting, feeding, etc., and are seen in infants and toddlers while inadequate limit settings are seen in preschool and school age children and include active resistance to bedtime by refusing to go to bed with verbal and aggressive protests and demands at bedtime.

Sleep Disorders

Table 1: Characteristic sleep problems in common neurodevelopmental disorders.

Disorder	Common sleep issues
Down syndrome	OSA, brainstem dysfunction, and sleep-related movement disorders
Angelman syndrome	Disorders of initiating and maintaining sleep, parasomnias, and characteristic EEG pattern (1–3 Hz bursts)
Prader–Willi syndrome	OSA and reduced N-REM sleep
Smith–Magenis syndrome	EDS (inverted melatonin secretion)
Fragile X syndrome	Sleep-onset difficulties and frequent night awakenings
Rett syndrome	Irregular sleep/wake pattern, EDS, problematic night-time behaviors
Autism spectrum disorder	Bed-time resistance, insomnias, parasomnias, day-time sleepiness, and sleep-related breathing disorders
Cerebral palsy	OSA, disorders of initiation, and maintenance of sleep
ADHD	EDS and sleep-related breathing disorders

(ADHD: attention deficit hyperactivity disorder; EDS: enveloping distribution sampling; EEG: electroencephalogram; OSA: obstructive sleep apnea; N-REM: non-rapid eye movement)

These behaviors if not handled well may result in prolonged sleep latency thus delaying sleep and insufficient sleep hours. Insomnia is commonly reported with problem in initiating and maintaining sleep, resistance to bedtime, or early awakenings. Though the sleep problems may seem similar to typically developing children, children with NDDs show multiple types of sleep problems in the same child with interplay of multiple factors in the child and the environment as well, thus necessitating a more individualized intervention plan.

EVALUATION

There is no ideal/universal sleep duration. Recommended sleep times at different ages are given in **Table 2**.

A detailed history is the most important step in evaluation of a child suspected of having a sleep disorder which should include detailed daily activity schedule, developmental, family, and medication history (if any). The sleep history should include the bedtime, waking up time, naps in the day, awakenings at night with details of duration, and behavior. A sleep screening tool should be used in all suspect cases, e.g., BEARS (Bedtime problems, EDS, night awakenings, regularity of sleep, and snoring) **(Flowchart 1)**. Once a sleep problem is identified, sleep routine, sleep habits, and sleep patterns of

Table 2: Recommended sleep durations at different ages over 24 hours cycle.

Age	Recommended sleep duration (in 24 hours)
Infant (4–12 months)	12–15 hours
Toddler (1–2 years)	11–14 hours
Preschool children (3–5 years)	10–13 hours
Preadolescent (5–12 years)	9–12 hours
Adolescents–adults	7–9 hours (varies widely)

Source: National Sleep Foundation, American Academy of Sleep Medicine, Sleep Research Society.

Flowchart 1: Algorithm for approach to sleeping disorders in children with NDDs.

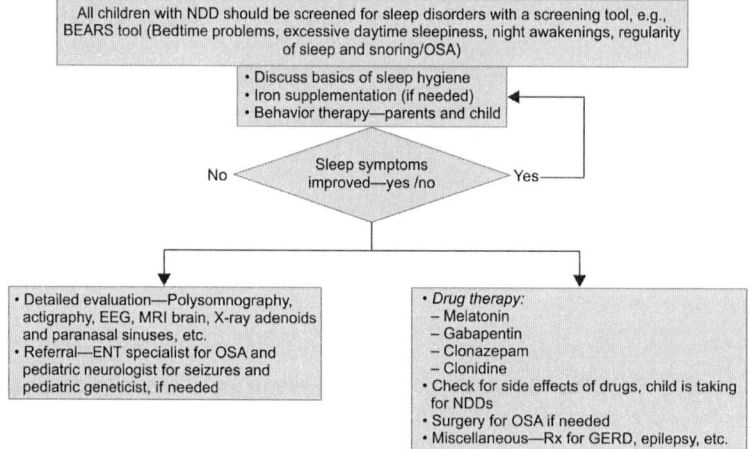

(EEG: electroencephalography; ENT: ear, nose and throat; GERD: gastroesophageal reflux disease; MRI: magnetic resonance imaging; NDDs: neurodevelopmental disorders; OSA: obstructive sleep apnea; Rx: a medical prescription)

the child as well as the family should be looked at to find whether the child has difficulty in falling asleep, maintaining sleep, or other sleep-associated problems.

A sleep diary usually consists of a 1–2 weeks record of child's sleep by the parents and includes details such as bedtime routine, time to fall asleep (sleep latency), night awakening, morning rise time and daytime naps, and total sleep time. All children suspected of a sleep disorder should also undergo a behavioral assessment to identify problematic behaviors. With the availability of smartphones and smartwatches and many sleep apps, it is possible to digitally track a child's sleeping pattern. Actigraphy is a method which tracks a child's sleep using a wearable device similar to a watch and can be used along with a sleep diary. All children suspected of having nocturnal seizures, parasomnias, OSA should undergo an overnight polysomnograph test in a sleep laboratory.

DIFFERENTIAL DIAGNOSIS

Nocturnal seizures, behavior disorder, mood disorder, anxiety disorder, medical issues that can disturb sleep-like GER, constipation, eczema, wheezing, dental problems, oversensitivity in children with autism to the environment causing discomfort.

MANAGEMENT

A healthy sleep requires adequate duration, appropriate timing, regularity, and quality to keep the body healthy. Management mainly consists of non-pharmacological and pharmacological measures with nonpharmacological measures being the first choice. Iron supplementation has been found to improve sleep and should be used along with nonpharmacological measures.

Nonpharmacological Measures

Parental sleep education: This is the most useful tool in the management plan. Parents should be counseled about sleep hygiene with discussion about day and evening schedule, bedtime routine, and sleep environment. Daytime schedule should include adequate physical activity, avoiding caffeinated drinks, and the amount of daytime naps should be noted. Evening schedules should be with minimal use of gadgets and electronic media with less stimulating activities toward late evening. Bedtime routines should be discussed with dimly lit, cool, and comfortable sleep environments taking into consideration the child's needs, e.g., a child with autism may benefit with an accompanying visual schedule. Ideally, the infant or young child should be placed on the bed when drowsy but awake avoiding the use of rituals such as rocking, etc. If practiced early in life the infant or child will learn to self soothe himself to sleep.

Behavioral Plan

Unmodified extinction: The child is placed in bed and all the calling to parents, crying, and tantrums are ignored till the next morning to avoid reinforcement of negative behaviors in sleep time. Care should be taken that pain or illness and such medical causes for the crying are ruled out. Parents may find this strategy quite stressful and the negative behaviors may escalate initially on enforcement of this strategy thus appropriate parental counseling is essential.

Graduated extinction: The strategy is principally similar to the earlier one with intermittent check-ins or positive, and calming brief interactions with the child which are gradually weaned off. This gives the child time to self-soothe.

Positive bedtime routines: Calm bedtime routines such as reading a story may be used.

Faded bedtimes: The family usually chooses a preferred or target bedtime which is then gradually delayed or faded into the time of natural onset of sleep to avoid the child from spending long periods of time in bed before falling asleep.

Friman has described a useful strategy of bedtime pass in older children who can understand action and consequences. The child is given a pass entitling him to one check-in. If he does not use it, then he gets reinforced in exchange of his pass in the morning.

Behavioral strategies may need to be individualized to a child and family's needs. Weighted blanket and sensory strategies used in children with autism lack empirical evidence presently.

Drug Therapy

Pharmacotherapy is needed for children not responding to nonpharmacological measures and consists mainly of melatonin, sedative-hypnotics, and other miscellaneous drugs. Drug choice is determined on a case-to-case basis. Melatonin should be the first choice in younger children while sedative-hypnotics and other miscellaneous drugs can be used in older children based on the clinical profile and associated comorbidities.

Melatonin: Melatonin secretion in preterm born children and those with neurodevelopment disorders is either reduced or the circadian pattern is not well-established resulting in sleep disorders in these children. Supplementation of melatonin in these children helps in establishing the sleep-wake pattern and improvement in daytime behavior/activity of the child. Melatonin is available as drops and tablets either alone or in combination with vitamins or other sedatives. Both immediate release and prolonged release formulations of melatonin are available; the prolonged release melatonin pharmacokinetics closely resemble to the physiological melatonin cycle. For children aged 1 month to 18 years, the starting dose can be 2–3 mg daily given 2 hours before bedtime. Dosage can be increased to 10 mg (maximum) slowly by doubling the dose every 2–3 weeks. The drug is usually well-tolerated, reduces sleep latency, improves sleep efficiency, and child has fewer night-time awakenings. There are no significant adverse effects reported with melatonin.

Sedative-hypnotics—clonazepam and zolpidem.

These drugs are commonly used as sleep-inducing agents in adults and act by facilitating inhibitory neurotransmitter gamma-aminobutyric acid (GABA) in the brain. The main concern about their use in children is for cognitive impairment, increased daytime sleepiness, and dependence risk.

Miscellaneous Drugs

Clonidine: It is a centrally acting adrenergic agonist and is mostly used in children with NDDs with behavioral disorders and sleep issues.

Table 3: Medications in sleep disorders.

Drug	Dose	Adverse effects
Melatonin	2.5–10 mg (Start at 2.5 mg for child <6 years)	No significant side effects
Clonidine	0.025–0.3 mg	Hypotension and bradycardia
Gabapentin	5–15 mg/kg	No significant side effects
Clonazepam	0.25–0.75 mg	Day-time sleepiness and habituation

Gabapentin: It is a precursor of inhibitory neurotransmitter GABA in the brain commonly used in management of partial seizures. It has a role in children with NDDs who have epilepsy as a comorbid disorder. The beneficial actions of gabapentin are seen at a much lower dose as compared to its anticonvulsant dose **(Table 3)**.

Trazodone, antihistaminics, chloral hydrate, etc., are other drugs used but their efficacy and safety in pediatric population is not established.

Sleep is the best meditation.
Dalai Lama

FURTHER READING

1. Angriman M, Caravale B, Novelli L, Ferri R, Bruni O. Sleep in children with neurodevelopmental disabilities. Neuropediatrics. 2015;46(3):199-210.
2. Arlington VA. American Psychiatric Association: Diagnostic and Statistical Manual of Mental Disorders, 5th edition. American Psychiatric Association; 2013.
3. Blackmer AB, Feinstein JA. Management of sleep disorders in children with NDDs: A review. Pharmacotherapy. 2016;36(1):84-98.
4. Chaput JP, Dutil C, Sampasa-Kanyinga H. Sleeping hours: What is the ideal number and how does age impact this? Nat Sci Sleep. 2018;10:421-30.
5. El Shakankiry HM. Sleep physiology and sleep disorders in childhood. Nat Sci Sleep. 2011;3:101-14.
6. Mindell JA, Kuhn B, Lewin DS, Meltzer LJ, Sadeh A; American Academy of Sleep Medicine. Behavioral treatment of bedtime problems and night wakings in infants and young children. Sleep. 2006;29:1263-76.
7. Narasimhan U, Anitha FS, Anbu C, Abdul Hameed MF. The spectrum of sleep disorders among children: A cross-sectional study at a South Indian tertiary care hospital. Cureus. 2020;12(4):e7535.
8. Paruthi S, Brooks LJ, D'Ambrosio C, Hall WA, Kotagal S, Lloyd RM, et al. Recommended amount of sleep for pediatric populations: A Consensus Statement of the American Academy of Sleep Medicine. J Clin Sleep Med. 2016;12(6):785-6.
9. Reynolds AM, Malow BA. Sleep and autism spectrum disorders. Pediatr Clin N Am. 2011;58(3):685-98.

Chapter 25

Feeding Disorders

Leena Deshpande

"Feeding my children is not like feeding myself: it matters more!"
Jonathan Safran Foer

INTRODUCTION

Feeding one's child is a very emotional issue in most families and can be quite a dramatic event in some families. It is affected by cultural setting, parental experience as well as temperament of the child and parent. Eating provides nutrition but the act of feeding also shapes emotional and social development of the child.

Feeding difficulties are an umbrella term used to describe problems in feeding the child irrespective of the etiology, severity, or consequences.

It can range from mild deviation like picky eating which is very common and may be seen in normal children to severe form of difficulties which is then labeled "feeding disorder".

Prevalence of feeding difficulties is around 25–35% in young children. In children with neurodevelopmental disorder (NDD), the prevalence is much higher around 40–80%. The difficulties also tend to be severe in these children causing significant psychosocial disturbance.

CLINICAL FEATURES

Aberrant feeding behaviors in children with NDD can be grouped in three categories:
1. Children eating too little
2. Children eating a restricted number of foods
3. Children displaying a fear of eating.

Diagnostic and Statistical Manual (DSM) 5 criteria groups these early childhood feeding disorders under the umbrella term—"avoidant restrictive food intake disorder". It looks only at psychological aspects **(Box 1)**.

> **Box 1:** Diagnostic and Statistical Manual of Mental Disorders (DSM-5).
>
> Diagnostic and Statistical Manual (DSM) 5 criteria groups these early childhood feeding disorders under the umbrella term—avoidant restrictive food intake disorder criteria:
> - Disturbance in eating or feeding as evidenced by one or more of substantial weight loss or absence of expected weight gain, nutritional deficiency, dependence on feeding tube or dietary supplements and significant psychosocial interference
> - Disturbance is not due to limitations in food availability
> - Disturbance is not due to anorexia nervosa or bulimia
> - Disturbance is not explained by any other medical conditions or mental disorders, or is not occurring concurrently with another condition
>
> *Source:* American Psychiatry Association, 2013.

However, children with NDD will have feeding difficulties due to a combination of organic or neurological causes and behavioral causes.

MANAGEMENT

The etiology of feeding difficulties in NDD is complex and multifactorial and hence, its management requires a stepwise and a multidisciplinary team approach coordinated by a developmental pediatrician including a pediatric neurologist, physiotherapist, occupational therapist, speech and language pathologist, psychologist, and a nutritionist.

Step-wise approach:
- The first step is to obtain a detailed history to determine if there are organic symptoms like dysphagia, pain while feeding, chronic respiratory symptoms suggesting aspiration or gastroesophageal reflux, failure to thrive which needs medical or surgical intervention **(Flowchart 1)**. These may be seen in children with cerebral palsy. It needs in depth evaluation including swallowing studies. These children will need help with optimum positioning during feeding, changing the consistency of feed offered, and use of adaptive cutlery. In severe cases, the child may need nasogastric tube feeding.
- The next step is to ascertain the severity of the feeding problem. This can be done by analyzing the child's growth chart and nutritional status **(Flowchart 2)**. Use of Feeding Behaviors' Rating Scales can help quantify the problem from the caregiver's point of view.
- Irrespective of the underlying NDD, neurological issues contributing to feeding problems are due to oromotor difficulties (the function of the muscles of the mouth, their tone, power, coordination which is needed to manipulate the food in the mouth), and orosensory difficulties (how oral tissues perceive sensory information such as taste, texture, and

130 Feeding Disorders

Flowchart 1: Neurological basis of feeding disorder.

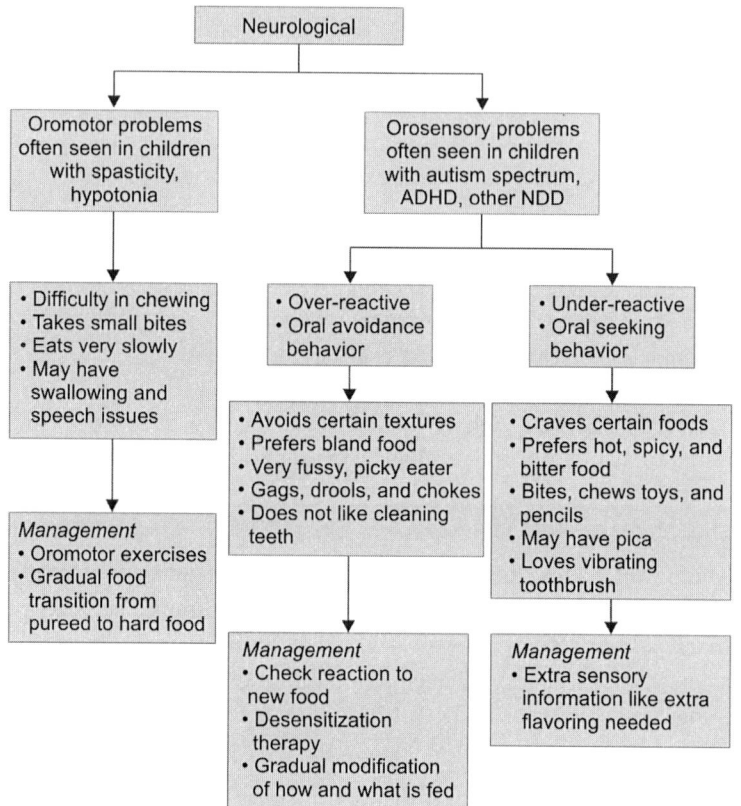

(ADHD: attention-deficit hyperactivity disorder; NDD: neurodevelopmental disorder)

Flowchart 2: Behavioral basis of feeding disorder.

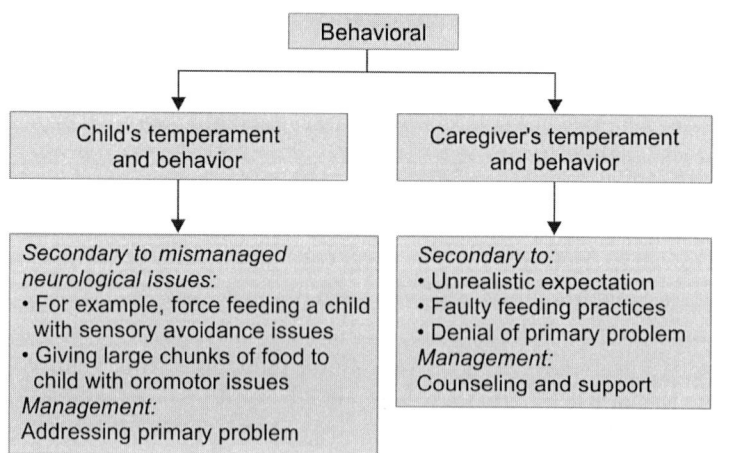

temperature of food). Apart from this, primary and secondary behavioral issues will contribute substantially to the feeding disorder. In many children, all the above difficulties may coexist.

Flowcharts 1 and 2 mention some of the symptoms and the management of these difficulties.

Awareness about these multiple and complex aspects of feeding disorders in children with NDD is crucial. As prevalence of feeding disorders is high in children with NDD, anticipatory guidance will minimize problems. Timely recognition and management will go a long way in improving the child's general condition and decreasing parental anxiety and stress.

FURTHER READING

1. Kerzner B, Milano K, MacLean WC Jr, Berall G, Stuart S, Chatoor I. A practical approach to classifying and managing feeding difficulties. Pediatrics. 2015135(2):344-53.
2. Yang HR. How to approach feeding difficulties in children? Korean J Pediatr. 2017;60(12):379-84.

Chapter 26

Elimination Disorders

Kawaljit Singh Multani

"The more risks you allow children to take, the better they learn to look after themselves."

Roald Dahl

INTRODUCTION

As an infant grows into a toddler, his understanding of self and his surroundings increases. It is during this stage that children begin to learn the control of their bowel and bladder and this is why initiation of toilet training should be done around 18–24 months of age. The sequence of control is—night-time bowel control followed by day-time bowel control followed by day-time bladder control and finally, night-time bladder. Earlier attempts to achieve control and subsequent failure may lead to frustration, anger and anxiety in both the child and the parents. Absence of bladder control (enuresis) or bowel control (encopresis) in a child that is expected based on child's age/stage of development is termed as elimination disorder. Enuresis is more common than encopresis. Both the conditions are more common in males compared to females and suffer significant emotional and behavioral issues, as these are often hidden by the parents or reported late. Both require counseling and training of the whole family and their whole-hearted participation for successful outcomes.

CLINICAL FEATURES

Encopresis (Fig. 1)

The term "encopresis" is derived from the Greek word "kopros" which means feces or dung. More than 95% of children are bowel continent by 4 years of age. Although encopresis is less common than enuresis, it is more impairing for both the child and the family.

Encopresis is characterized by repeated defecation in inappropriate places (in clothes or on the floor) in children above 4 years of age with

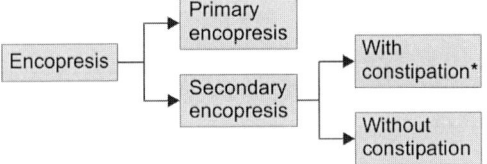

Fig. 1: Classification of encopresis.
Note: *Most common type.

episodes occurring at least once a month for 3 months. Though the voiding is regarded as involuntary, it may be volitional at times. The behavior must not be attributable to any medical illness/condition, other than constipation, or medication like laxatives.

The condition is seen in 1.5–7.5% of school-aged children and is more common in boys (3:1). It can be classified as primary or secondary. Primary encopresis is the term used for children who have never acquired bowel control for a period of 6 months or more. Secondary encopresis is the more common variety and seen in children who had earlier become bowel continent. It has two main subtypes—one with constipation and overflow incontinence (retentive type) which is the most common type seen and the other without constipation. Most of these children have an early history of constipation with a long-standing habit of withholding stools which results in acquired megacolon and over stretched rectum and poor muscle tone that in turn reduces the child's ability to feel the urge for defecation, thereby resulting in overflow fecal incontinence. Some children have paradoxical contraction of external anal sphincter or may have failure of relaxation of the sphincter in response to the urge to pass stool. These children have a fear of going to the toilet, aversion to public places, or unfamiliar toilets. Most of the episodes happen during the day and hence affect the child's school performance and may result in low self-esteem and peer rejection/teasing. The stools in cases with constipation are poorly formed and the soiling happens continuously while in cases without constipation, the feces are well formed and soiling is intermittent. The cases without constipation are associated with stressors like child abuse, parental discord/divorce, etc. and in conditions like oppositional defiant disorder (ODD), conduct disorder, and mental subnormality.

Enuresis (Flowchart 1)

Enuresis is a term derived from a Greek word meaning "to void urine" and refers to repeated involuntary passage of urine in bed or clothes in children of age 5 years or more, at least twice a week for at least three consecutive months. One-third of the cases have constipation as well. Around 10% of the children of the age group 6–7 years suffer from this condition, and this incidence reduces with increasing age most likely due to delayed maturation

Flowchart 1: Classification of enuresis.

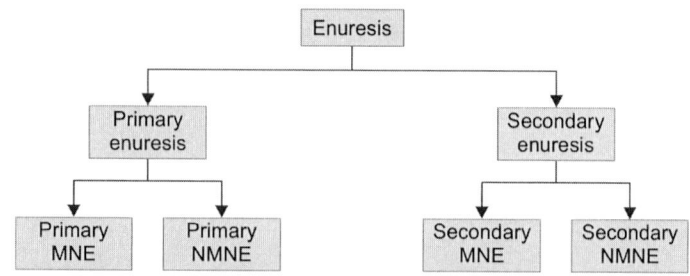

(MNE: monosymptomatic enuresis; NMNE: nonmonosymptomatic enuresis)

Table 1: Features of lower urinary tract symptoms (suggestive of a urinary bladder dysfunction) adapted from guidelines by ICCS 2017.

Symptom	Yes/No
Leakage of urine during daytime	
Urinary frequency (>8/day)	
Infrequent voiding (<3/day)	
Urgency symptoms	
Holding behaviors like crossing legs, etc.	
Poor or interrupted urinary stream	
Past history of UTI	
Constipation symptoms	
Known malformation of urogenital tract or known renal illness	

(ICCS: International Children's Continence Society; UTI: urinary tract infection)

of achieving bladder control. Spontaneous remission rate of 15% per year is seen in affected children; by adolescence, 1–2% of all children still suffer from enuresis. 20–30% children with enuresis suffer from behavioral issues.

The condition can be termed primary or secondary based upon whether the child had achieved bladder control for a period of 6 months or more anytime. The International Children's Continence Society (ICCS) categorizes enuresis into monosymptomatic enuresis (MNE) and non-NMNE based on the presence or absence of day-time lower urinary tract symptoms **(Table 1)**. NMNE is a heterogeneous group of disorders involving day-time wetting, excessive voiding frequency, dribbling, and holding.

MANAGEMENT

Encopresis

It is essential to treat any underlying disorder that is suspected. Whenever an identifiable organic cause can be determined, it should be treated appropriately. The parents should be advised to increase fluid intake and fiber in the child's diet and reduce milk intake. Older children should be encouraged to exercise more frequently. Regular bathroom times/best times are after meals for up to 15 minutes, improved access to the toilet, star charts/small rewards, timed sitting, and asking the child to assist in cleaning-soiled clothing also help.

Cognitive behavioral therapy (CBT) and psychodynamic therapy can help decrease symptoms of anxiety and depression associated with encopresis. Biofeedback can be beneficial in the treatment of pelvic floor dysfunction and can also teach the child sphincter control.

In cases with constipation, it is essential to clear the colon of the retained fecal matter using osmotic laxatives like lactulose and polyethylene glycol or stool softeners like docusate in order to break the cycle of constipation and painful defecation. Enemas are used in cases not responding to laxatives. Tricyclic antidepressants like imipramine and loperamide have been used in nonretentive encopresis as they improve the tone of external anal sphincter.

Enuresis

Treatment of enuresis is indicated in children above 5 years of age. A detailed medical history, including detailed developmental and family history, along with details of fluid intake and voiding patterns (voiding diary including star charting) is important to classify the type of enuresis and look for comorbid conditions. A detailed physical examination of the patient including growth parameters, blood pressure, spine, genitalia, and lower limbs needs to be undertaken. Urinalysis, urine culture, ultrasound examination of urinary bladder with assessment of bladder capacity [expected bladder capacity (EBC) = (age + 1) × 30 mL)], postvoid residual volume, bladder wall thickness need to be carried out. Urodynamic studies are needed in resistant cases. Conditions like congenital anomalies of urogenital tract, chronic kidney disease, posterior urethral valves, and spina bifida need to be excluded.

Management includes reassurance of parents (including information about spontaneous resolution), nonpharmacological, and pharmacological methods. Nonpharmacological methods include behavior therapy, dry-bed training, hypnotherapy, and use of urine alarms. Although urine alarms are effective therapy with success rates of 60–70% (though some brands are now available on e-market sites like Amazon), they require considerable time, involvement, and efforts from the whole family. Dry-bed training involves waking up the child at night on a fixed schedule after he/she has gone to sleep as well as use of positive parenting practices and can be used along with a urine alarm. Medications used in enuresis include desmopressin (tablet 0.2 mg and nasal spray 0.1 mg/mL), oxybutynin, and imipramine. Of the three, desmopressin is the most commonly used and has a good safety profile in cases with nocturnal enuresis. The tablet is taken 30–60 minutes before bedtime and treatment is continued for 3–6 months; relapses are known to occur after stopping treatment. Hyponatremia is a known complication and can be prevented by reducing fluid intake from 1 hour to 8 hours after taking medication. Oxybutynin in a dose of 0.3–0.6 mg/kg body weight/day (maximum 15 mg/day) is used in cases with features of overactive bladder (small maximum voided volume, i.e., <65% of EBC or nocturnal polyuria, i.e., total night-time urine volume > 130% of EBC and thickened bladder wall > 2 mm) as it improves the bladder capacity, thereby reducing urgency and frequency while imipramine has a role in cases of dysfunctional voiding and those with comorbid conditions like attention-deficit/hyperactivity disorder (ADHD). Other anticholinergic medicines like tolterodine have been used with similar success. Biofeedback treatment and electrostimulation [transcutaneous electrical nerve stimulation (TENS)] treatment using electrodes placed over the sacral surface have been tried and found useful in difficult cases. Constipation, if associated, needs to be treated using laxatives or stool softeners.

FURTHER READING

1. American Psychiatric Association. Diagnostic and Statistical Manual of Mental Disorders, 5th edition, text rev. Arlington, Virginia: American Psychiatric Publishing; 2013.
2. Cox DJ, Sutphen J, Borowitz S, Kovatchev B, Ling W. Contribution of behavior therapy and biofeedback to laxative therapy in the treatment of pediatric encopresis. Ann Behav Med. 1999;20(2):70-6.
3. Gontard AV, Kuwertz-Broking E. The diagnosis and treatment of enuresis and functional daytime urinary incontinence. Dtsch Arztebl Int. 2019;116(16):279-85.
4. Reddy NM, Malve H, Nerli R, Venkatesh P, Agarwal I, Rege V. Nocturnal enuresis in India: Are we diagnosing and managing correctly? Indian J Nephrol. 2017;27(6):417-26.
5. Vande Walle J, Rittig S, Tekgül S, Austin P, Yang SS, Lopez PJ, et al. Enuresis: Practical guidelines for primary care. Br J Gen Pract. 2017;67(660):328-9.

Chapter 27

Seizures and Epilepsy

Sarbani Raha, Vrajesh Udani

INTRODUCTION

The lifetime risk of a single seizure in any individual is around 8–10%—many occurring in infancy and childhood. Though epilepsy is much less common it still remains one of the most common neurological disorders with an incidence in India ranging from 20 to 60/100,000 and a prevalence of 3–11/1,000 population. Febrile seizures have an estimated prevalence of 2–5% of children.

DEFINITIONS

Seizure: This is defined as "transient occurrence of signs and/or symptoms due to abnormal excessive or synchronous neuronal activity in the brain."

Provoked (acute symptomatic) seizures: These occur in temporal relation to a systemic (e.g., hypoglycemia) and/or brain insult (e.g., perinatal asphyxia and traumatic brain injury).

Epilepsy: Epilepsy is a disease characterized by an enduring predisposition to generate epileptic seizures and by the neurobiological, cognitive, psychological, and social consequences of this condition. A diagnosis can be made if (1) at least two unprovoked (or reflex) seizures occur >24 hours apart; (2) one unprovoked (or reflex) seizure and a probability of further seizures similar to the general recurrence risk (at least 60%) after two unprovoked seizures, occurring over the next 10 years. The probability is based on clinical (e.g., seizures in cerebral palsy) or presence of epileptic discharges on electroencephalogram (EEG) or lesions on neuroimaging.

Febrile seizures: A seizure occurring in childhood after 1 month of age, associated with a febrile illness not caused by an infection of the central nervous system without previous neonatal seizures or a previous unprovoked seizure.

Status epilepticus: A seizure with 5 minutes or more of continuous clinical and/or electrographic seizure activity, or recurrent seizure activity without recovery between seizures.

CLINICAL FEATURES

The first task of a clinician is to determine the event is a seizure or a seizure mimic. A careful history from an eye-witness supplemented by a video of the event if possible is the only way to reach this very important conclusion. Though tests may help, they should be used as a substitute for the history. Seizure-mimics differ with age (e.g., neonatal: benign sleep myoclonus, infant: shuddering attacks, breath-holding spells; tics, migraine in school children and syncope, psychogenic nonepileptic seizures in teenagers). Clinical features favoring true seizures are an aura, lateral tongue bite, stereotyped movements, open eyes, incontinence, and a recognizable postictal lethargy or deficits are characteristic but not mandatory.

As per the 2017 International League Against Epilepsy (ILAE) revised classification **(Fig. 1)**, seizures can be now classified as focal (earlier partial), generalized, or unknown in onset. Focal seizures may or may not be associated with impaired awareness (earlier simple and complex partial); motor seizures may be clonic, tonic, myoclonic spasms have prominent automatisms, etc., **(Fig. 2)**. Nonmotor focal seizures may manifest as behavioral arrest or with sensory, cognitive, and other symptoms. Focal seizure can evolve into bilateral tonic-clonic seizures (earlier secondarily generalized tonic-clonic

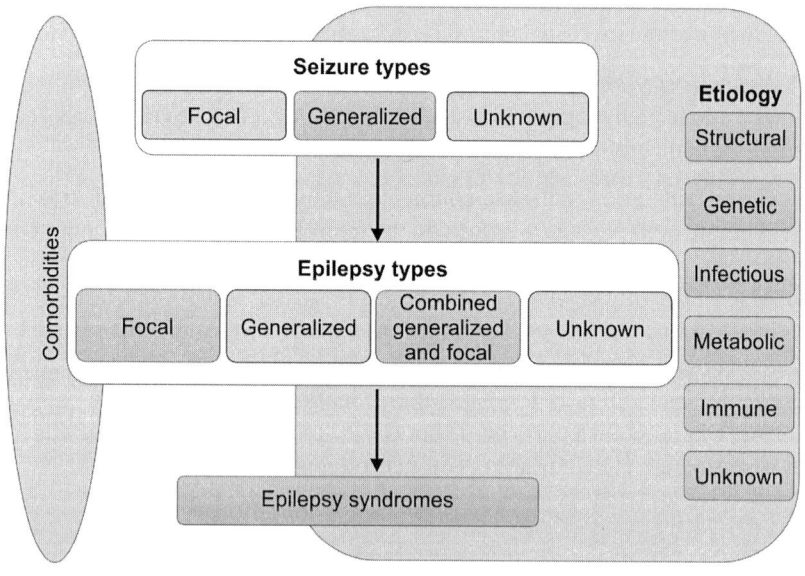

Fig. 1: Classification of seizures.

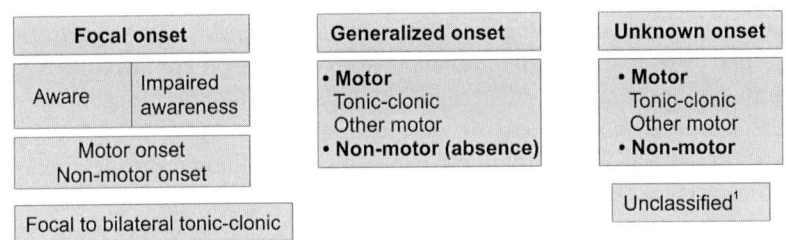

Fig. 2: ILAE 2017 classification of seizure types basic version[2].
[1]Due to inadequate information or inability to place in other categories.
[2]Definitions, other seizure types and description are listed in the accompanying paper and glossary of terms.

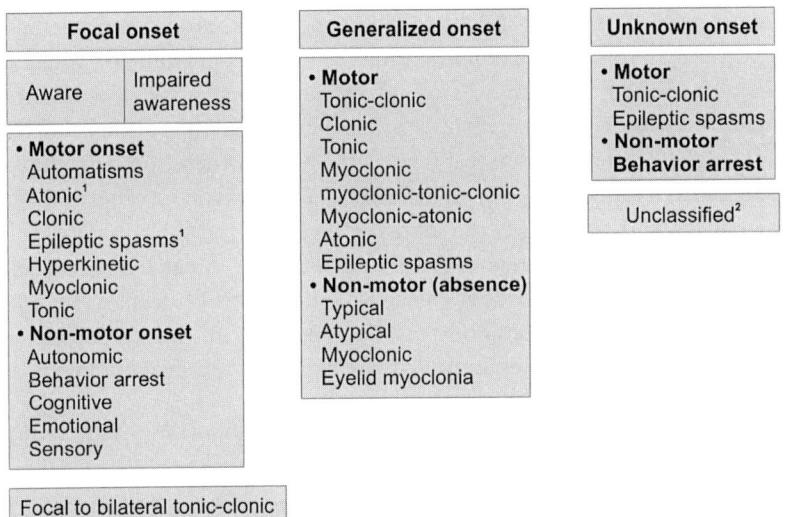

Fig. 3: ILAE 2017 classification of seizure types expanded version[3].
[1]Degree of awareness usually is not specified.
[2]Due to inadequate information or inability to place in other categories.
[3]Definitions, other seizure types and descriptors are listed in the accompanying paper and glossary of terms.

seizures). Generalized seizures always have impaired awareness and could be motor tonic-clonic, myoclonic, atonic seizures as well as epileptic spasms. Absence seizures are classified as nonmotor generalized seizures.

If epilepsy is diagnosed, the initial exercise is to classify the epilepsy into focal, generalized, combined focal, and generalized and unknown based primarily on the predominant seizure types as well as EEG and neuroimaging data **(Fig. 3)**. The diagnosis of epilepsy should be in three levels: seizure type, epilepsy type, and epilepsy syndrome.

Grouping patients into epilepsy syndromes using age at presentation and common clinical features helps in etiological diagnosis as well as prognostication. For instance, West syndrome presents with epileptic spasms in infants associated with severe EEG abnormalities and often secondary to structural or genetic etiologies with responses to steroids or vigabatrin and a guarded prognosis for both the epilepsy and cognitive outcomes. On the other hand, self-limiting (earlier "benign") epilepsy of childhood focal epilepsies with centrotemporal spike or occipital spikes are pharmacoresponsive and have an excellent prognosis. Generalized childhood absence epilepsy similarly do well while in adolescents with juvenile myoclonic epilepsy (JME) usually do not remit in the long-term. It is important to note that many of the epilepsies do not neatly fit into any specific epilepsy syndrome.

Epilepsy etiologies are diverse and can include genetic causes [e.g., early infantile epileptic encephalopathies, JME, tuberous sclerosis (TS), etc.], structural causes [perinatal brain injury, TS, focal cortical dysplasia (FCD), hippocampal sclerosis (HS), etc.], infectious causes [neurocysticercosis (NCC), etc.], immune disorders (autoimmune encephalitis), metabolic disorders (Glut-1 deficiency, biotinidase deficiency, etc.), and finally an unknown group which has a sizable numbers of patients. Though the EEG remains the most important test for seizure-type and syndrome diagnosis, a single normal awake EEG is seen in ~50%; sleep deprivation, other activation procedures, and repeat EEG will increase the yield.

Neuroimaging [read high resolution magnetic resonance imaging (MRI) with specific protocols] have increased the diagnosis of structural diseases notably HS and FCD. Metabolic testing is helpful in infantile epilepsy. It should be noted that the epilepsy may be classified into two etiologies, e.g., TS is structural and genetic.

Neuropsychologic comorbidities often accompany especially if drug-resistant epilepsy (DRE) and include learning and intellectual disabilities, behavior disorders (attention deficit hyperactivity disorder, autistic spectrum disorder (ASD), etc). There might be an underlying neurological disorder causing both though DRE may cause/worsen the disability [e.g., ASD following West syndrome].

MANAGEMENT

Acute care: Most seizures terminate spontaneously within a few minutes. Caregivers of patient with epilepsy should be trained in emergency care of seizures (turn patient on the side, do not insert objects into the mouth, prevent injury, keep airway open, note time of episodes, etc.). Intranasal midazolam spray is available for use in aborting a seizure at home.

Status epilepticus: IV Lorazepam (LZP) or nasal, buccal, IM/IV midazolam (MDZ) form the mainstay in treating a prolonged seizure, depending on where the patient is. MDZ has the advantage that it can be used easily at home and the clinic setting. Fosphenytoin and levetiracetam (LEV) are the preferred IV antiepileptic drugs (AEDs), if seizures continue even after two doses of benzodiazepines (BZDs). Failure of these first two lines of treatment suggest refractory status epilepticus (SE) and should be managed in an intensive care unit (ICU) setting with third line drugs and/or coma producing therapies (MDZ infusions, barbiturates, etc.).

Provoked seizures like febrile seizures or seizures with meningoencephalitis rarely warrant long-term AEDs beyond a few days to weeks.

Long-term AED therapy is used once the diagnosis of epilepsy (discussed earlier) is secure and there seems to be >60% chance of recurrence. Most AEDs are symptomatic treatments and are not disease-modifying. First seizures usually do not warrant therapy beyond acute care advice.

Choice of AED depends on the seizure type and epilepsy syndrome. For instance, generalized seizures may not respond to narrow-spectrum AEDs like carbamazepine (CBZ), oxcarbazepine (OXZ), phenytoin, etc. Absence seizures need ethosuximide, valproate or lamotrigine, and often worsen with narrow-spectrum agents.

Though there are >25 AEDs to choose from, efficacy broadly is the same for the old and new drugs, with ~60–70% of children getting controlled. Comorbidities and risk of adverse events (AE) decide treatment choices. For instance, many neurodevelopmental disorders where behavior issues are common will worsen with LEV, phenobarbital (PB), and the BZDs. CBZ for focal epilepsy and valproate (VPA) for generalized epilepsy are still the bedrock of treatment in new-onset epilepsies primarily because they usually do not cause major neuropsychiatric AE. Non-neurologic morbidities are also important, e.g., obese teenage should avoid VPA because of increased risk of weight gain, menstrual irregularities, and teratogenic potential. Certain principles like "Start low, Go slow", monotherapy, and when needed rational combination therapy, using appropriate doses and formulations, keeping seizure diaries, monitoring AE, parent education, and counseling are useful in successful treatments. About 70% of childhood-onset epilepsy remits in about 2 years and is the basis for the usual duration of treatment once seizure freedom is attained. However, the rest may need longer periods depending on the syndrome or etiology or difficulties in control.

POINTS TO REMEMBER

> Always prefer a first-hand witness account of the event which should form the basis of diagnosis.
> Electroencephalogram and imaging should be used as supplementary aids to diagnosis and cannot replace the history.
> When in doubt, keep the diagnosis open without starting long-term AED.
> Seizure-type, epilepsy type, epilepsy syndrome, and etiological diagnosis should follow a methodological approach and often helps in management decisions.
> Choice of AED depends on consideration of AE and comorbidities rather than efficacy.

FURTHER READING

1. Fisher RS, Cross JH, French JA, Higurashi N, Hirsch E, Jansen FE, et al. Operational classification of seizure types by the International League Against Epilepsy: Position Paper of the ILAE Commission for Classification and Terminology. 2017;58(4):522-30.
2. Perucca P, Scheffer IE, Kiley M. The management of epilepsy in children and adults. Med J Aust. 2018;208(5):226-33.
3. Pina-Garza JE, James KP. Fenichel's Clinical Pediatric Neurology: A Signs and Symptoms Approach, 8th edition. Philadelphia, PA: Elsevier; 2019.
4. Scheffer IE, Berkovic S, Capovilla G, Connolly MB, French J, Guilhoto L, et al. ILAE Classification of the Epilepsies: Position Paper of the ILAE Commission for Classification and Terminology. Epilepsia. 2017;58(4):512-21.

Chapter 28

Cerebral Palsy

Anaita Udwadia-Hegde, Omkar Pradip Hajirnis

"Listen to the silliest complaint of the patient, a good medical history is half the battle won, and also the family's heart"

PK Mullaferoze

(Founder President of Indian Academy of Cerebral Palsy), a champion of nobility, on whose birthday (3rd October) is celebrated as the National Cerebral Palsy Day.

INTRODUCTION

Cerebral palsy (CP) refers to a nonprogressive, static impairment in neuromotor control (namely movement and posture) due to deficit/lesion in the developing brain which can occur in the prenatal, perinatal, or postnatal period. Injury occurs before the brain has matured. There is no neuroregression/loss of skills but only delay in development.

Children with CP are usually diagnosed by the age of 2 years. Their primary abnormality is motor impairment with problems such as muscle weakness, stiffness/spasticity, slowness, and difficulty with balance. These range from mild to severe. About 70% have additional comorbidities like seizures, intellectual disability, speech and language impairment, vision deficits, and hearing loss among the few to name.

Worldwide incidence of CP is in the range of 2–2.5 per 1,000 live births. While exact figures are unavailable in India, it can be safely estimated that the figures may be staggeringly higher. Prevalence has increased due to higher numbers of preterm survival where the chances of CP are higher than term born babies.

Classification of CP is based on the type of motor dysfunction, its anatomical distribution, timing of the brain insult (prenatal, perinatal, or postnatal period) and associated impairments. Accordingly, as per motor dysfunction it could be spastic, ataxic, dyskinetic (dystonic or athetoid) or a mixed type. Anatomically, it could be classified as diplegic, hemiplegic, quadriplegic, etc.

The causative factors/risk factors for CP are myriad. They may be divided into prenatal, perinatal, and postnatal factors. The commonly seen prenatal risk factors are prematurity, low birth weight, multiple gestations, maternal systemic disorders such as thyroid problems, intrauterine infections, and genetic disorders to name a few. Perinatal asphyxia, neonatal hypoglycemic brain injury, sepsis, and kernicterus are some of the common perinatal risk factors. Postnatal factors include meningitis, encephalitis, traumatic brain injury, stroke, etc.

CLINICAL DIAGNOSIS

Cerebral palsy is essentially a clinical condition and the cause for it needs to be sought from a thorough history and examination along with requisite investigations to aid in it. **Table 1** depicts the common presentations of CP as per the tone and anatomical distribution.

The Gross Motor Function Classification System (GMFCS) is a method of describing the range of gross motor dysfunction. The GMFCS describes five levels of motor function with emphasis on abilities and limitations in areas of sitting, standing, and walking. They are as follows:

Level I—walks without limitations
Level II—walks with limitations
Level III—walks using a handheld mobility device
Level IV—self-mobility with limitations; may use powered mobility
Level V—transported in a manual wheelchair

MANAGEMENT

Management includes investigations for the causative factors and screening for the associated comorbidities. This includes neuroimaging where a magnetic resonance imaging (MRI) brain is preferred over a computed tomography (CT), especially if the etiology is not established. An electroencephalogram (EEG) is advocated if history suggests seizures. Metabolic and genetic studies are done if a causative reason is otherwise not found for the condition.

Comorbidities which are seen and also anticipated are screened namely vision and hearing assessment, orthopedic abnormalities such as dislocations, osteoporosis, etc. The clinician must be always wary to rule out disorders which mimic CP but are not.

Treatment is multidisciplinary. Early detection and intervention are the most pivotal part. Physical therapy, occupational therapy, speech therapy, and orthoses form a part of this teamwork under appropriate-supervised guidance. Similarly, psychosocial and educational support is of utmost importance.

Table 1: Presentations of cerebral palsy.		
CP type	Clinical presentation	Usual causative factors
Diplegic CP (spastic)	• Weakness/spasticity of all four limbs, but lower limbs affected more than upper • Commonly seen features on examination are spasticity in lower limbs with hyper-reflexia and clonus, scissoring in ventral suspension, and crossed adductor response • Cognition usually preserved	Prematurity
Hemiplegic CP (spastic)	• Weakness on one side of the body • Commonly seen features are early hand dominance with hand fisting on nondominant side and hemiplegic gait later	• Neonatal stroke • Cerebral malformations
Quadriplegic CP (spastic)	• Weakness of all four limbs and legs usually more affected than hands • Commonly seen features are severe developmental delay with intellectual disability • Characteristic supine posture with head retracted, legs extended with flexed elbows and clenched hands	• Perinatal asphyxia • Intrauterine infections
Ataxic (hypotonic)	• Truncal hypotonia with brisk reflexes • Commonly seen features are ataxic signs (titubations, tremors, and wide-based gait)	Genetic factors
Athetoid/ dyskinetic	• Dystonia and spasticity with dyskinesias • Commonly seen features include dystonic posturing appearing in infancy with hypertonia and involuntary movements gradually increasing overtime	• Kernicterus • Hypoxic injury to basal ganglia

(CP: cerebral palsy)

Antispasticity medications usually used are baclofen and benzodiazepines like clonazepam. Medications for dystonia like trihexyphenidyl which is an anticholinergic is used in patients with significant dystonia which also benefits to prevent excessive drooling. Antiepileptic medications for seizures and medications for other comorbidities may be needed. Injectable botulinum toxin A is used for relief in localized spasticity. Surgical options are tenotomy for gait correction and osteotomy for secondary bone deformities.

The prognosis is variable and difficult to explain to parents. Independent sitting by 2 years is clinically a good prognostic indicator of independent ambulation. In terms of type of CP, some types of ambulation are seen in about 80% of diplegic, 70% of dyskinetic, and 50% of quadriplegic CPs. Hemiplegic CPs usually walk by 2-3 years of age. The associated comorbidities play a huge role in prognosticating CP.

FURTHER READING

1. Ashwal S, Russman BS, Blasco PA, Miller G, Sandler A, Shevell M, et al. Practice parameter: Diagnostic assessment of the child with cerebral palsy: Report of the Quality Standards Subcommittee of the American Academy of Neurology and the Practice Committee of the Child Neurology Society. Neurology. 2004;62(6):851-63.
2. Moreno-De-Luca A, Ledbetter DH, Martin CL. Genomic insights into the causes and classification of cerebral palsies. Lancet Neurol. 2012;11(3):283-92.
3. Piña-Garza JE, James KC. Fenichel's Clinical Pediatric Neurology: A Signs and Symptoms Approach, 8th edition. Philadelphia, PA: Saunders Elsevier; 2019.
4. Swaiman KF, Ashwal S, Ferriero DM, Schor NF, Finkel RS, Gropman AL, et al. Swaiman's Pediatric Neurology: Principles and Practice, 6th edition. Philadelphia, PA: Elsevier Saunders; 2017.
5. Taft LT. Cerebral palsy. Pediatr Rev. 1995;16(11):411-8.

Chapter 29

Movement Disorders in Children with Neurodevelopmental Disorders

Abhishek R Jain, Lokesh Lingappa

INTRODUCTION

Children with neurodevelopmental disorders frequently manifest movement disorders, which can be either hyperkinetic or hypokinetic. The common movement disorders reported in children with neurodevelopmental disorders include ataxia, akinesia, dyskinesia, bradykinesia, Tourette syndrome, and catatonic-like symptoms which may be present at all times or episodic **(Table 1)**. Some of these movement disorders may lead to complications like contractures and falls which may cause further problems. Pathophysiology of most of these movement disorders involves dysfunction of cerebellum and basal ganglia, either due to the illness itself or due to the drugs used in their treatment **(Tables 2 and 3)**.

CLINICAL FEATURES

Hyperkinetic movement disorders are far more common than hypokinetic disorders.

Hyperkinetic movement disorders, also known as dyskinesias, are repetitive involuntary movements commonly seen in children including tics, chorea, dystonia, myoclonus, stereotypies, and tremor.

Table 1: Characteristics of common movement disorders in childhood.

	Rhythmic	Stereotyped movements	Repeated posture	Speed	Suppressible
Tics	No	Yes	Yes	Jerky	Usually
Chorea	No	Rarely	No	Jerky	No
Athetosis	No	No	No	Nonjerky	No
Myoclonus	Occasionally	Usually	Occasionally	Jerky	No
Tremor	Yes	Yes	No	Nonjerky	Sometimes briefly
Dystonia	Rarely	Occasionally	Yes	Nonjerky	Partial or only briefly

Table 2: Etiology of the various movement disorders.

Type of movement disorder	Etiology
Chorea	Sydenham's, SLE, thyrotoxicosis, hypoparathyroidism, disorders of sodium/glucose, renal failure, basal ganglia infarction/hemorrhage, postpump chorea, inherited, and drugs
Dystonia	Perinatal hypoxia/trauma, genetic, encephalitis, basal ganglia stroke/tumor, juvenile Wilson's disease, mitochondrial encephalopathy, DOPA responsive, and drugs
Myoclonus	Epileptic, mitochondrial (MERRF), GM2 gangliosidosis, biotinidase/carboxylase deficiency, renal/hepatic failure, hyperglycemia, SSPE, opsoclonus-myoclonus syndrome, posthypoxia, spinal cord tumor, and drugs
Tremor	Essential, hypoglycemia, hypocalcemia, hypomagnesemia, perinatal hypoxia, hyperthyroidism, and drugs
Tics	PANS, Tourette syndrome, and drugs
Stereotypies	Autism, mental retardation, PDD, Rett syndrome, and healthy children
Athetosis	Perinatal hypoxia/trauma and kernicterus

(DOPA: L-3,4-dihydroxyphenylalanine; DYT1: early-onset primary dystonia; MERRF: myoclonic epilepsy with ragged red fibers; PANS: pediatric acute-onset neuropsychiatric syndrome; PDD: pervasive developmental disorder; SLE: systemic lupus erythematosus; SSPE: subacute sclerosing panencephalitis)

Table 3: Drug-induced hyperkinetic movement disorders.

Type of movement disorder	Drugs
Chorea/athetosis	Phenytoin, carbamazepine, valproic acid, dopamine receptor blocking agents, tricyclic antidepressants, theophylline, oral contraceptives, steroids, and stimulants
Dystonia	Typical neuroleptics, antipsychotics, and metoclopramide
Myoclonus	Epileptic myoclonus can be aggravated by some antiepileptics
Tremor	Salbutamol, tricyclic antidepressants, valproic acid, phenytoin, carbamazepine, and theophylline
Tics	Lamotrigine, central nervous system stimulants, levodopa, and neuroleptics

These movement disorders occur more commonly in children than in adults. These movements can be characterized according to their:
- Speed (slow or rapid)
- Volition (involuntary or voluntary)

- Repetition (stereotypical or nonstereotypical)
- Rhythmicity (rhythmic or nonrhythmic)
- Purpose of the movement (purposeful, nonpurposeful, or semipurposeful).

They are further evaluated on the involvement of muscle groups (distal or proximal, either manifesting in the upper or lower limbs, or the face).

Tics

Tics are the most common movement disorder in children. Tics are also a common comorbidity in many neurodevelopmental disorders, especially attention deficit hyperactivity disorder (ADHD) and many genetic disorders associated with intellectual delay. They may be seen with pediatric autoimmune neuropsychiatric features due to streptococcal infection [pediatric acute-onset neuropsychiatric syndrome (PANS)] which is triggered by streptococcal infection is associated with regression of speech, florid onset of tics, along with other movement disorders. Any child with acute/subacute onset of regression of speech with motor tics mandates the pediatrician to consider the diagnoses of PANS as the management and outcomes of the condition are much better when intervened early.

Tremor

It is an involuntary, rhythmic, and sinusoidal alternating movement of one or more body parts. It can affect a limb, or any body part, including the head, chin, and soft palate. Tremors can be classified in various ways:

Resting tremor: When the affected body part has tremors at rest, with gravity eliminated. The tremor usually disappears during voluntary actions. It has a frequency of 4–5 Hz. Rest tremor is a characteristic feature of Parkinson's disease which is exceptionally uncommon in children.

Postural tremor is seen when the limb is static but held against gravity, such as when the arms are held outstretched in front, or held in a wing beating position. It has a frequency of 6–12 Hz. It is commonly seen in basal ganglia disorders.

Intention tremor, characterized by worsening of tremor on approaching a target, is characteristically seen in cerebellar disorders. The tremors have a slower frequency of 2–4 Hz.

Dystonic tremors when dystonia is a prominent feature along with tremor, the condition is called dystonic tremor. This type of tremor can also be seen in basal ganglia and thalamic involvement.

Chorea

Chorea, in Greek, means "dance". These movements are abrupt, involuntary, nonrepetitive, nonrhythmic, often occurring in proximal extremities, neck, trunk, and facial muscles resulting in a continuous random flow of muscle contractions, with a variable frequency and intensity. Often the movement can merge into a purposeful movement, giving it a dance-like appearance. Seen with involvement of the caudate nucleus.

Myoclonus

Myoclonic movements are sudden, shock like, brief, and involuntary movements which are usually positive (caused by muscle contraction).

The distribution of myoclonus can be focal, multifocal, segmental or generalized. Etiologically, myoclonus is subdivided into physiological myoclonus (e.g., sleep myoclonus), essential myoclonus (idiopathic or hereditary), epileptic myoclonus, or symptomatic myoclonus in cases where the myoclonus is secondary to an underlying disorder.

Physiologically, myoclonus is subdivided into cortical, subcortical, spinal and peripheral types.

Athetosis

Athetosis is a slow, continuous, and involuntary writhing movement that prevents maintenance of a stable posture. Athetosis involves continuous smooth movements that appear random and are not composed of recognizable submovements or movement fragments.

Athetosis can worsen with attempting movements or while maintaining certain posture, as is seen in dystonia and chorea, but can also occur at rest. Athetosis characteristically involves the distal extremities (hands or feet) more than the proximal ones, and it can also involve the face, neck, and trunk.

In children, a combination of chorea and athetosis is called "*choreoathetosis*", most often caused by the dyskinetic form of cerebral palsy in which dystonia is a frequently associated movement disorder. Choreoathetosis also occurs due to kernicterus and other causes of basal ganglia injury.

Dystonia

Dystonia is characterized by sustained or intermittent muscle contractions causing abnormal, often repetitive movements, postures, or both. The movements are typically patterned, twisting, and may be tremulous. Dystonia is often initiated or worsened by voluntary action and is associated with overflow muscle activation.

Dystonia typically diminishes or disappears with distraction and sleep. Characteristic feature of dystonia is the presence of "sensory tricks" or "geste-antagoniste" (proprioceptive or tactile) that ameliorate the dystonic movement, although this is not seen in all types of dystonias.

Hypokinetic Disorders in Children

Hypokinetic disorders are uncommon in children. They are well described and studied in adults. Parkinsonism is the most described entity in this group of children.

Parkinsonism in Children

The key motor features (bradykinesia, rigidity, rest tremor, and postural instability) of idiopathic Parkinson disease can also be present in children. Pure Parkinsonism is often not seen in children, but can be present with few monogenic disorders. Secondary Parkinsonism features are commonly due to tuberculous meningoencephalitis and post-Japanese encephalitis.

NEURODEVELOPMENTAL DISORDERS WITH MOVEMENT DISORDERS

Syndromic autism refers to the presence of comorbid autism in people with a distinct genetic developmental disorder with syndromic autism being particularly prevalent in Angelman (up to 80%), tuberous sclerosis complex (TSC) (up to 60%), fragile X syndrome (FXS) (up to 50%), Rett's syndrome (40–97% depending on subtype), CHARGE syndrome (up to 50%) and Down syndrome (up to 39%).

Fragile X syndrome-autism spectrum disorder (ASD) occurs in 21–50% of males with FXS with ASD being more likely to be identified in individuals with a greater degree of intellectual disability. Ataxia is the most common movement disorder associated with FXS and is usually present as the predominant clinical feature throughout the course of illness. This is characterized by intention tremor, dysmetria, asynergia, dysdiadochokinesis, gait ataxia, and dysarthria and is present in 80–90% of patients.

Children with Rett's syndrome (RS) have hand stereotypies which are the hallmark of this condition, with typical movements of both hands (clapping, tapping, wringing, and hand mouthing). These are continuous, repetitive, and compulsive automatisms which disappear during sleep and may aggravate with anxiety. Other movement disorders noted in Rett's syndrome are dystonia, rigid akinetic syndrome, chorea and athetosis. These work as handles toward diagnoses as well. The prevalence of ASD in RS ranges from 25 to 40% and up to 97% in individuals with the preserved speech variant of RS. ASD is also the most common initial misdiagnosis in children with RS, with 18% of individuals being diagnosed with ASD before receiving a diagnosis of RS. Important to keep in mind is the characteristic repetitive hand movements in RS are very different from the motor stereotypes observed in individuals with ASD.

Children with Angelman syndrome (AS) have a small head and a specific dysmorphology, delayed development, severe intellectual disability, speech abnormalities, balance and movement problems, seizures, and sleep problems. The prevalence of ASD in AS ranges from 50 to 80%. The reported prevalence of ataxic/jerky movements in AS varies up to 72.7%. Ataxic/jerky gait is more prevalent in AS; whereas a greater proportion of people with Rett syndrome experience tremor.

CHARGE syndrome occurs in approximately 1 in 10,000–12,000 live births. The syndrome's acronym, CHARGE, refers to the characteristic physical deficits: Coloboma of the eye, heart defects, atresia of the choanae, retardation of growth and/or development, genital and/or urinary abnormalities, and ear abnormalities and deafness, hyperactivity, obsessions, compulsions, and tic disorders have been noted. Autism-like behaviors have been described in several case reports. Studies suggest that the prevalence of ASD ranges from 15 to 50%.

DYRK1A-dual specificity tyrosine phosphorylation-regulated kinase heterozygous mutation leads to intellectual delay, severe speech delay/absent speech, epilepsy, and primary microcephaly. 21q22.13 (located within the Down syndrome critical region) with distinct facial features: sparse scalp hair, deep-set eyes, hooded eyelids, prominent nasal root, pointed nasal tip, and short chin. Magnetic resonance imaging (MRI) brain demonstrates cerebral atrophy and they have significant seizures. Those who achieve ambulation have significant ataxia.

Movement disorders in genetic syndromes associated with syndromic autism are limited by the small number of patients in each syndrome. Examples include CHARGE syndrome, Cohen syndrome, Cornelia de Lange syndrome, TSC, etc.

MANAGEMENT

Management of movement disorders should consider the amount of disability secondary to the movement itself. Conditions causing impairment in functioning need to be managed with pharmacotherapy **(Table 4)**. As many of these conditions may not cause much impairment in functioning, they can be followed up without pharmacological intervention, e.g., motor tics, mild chorea, or tremors can be managed without drug intervention along with appropriate therapy like occupational therapy. Appropriate scales need to be used to assess the severity of the movement disorder for long-term follow-up and to assess the effect of intervention.

A reference to a pediatric neurologist is indicated for the following:
- Suspect fragile X syndrome in a male child who has dysmorphology like a long face, prominent forehead, large ears and prominent jaw, and who has either ataxia or tremor, along with features of autism.

Table 4: Drugs used in treatment of movement disorders.	
Repetitive and stereotypic disorder	Risperidone and sertraline
Selfinjurious behavior	Clomipramine, olanzapine, and divalproex sodium Others—beta blockers and anxiolytics
Dystonia	Trihexyphenidyl, tetrabenazine, gabapentin, and clonazepam
Chorea	Tetrabenazine, sodium valproate, and carbamazepine
Tics	Risperidone, clonidine, and tetrabenazine

- A girl child with acquired microcephaly with repetitive stereotypic movements along with features of ASD-suspect Rett's syndrome.
- A child who presents with epileptic spasms, always look for ash leaf macules. TSC can often present with varied behavioral problems in children.
- Any child with movement disorder with a neurodevelopmental disability should undergo a thorough neurological evaluation.

FURTHER READING

1. FitzGerald PM, Jankovic J, Glaze DG, Schultz R, Percy AK. Extrapyramidal involvement in Rett's syndrome. Neurology. 1990;40:293-5.
2. Hagberg B. Clinical criteria, stages and natural history. In: Hagberg B, Anvret M, Wahlstrom J, (Eds). Rett Syndrome—Clinical and Biological Aspects. London: MacKeith Press; 1993. pp. 4-20.
3. Moss J, Howlin P. Autism spectrum disorders in genetic syndromes: Implications for diagnosis, intervention, and understanding the wider autism spectrum disorder population. J Intellect Disabil Res. 2009;53(10):852-73.
4. Temudo T, Ramos E, Dias K, Barbot C, Vieira JP, Moreira A, et al. Movement disorders in Rett syndrome: An analysis of 60 patients with detected MECP2 mutation and correlation with mutation type. Mov Disord. 2008;23(10):1384-90.
5. Williams CA, Beaudet AL, Clayton-Smith J, Knoll JH, Kyllerman M, Laan LA, et al. Angelman syndrome 2005: Updated consensus for diagnostic criteria. Am J Med Genet A. 2006;140(5):413-8.

Chapter 30

Neuroregressive Disorders

Shekhar Patil

INTRODUCTION

Regression in simple terms means a return to a former or a less developed state. Neuroregression is a term that implies reversal of the developed state of the brain to a lesser developed or a lower level of functioning. This may include loss of previously acquired skills pertaining to motor, visual, hearing, intellectual, and cognitive domains; either singly or across multiple domains. However, the use of the term "neuroregression" implies reversal of skills primarily in the cognitive domain with other domains involved in various combinations. Though inborn errors of metabolism (IEM) are the most commonly encountered diagnosis, one should be aware of toxic, inflammatory, infectious, and neoplastic disorders as a differential to inherited/sporadic variety of neuroregressive disorders.

CLINICAL FEATURES

In this era of genomics, the classification of neuroregressive disorders would be driven by the genetic defect; yet, for the clinician it may be prudent to categorize these disorders on the basis of affection of the neuraxis; preferential cortical involvement will be poliodystrophies, white matter involvement would be leukodystrophies, the basal ganglia diseases would be corencephalopathies and lastly, spinocerebellar diseases involving brainstem, spinal cord, and cerebellum or only the cerebellar hemispheres.

In a broader sense, prominence and presentation of certain symptoms can help categorize, plan appropriate tests, and management such as:

Poliodystrophies: Cognitive decline, epilepsy and visual impairment.

Leukodystrophies: Pyramidal tract dysfunction and visual impairment.

Corencephalopathies: Movement disorders.

Key questions to be asked:
- Age at onset and pattern of clinical presentation
- Inheritance and family history
- Localization of symptoms within the neuraxis
- Extraneural involvement
- Course and severity of the condition
- Exposure to toxins
- Behavioral and language dysfunction
- Epilepsy
- Visual symptoms/progressive visual impairment
- Nutrition status
- Identify any treatable conditions.

SYMPTOM-BASED APPROACH TO DIAGNOSIS

Epilepsy: Neonatal/infantile or progressive myoclonic epilepsies:

Glycine encephalopathy, molybdenum co-factor deficiency, maple syrup urine disease (MSUD), Alper's disease (*POLG* related), phenylketonuria (PKU), biotinidase deficiency, Menke's disease, neuronal ceroid lipofuscinosis, Niemann-Pick type C, Gaucher disease, subacute sclerosing panencephalitis (SSPE), cherry red spot myoclonus, and myoclonus, epilepsy, ragged-red fibers (MERRF).

Pyramidal dysfunction: Spastic paraparesis/quadriparesis ± peripheral neuropathy:

Metachromatic leukodystrophy, Krabbe's disease, urea cycle defects, biotinidase deficiency, adrenoleukodystrophy, adrenomyeloneuropathy, hyperhomocysteinemia, and hyperornithinemia-hyperammonemia-homocitrullinemia (HHH) syndrome.

Movement disorder: Chorea/dystonia or Parkinsonism:

Wilson's disease, neurodegeneration with brain iron accumulation, glutaric aciduria, Leigh's disease, Lesch–Nyhan disease, and organic acidemia.

Behavioral difficulties: Anxiety/psychosis/aggression:

X-linked adrenoleukodystrophy, Wilson's disease, and Sanfilippo disease.

Any classification of this group of disorders as gray matter diseases or white matter diseases is over simplification of the approach. In reality, the clinician is always faced with a mixed bag of symptoms that may not conform to the accepted concept of classification. Newer approaches to these conditions based on information collected through clinical signs/symptoms, neuroimaging, and genetic tests may be the way forward because this may offer hope of a therapeutic option.

Investigations

Complete blood count, liver function tests, ammonia, lactate, tests for vitamin B12 metabolism, toxin screen, metabolic profile including blood spot for tandem mass spectrometry (TMS) and urine sample for gas chromatography mass spectrometry (GCMS), ceruloplasmin, oligosaccharides, glycosaminoglycans, and cerebrospinal fluid (CSF) tap.

Electrophysiological studies such as visual-evoked potential, electroretinography, brainstem evoked response audiometry, nerve conduction study, and most importantly neuroimaging [magnetic resonance imaging (MRI) brain with additional spectroscopy and diffusion tensor imaging as indicated].

Tests for enzyme activity, endocrine dysfunction, neoplastic etiologies, and autoimmune diseases as deemed appropriate.

Genetic testing such as chromosomal microarray, clinical/whole exome sequencing based on the results of the routine blood tests and neuroimaging.

MANAGEMENT

Most of the neuroregression cases are due to neurometabolic causes/IEM.

In general, the manifestations of the IEM are due to intoxication (accumulation of organic acids, phenylalanine, etc.) or due to energy failure (mitochondrial diseases, glycolytic pathway affection, etc.) or storage disease such as lysosomal diseases.

Some of the interventions are:
- Dietary advice or restriction of offending agent, e.g., diet for PKU/MSUD
- Enzyme blockage in the initial part of the pathway
- Increasing the substrate/use of alternative substrate
- Use of hemodialysis or peritoneal dialysis in the acute phase of intoxication
- Replacement such as enzyme replacement therapy or bone marrow transplantation
- Gene therapy
- Appropriate medications for epilepsy, spasticity, and dystonia
- General care and nutritional support
- Supportive care—physiotherapy, occupational therapy, orthotic use, psychological support to the family and caregivers, and patient support groups
- Counseling in the antenatal period for subsequent pregnancies.

FURTHER READING

1. Cassis L, Cortes-Saladelafont E, Molero-Luis M, Yubero D, González MJ, Ormazabal A, et al. Review and evaluation of the methodological quality of the existing guidelines and recommendations for inherited neurometabolic disorders. Orphanet J Rare Dis. 2015;10:164.

2. Helbig I, von Deimling M, Marsh ED. Epileptic encephalopathies as neurodegenerative disorders. Adv Neurobiol. 2017;15:295-315.
3. Kovacs GG. Concepts and classification of neurodegenerative diseases. Handb Clin Neurol. 2017;145:301-7.
4. Mastrangelo M. Clinical approach to neurodegenerative disorders in childhood: An updated overview. Acta Neurol Belg. 2019;119(4):511-21.
5. van der Knaap MS, Bugiani M. Leukodystrophies: A proposed classification system based on pathological changes and pathogenetic mechanisms. Acta Neuropathol. 2017;134(3):351-82.

Chapter 31

Inborn Errors of Metabolism: Developmental and Behavioral Outcomes

Shibani Kanungo, Neelkamal Soares

INTRODUCTION: CELLULAR TO CLINICAL PERSPECTIVE

Inborn errors of metabolism (IEM) are rare genetic or inherited disorders resulting from impaired cellular digestion or recycling of nutrients such as proteins, fats, carbohydrates, vitamins, and cofactors or impaired organelle function affecting normal cellular functions of survival and or growth. The cellular digestion or recycling involves multiple biochemical processes organized into specific biochemical pathways, which are dependent on several enzymes degrading a specific substrate. Enzymes are proteins and their function determined by a specific gene/genetic code. This multitude of complex cellular biochemical events or metabolism is affected by a dysfunctional enzyme, and can result in excess or paucity of a substrate or create alternate toxic substrates affecting cellular growth and survival. A gene mutation providing abnormal coding message results in enzyme dysfunction or deficiency.

Saudubray's classification of IEMs includes three main diagnostic groups—intoxication, energy metabolism, and complex molecules.

Intoxication group includes:
- Inborn error of intermediary metabolism *(*amino acid disorders, organic acid disorders, urea cycle defects, carbohydrate intolerance disorders, vitamin disorders, metal disorders, and porphyrias)
- Inborn error of neurotransmitter synthesis and catabolism
- Inborn error of amino acid synthesis.

Energy metabolism group includes:
- Mitochondrial energy defects (congenital lactic acidemias, respiratory chain disorders, fatty acid oxidation disorders, and ketone body defects)
- Cytoplasmic energy defects (disorders of glycolysis, glycogen metabolism and gluconeogenesis, hyperinsulinism, pentose phosphate pathway defects, and creatine metabolism defects).

Complex molecules group includes:
- Cellular organelle (lysosome, peroxisome, Golgi apparatus, endoplasmic reticulum, and mitochondria) involvement in synthesis, remodeling, recycling, trafficking, and catabolism presenting as lysosomal storage disorders (LSD), congenital disorders of glycosylation (CDG), and peroxisomal biogenesis disorder (PBD)
- Complex lipids and fatty acids (defects of phospholipids, triglycerides, sphingolipids, isoprenoids, cholesterol, bile complex, very long chain fatty acids, plasmalogens, dolichol, and ubiquinone).

CLINICAL FEATURES

Based on severity of a specific enzyme dysfunction/defect and organ system affected, IEMs can have heterogeneous clinical presentation from growth delay, failure to thrive, feeding problems, hypoglycemia, unusual body odor, gut dysmotility, anemia, seizures, encephalopathy, hypotonia, cerebral palsy, quadriplegia, dystonia, strokes, neuropathy, cardiomyopathy, arrhythmias, rhabdomyolysis, cholestasis, liver dysfunction, hepatomegaly, liver failure, liver cancer, splenomegaly, cataracts, corneal clouding, retinopathy, kidney stones, tubular dysfunction, renal failure, developmental delay, hearing loss, speech delay, apraxia, learning disabilities, intellectual disabilities, hyperactivity, self-mutilatory behavior, aggression, autism, schizophrenia, depression, tremors to dysmorphism, skin rashes, skeletal abnormalities, brain anomalies, genitourinary anomalies, or normal appearance. They can present at any time—in utero to adulthood, leading to multiple comorbidities, and sometime mortalities acutely even during common illnesses.

Biochemical analyte analysis in blood, urine, and cerebrospinal fluid (CSF); enzyme activity in leukocyte, fibroblasts, or liver tissue with molecular analysis of specific gene can help diagnosis, genetic counseling, and prognosis of each IEM. Technological advances such as tandem mass spectrometry, liquid chromatography, and easy detection of enzyme activity in asymptomatic newborn with successful treatment using metabolic nutrition, cofactor or vitamin supplementation, enzyme or substrate therapy, and hematopoietic stem cell transplantation (HSCT) have helped inclusion of 50+ disorders in the newborn screening panel.

DEVELOPMENTAL AND BEHAVIORAL PERSPECTIVES

Developmental and behavioral problems can be seen in all IEMs. In determining developmental functioning and outcomes, it is important to understand the natural history of specific IEM, as well as disease attenuation as a result of newborn screening-related early detection, treatment, and secondary comorbidities. A good understanding of cognitive and developmental testing tools, to determine when and on which age ranges to use helps provide best intervention, in tandem with IEM treatment. It is also important to distinguish changes resulting from natural history (and treatment of) IEM from normal progression of childhood development. Since, there are a wide variety of IEMs affecting multiple organ systems, only general statements are made in this chapter about developmental perspectives. In general, developmental delays can be seen in all untreated IEM.

Notably, phenylketonuria has long been known to have significant intellectual disability and/or self-mutilation behaviors (when untreated), though if treated, there can still be learning disorders or attention-deficit/hyperactivity disorder (ADHD) symptoms. Amino acid disorders such as maple syrup urine disease (MSUD), glutaric aciduria, and nonketotic hyperglycinemia (NKH) can present with severe psychomotor delay. Usually such presentation can occur acutely after a single common childhood illness, in an otherwise previously-diagnosed asymptomatic patient.

Smith–Lemli–Opitz, a disorder of cholesterol metabolism, has been associated with intellectual disability, language deficits, sensory hyper-reactivity, irritability, sleep problems, self-injurious behavior, and even behaviors consistent with autism spectrum disorder.

Galactosemia can manifest as irritability, developmental delay if untreated and with treatment often as expressive verbal dyspraxia.

Fatty acid oxidation disorders can present as irritability and mood changes in the setting of common childhood illness and resulting hypoglycemia. Glycogen storage disorders (GSD) generally cause systemic and not developmental disorders, though, a generalized form (Lafora) can lead to myoclonic epilepsy and progressive dementia. In IEMs presenting with hypoglycemia involved with energy metabolism, long-term and recurrent episodes of subclinical hypoglycemia without severe presentation of hypoglycemic seizures, can show reversible learning and cognitive delay as well can reversible gray and white matter changes in magnetic resonance imaging (MRI). As with any chronic illnesses, depression can be seen in adolescence and adulthood.

Mitochondrial disorders can present with autism spectrum disorder symptoms, particularly with regressive features, learning delays, dementia, delirium with stroke like illness. LSD can present with neuropathic symptoms and can present with psychomotor delays and if severe causes regression of motor and intellectual functioning (as in Niemann-Pick forms). Some forms (such as type I GM1-gangliosidosis) present early in life with hypotonia, feeding challenges, and neurological regression with seizures progressing to early death. Other forms may present with developmental and intellectual delays.

Neurotransmitter disorders can present with severe persistent global delay and hypotonia.

Urea cycle defects can present with developmental delays when younger, but in older presentations can have behavior issues (aggression and irritability) with fluctuation depending on ammonia load (depending on treatment compliance).

Metal disorders can present with only liver failure or with a range of developmental delay to severe intellectual disability or with psychiatric symptoms as general as behavior problems such as impulsivity and irritability to psychosis.

MANAGEMENT

Given clinical heterogeneity, high index of suspicion in context of multiorgan involvement with growth failure, neurodevelopmental issues, or rapid deterioration after common illnesses or extreme avoidance or preference of specific food nutrient (proteins or simple carbohydrates or fats) can help with IEM diagnosis. Effective treatments include metabolic nutrition, cofactor or vitamin supplementation, enzyme or substrate therapy and HSCT, and gene therapy along with early detection through newborn screening has made this individually rare disorders when grouped as IEM to be more common than diabetes.

Successful management is best achieved with a metabolic genetics clinic. A multidisciplinary approach is necessary to serve the unique needs of these patients and their families.

Supportive educational and rehabilitative management are usually required for developmental and behavioral consequences of IEM. Educational interventions include specialized instruction for developmental and cognitive impairments. Specific monitoring of neurological regression (with caution for seizures and motor deterioration) will require collaborative care with neurology colleagues. Behavioral issues should be managed by addressing the underlying substrate accumulation (likely reversible), but may need behavioral interventions and medications (as indicated).

FURTHER READING

1. Annals of Translational Medicine. (2018). Focused Issue; Inborn Errors of Metabolism. [online] Available from: https://www.ncbi.nlm.nih.gov/pmc/issues/327511/(Last accessed December, 2021).
2. Kline MW. Rudolph's Pediatrics, 23rd edition, Section 11: Inherited Disorders of Metabolism. McGraw Hill.
3. Saudubray JM, Baumgartner MR, Walter J. Inborn Metabolic Diseases: Diagnosis and Treatment. Switzerland AG: Springer Nature; 2016.
4. Scriver's OMMBID. The Online Metabolic and Molecular Bases of Inherited Disease. [online] Available from: https://ommbid.mhmedical.com/(Last accessed December, 2021).

Chapter 32

Traumatic Brain Injury

Prameela Joji

INTRODUCTION

Traumatic brain injury (TBI) is the leading cause of pediatric trauma death and disability and affects up to 280 of 100,000 children worldwide. Approximately, 5,000 children are disabled due to TBI each year. In developed countries, TBI is the most common cause of trauma-related death and disability in childhood. Overall, falls and motor vehicle crashes account for the majority of injuries.

Various mechanisms result in TBI severe enough to require hospitalization. Inflicted head injury is a significant mechanism, particularly for infants younger than 1 year of age.

The highest pediatric morbidity and mortality is reported in children younger than 4 years of age, and in those with hypotension, low Glasgow Coma Scale (GCS) scores at initial presentation, coagulopathy, or hyperglycemia. Despite the higher survival in children with TBI, disability is significant with the functional long-term outcome associated with the initial injury severity.

CLINICAL FEATURES

According to the Centers for Disease Control and Prevention, the severity of TBI is typically defined by the initial GCS or pediatric GCS score:
- Mild (GCS Score 13–15)
- Moderate (GCS Score 9–12)
- Severe (GCS Score <9)

The pathophysiology of TBI involves two insults:
- Primary injury is the direct trauma to the brain
- Secondary injury is the result of a cascade of biochemical, cellular, and metabolic responses to direct injury, which worsens in patients who develop hypoxia, hypotension, or both.

EVALUATION

- All baseline hematological investigations should be done.
- *Neuroimaging*—All pediatric patients with severe TBI should undergo computed tomography (CT) scan of the head.
  Any lesion that requires emergent surgery (e.g., epidural hematoma) is reliably identified by CT.

MANAGEMENT

Initial assessment: During the primary survey, neurologic disability should be assessed as follows:
- Assign GCS score—GCS score provides a global assessment of consciousness and indicates need for intervention:
  - Any patient with a GCS ≤ 12 or higher GCS with an abnormality on head CT scan warrants emergency consultation with and evaluation by a neurosurgeon.
  - In addition to neurosurgery consultation, any patient with a GCS ≤ 8 or a GCS that is rapidly falling warrants emergency endotracheal intubation by rapid sequence intubation (RSI).
- Identify signs of impending herniation.

Initial stabilization:
- When intracranial pressure (ICP) monitoring is in place, maintain cerebral perfusion pressure > 40 mm Hg
- Avoid hypocarbia.

Airway and breathing:
- The child who is lucid and has a normal blood pressure can be managed with supplemental oxygen alone.
- Advanced airway management, including tracheal intubation, is warranted in the following situations:
  - Decreasing level of consciousness (GCS ≤ 8) or rapidly falling
  - Signs of respiratory failure
  - Hemodynamic instability.

Circulation: Cerebral perfusion must be maintained to prevent secondary ischemic injuries.

Fluid management:
- Hypovolemic shock should be treated using isotonic solutions (e.g., isotonic saline) with a goal of attaining a state of normal, rather than excess, circulating volume.
- Excess intravascular volume may exacerbate the development of cerebral edema.

- The administration of hypotonic fluids, such as D5W, should be avoided because they deliver too much free water, which may exacerbate cerebral edema and cellular destruction.

Target blood pressure: Systolic blood pressures (SBP) should be maintained at least above the 5th percentile for age because outcomes such as mortality and neurologic disability for children with severe TBI who are hypotensive at the initial evaluation are typically poor.

Focal injuries that may require neurosurgical intervention must be quickly identified and surgically managed.

Manage raised ICP-elevate head end, minimize stimulation, adequate sedation, osmotic therapy, and antiepileptics. Surgical management is indicated, as needed. All neuroprotective measures to reduce morbidity must be initiated.

Regular follow-up post-treatment with extensive neuro rehabilitation is a must.

In patients whose brain injury is not amenable to surgical correction, further care is focused on preventing hypoxia or hypotension and monitoring for and treating intracranial hypertension.

POINTS TO REMEMBER

- Cervical spine motion restriction.
- In general, cuffed endotracheal tubes should be used for all major pediatric patients with major trauma.
- Procedures may result in increased ICP if patients are not adequately sedated. These procedures range from suctioning to more invasive procedures.
- Manual in line cervical immobilization throughout intubation.
- Early airway management and maintain normoxia and normocarbia.

Early and prompt management helps in reducing morbidity and mortality. Those who have recovered need regular follow-up from a multidisciplinary team under the guidance of developmental pediatrician and neurologist for optimal outcomes.

FURTHER READING

1. ATLS Subcommittee; American College of Surgeons Committee on Trauma; International ATLS working group. Advanced Trauma Life Support (ATLS), 9th edition. J Trauma Acute Care Surg. 2017;82(5):877-86.
2. Kochanek PM, Tasker RC, Carney N, Totten AM, Adelson PD, Selden NR, et al. Guidelines for the Management of Pediatric Severe Traumatic Brain Injury, 3rd edition: Update of the Brain Trauma Foundation Guidelines, Executive Summary. Pediatr Crit Care Med. 2019;20(3):280-9.
3. Krug EG, Sharma GK, Lozano R. The global burden of injuries. Am J Public Health. 2000;90:523.

4. Langlois JA, Rutland-Brown W, Thomas KE. Traumatic brain injury in the United States; emergency department visits, hospitalizations, and deaths. Atlanta: Centers for Disease Control and Prevention; 2006.
5. Lavoie M, Nance ML. An approach to the injured child. In: Fleisher and Ludwig's Textbook of Pediatric Emergency Medicine, 7th edition, Bachur RG, Shaw KN (Eds). Philadelphia: Lippincott Williams & Wilkins; 2015. p. 9.
6. Liang T, Roseman E, Gao M, Sinert R. The utility of the focused assessment with sonography in trauma examination in pediatric blunt abdominal trauma: A systematic review and meta-analysis. Pediatr Emerg Care. 2021;37(2):108-18.
7. Luerssen TG, Klauber MR, Marshall LF. Outcome from head injury related to patient's age. A longitudinal prospective study of adult and pediatric head injury. J Neurosurg. 1988;68:409.
8. Massagli TL, Michaud LJ, Rivara FP. Association between injury indices and outcome after severe traumatic brain injury in children. Arch Phys Med Rehabil. 1996;77:125.

Chapter 33

Neuromalignancies and Developmental Outcomes

Vasudha N Rao, Samir H Dalwai

> "You may have to fight a battle more than once to win it."
> **Margaret Thatcher**

> "The best way out is always through."
> **Robert Frost**

INTRODUCTION

Treatment of childhood cancer is one of the most remarkable success stories, which has evolved over the past four decades. Owing to early detection, evidence-based protocols of treatments and improvement in supportive care, majority of childhood cancers, including brain tumors, are treatable.

Pediatric brain tumors have a two-fold effect on normal developmental milestones. Primarily, brain tumors can present with developmental delay or regression especially in infants and toddlers. In children, between 0 and 4 years of age, nonspecific presentations such as irritability, drowsiness, failure to thrive, and delayed milestones may be the only manifestations of an underlying brain tumor.

Secondly, treatment of brain tumors do cause decline in cognitive abilities including intelligence, executive functioning, processing, and memory with a progressive decline for several years after treatment. Although subtle, these deficits often translate into difficulty in school, employment, and overall negatively affect the quality of life. Thus, minimizing the long-term toxicity of treatment and managing late effects fall in the realm of developmental and behavioral pediatrics.

If the success of the treatment is to parallel the quality of life and neurological outcome, it is imperative to work on interventions that may minimize or remediate the effect of residual disease as well as immediate and late effects of treatment. This chapter aims to delineate the neurocognitive effects, risk factors, and interventions to remediate these late effects.

CLINICAL DIAGNOSIS

Risk Factors

There is a host of variables impacting the neurocognitive effects during treatment of brain tumors. These include:

- *Individual factors related to the child:* Factors that contribute to the neurocognitive outcome are:
  - Age at diagnosis
  - Prediagnostic level of functioning
  - Environmental influences.

  Age of the child has a significant impact with younger children showing poorer outcomes as compared to their older peers.

  Additionally, children with higher levels of functioning capabilities at baseline tend to demonstrate greater declines in intellectual ability over time.

- *Factors related to the tumor:* Tumor size, tumor location, and to a lesser extent tumor histology have been found to be associated with outcomes in several studies. Posterior fossa tumors frequently cause hydrocephalus and are associated with neurocognitive deficits. Regardless of tumor type and treatment, presence of hydrocephalus negatively affects neurocognitive outcome.

- *Factors related to treatment:* Pediatric brain tumors are often treated with a multimodal approach of surgery, chemotherapy, and radiotherapy.

  Surgery: Despite refined neurosurgical techniques, as high as 30% children with infratentorial tumors experience "posterior fossa syndrome" after surgery. The acute effects of this syndrome include diminished speech, ataxia, and emotional lability, which improve over time. Children who do not exhibit this syndrome have a better outcome.

  Radiation: The most significant factor contributing to the development of neurocognitive decline is cranial radiation therapy. Most protocols avoid radiation therapy to children <3 years of age to limit the effects of cranial irradiation to the growing brain. Children treated with radiation often show:
  - A downswing in intelligence with a 2–4 point reduction in intelligence quotient (IQ) per year, most evident a year after treatment.
  - Additionally, working memory is also impaired due to decreased hippocampal volume.

  Chemotherapy: The effect of chemotherapy on neurodevelopmental outcomes is often difficult to deduce, since a combination of chemotherapeutic agents is frequently used. Specifically, several chemotherapeutic agents are known to cause ototoxicity.

  The use of folate antagonist methotrexate has been shown to result in a lower IQ compared to age-matched controls, but higher than children receiving radiation therapy.

- *Factors related to time since treatment:* Neurocognitive effects tend to be cumulative, with studies showing a progressive decline in neurocognitive functioning, from treatment until late adolescence.

NEURODEVELOPMENTAL OUTCOMES

The neurocognitive phenotype may vary with each individual child ranging between mild deficits in learning and memory to significant limitations in intellectual and adaptive functioning.

It is imperative to understand that intelligence is a composite of multiple core functions like attention, processing speed, and working memory. These core cognitive skills are affected more than the global intelligence in all pediatric brain tumor survivors and merit greater emphasis for intervention.

Further, studies have also shown deficits in visual-based tasks, nonverbal IQ, and visual spatial processing. Additionally, tumors in the cerebellum may contribute to speech and language deficits including dysfluencies and slowed speech.

It is indeed ironic to note that survivors may not have awareness of their deficits and often end up with an expectation and performance mismatch.

Key questions to ask:
- What was the age at diagnosis?
- How was the child's prediagnostic level of functioning?
- What were the type, location, and size of tumor?
- What were the treatment modalities: surgical, radiation, and chemotherapy?
- How is the behavior and speech at school and other community and social settings?

MANAGEMENT

Genomic studies and risk stratification in pediatric brain tumors have paved the way for less intensive treatment for several brain tumors; thus attempting to limit disruption and damage, and at the same time, preserve the developed and developing cognitive functions. The aim of management is to conserve and promote cognitive functions in children. This may include early identification, remediation, skill training, accommodation, family support, and pharmacological interventions.

Inclusion of neuropsychological care and transitioning services is also equally important to prevent late psychological sequelae.

Effective identification of children at risk followed by comprehensive neurocognitive, developmentally appropriate assessment is essential, both before and after completion of treatment. Audiology and vision assessments should be an integral component of evaluation.

Several interventions both nonpharmacologic and pharmacologic have been attempted depending upon the age and neurocognitive functioning of the child.

Nonpharmacologic interventions mainly attempt to accommodate the deficits and include cognitive/behavior-based skill acquisition. Since, these children miss considerable time at school, care should be taken to offer academic support which may include extra time in classroom to complete assignments, special education, audio books, preferential seating, etc. It is of utmost importance that parents should be aware of the child's special educative and psychosocial needs. In accordance with the deficits observed, various cognitive training programs have attempted to improve working memory, attention, and processing speed.

Pharmacological interventions have attempted to remediate the attention deficit experienced by pediatric brain tumor survivors and are similar to those for children with attention deficit hyperactivity disorder (ADHD). Use of methylphenidate was indeed associated with improvement in sustained attention among survivors in a double-blind randomized controlled trial (RCT).

FURTHER READING

1. Krull KR, Hardy KK, Kahalley LS, Schuitema I, Kesler SR. Neurocognitive outcomes and interventions in long-term survivors of childhood cancer. J Clin Oncol. 2018;36(21):2181-9.
2. Rey-Casserly C, Diver T. Late effects of pediatric brain tumors. Curr Opin Pediatr. 2019;31(6):789-96.
3. Scheinemann K, Bouffet E. Pediatric Neuro-oncology; Springer, 2014.
4. Stavinoha PL, Askins MA, Powell SK, Pillay Smiley N, Robert RS. Neurocognitive and psychosocial outcomes in pediatric brain tumor survivors. Bioengineering (Basel). 2018;5(3):73.

Chapter 34

Attention Deficit Hyperactivity Disorder

Samir H Dalwai, Hilla Sukhadwala

INTRODUCTION

Attention deficit hyperactivity disorder (ADHD) is one of the most common behavioral disorders of childhood and adolescence and may persist into adulthood. ADHD can profoundly affect academic achievement, well-being, and social interactions of children. It may be described as a complex syndrome of developmental impairments of executive function, i.e., the self-management system of the brain. The core symptoms of ADHD are inattention, hyperactivity, and impulsivity. ADHD has a genetic and biochemical basis. The role of environmental factors is not yet clear; they may influence symptoms of ADHD (subsyndromic) rather than "cause" the syndrome of ADHD.

CLINICAL DIAGNOSIS

Clinical subtypes are laid out in **Flowchart 1**. Common symptoms associated with ADHD are outlined in **Flowchart 2**.

Attention deficit hyperactivity disorder is diagnosed if the child meets the diagnostic and statistical manual of mental disorders, 5th edition (DSM-5). DSM-5 criteria and core symptoms impair function in academic, social, behavioral, and emotional or occupational activities.

Flowchart 1: Subtypes of attention deficit hyperactivity disorder (ADHD).

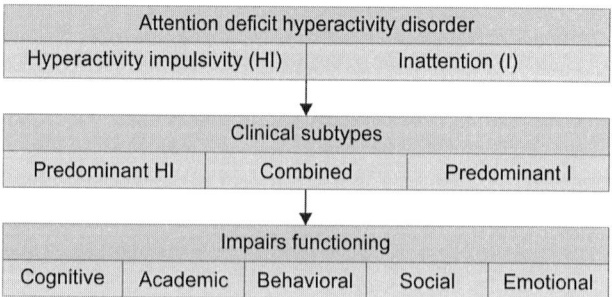

Flowchart 2: Symptoms of ADHD.

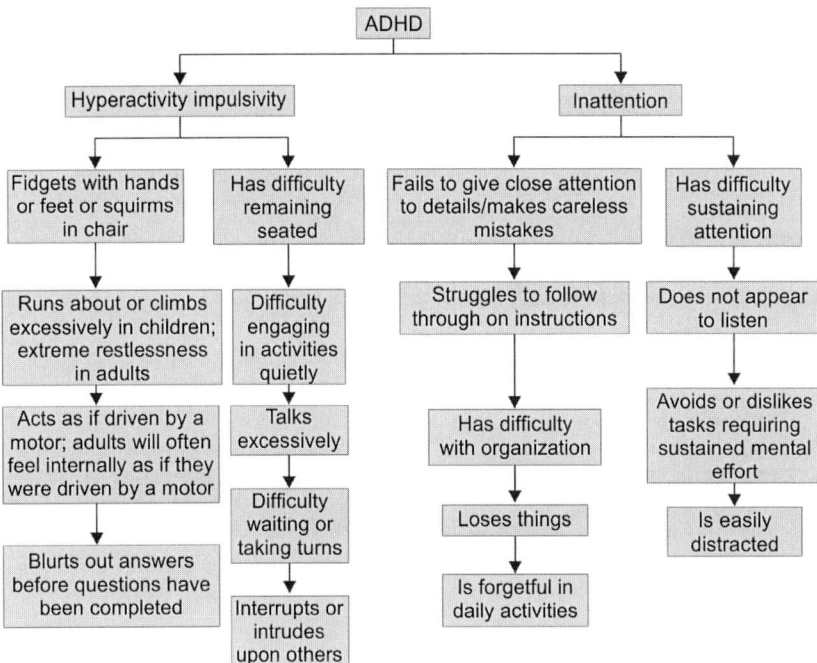

(ADHD: attention deficit hyperactivity disorder)

Attention deficit hyperactivity disorder can be diagnosed:
- If there is evidence that symptoms began before the age of 12 years.
- In those 17 years or older with fewer problem behaviors.

Comorbid conditions like:
- Oppositional defiant disorder
- Anxiety disorder
- Depression
- Learning disability
- Conduct disorder can worsen the outcome for the child.

Thus, comprehensive evaluation for ADHD requires comprehensive medical, developmental, educational, and psychosocial evaluation are listed in **Box 1** and **Table 1**.

The objectives of comprehensive evaluation of ADHD are given in **Box 2**.

This mandates the necessity of a team approach.

Attention deficit hyperactivity disorder evaluation does not require blood lead levels, thyroid hormone levels, neuroimaging, or electroencephalography unless these tests are indicated by the clinical evaluation.

Box 1: Comprehensive evaluation for ADHD.

History of prenatal exposures	Age of onset of the core symptoms of ADHD
Perinatal complications or infections	Duration of symptoms
Head trauma	Settings in which the symptoms occur
Recurrent otitis media	Degree of functional impairment and functional impact symptoms
Sleep disturbances	Developmental milestones, especially language milestones
Family history of similar behaviors	School absences
Observation of parent-child interactions	Psychosocial stressors

(ADHD: attention deficit hyperactivity disorder)

Table 1: Comprehensive evaluation of a child with attention deficit hyperactivity disorder (ADHD).

Medical	Developmental	Educational	Psychosocial
Medical history	Clinical interviews with parent and patient	Information about functioning in school	Evaluation for coexisting emotional disorders
Social and family history	Developmental evaluation	Information about functioning in day care	Evaluation for behavioral disorders
Investigations, if clinically indicated			

Box 2: Objectives of comprehensive evaluation.

- *Confirm core symptoms:* Presence, persistence, pervasiveness, and functional complications
- Exclude other explanations of core symptoms
- *Identify coexisting disorders:* Medical, emotional, and behavioral

Key Questions to ask

- How is your child doing at school? Is your child happy in school?
- Does your child have any behavioral problems at school or home or when playing with friends?
- Have you or the teacher noticed any problems with learning?
- Does your child have problems completing school assignments at school or home?
- Does your child display undue aggression or anxiety?

MANAGEMENT

"How do you solve a problem like Maria?" Oscar Hammerstein II, The Sound of Music.

Early diagnosis and effective multidisciplinary intervention are essential to prevent further compromise of functional achievement.

Aim of management:
- *Target functional outcomes*: It is very important to set and document functional outcomes such as decrease in hyperactivity, aggression, improvement in relationships, academic performance, etc. These are chosen in collaboration with the child, parents, and school personnel.
- Coexisting conditions must be treated concurrently with ADHD.

Hence, management of ADHD must begin with a documented program made by a Developmental Pediatrician that involves collaboration between the intervention team and the child, caregivers, and school personnel.

Modalities of Management

- Behavioral interventions—the first-line treatment for preschool children (below 6 years) with ADHD
- Medication—with or without behavioral interventions are the first-line therapy for school-aged children (≥6 years) and adolescents who meet the diagnostic criteria for ADHD
- Educational interventions
- Combination of the above.

Behavioral interventions are modifications in the physical and social environment that are designed to change behavior, via rewards and nonpunitive consequences. Behavior therapy, especially parent training in behavior management (PTBM), is recommended as:
- The first-line treatment for preschool children with ADHD (rather than medication)
- An adjunct to medication for school-aged children and adolescents with ADHD, and
- The intervention for children who have problems with inattention, hyperactivity, or impulsivity but do not meet criteria for ADHD (subsyndromic).

Medications: Medications may be added with care in an older preschool child if there is no benefit with behavioral intervention.

Methylphenidate is the first-choice medication for children and adolescents above 6 years of age. Initial dose is 5 mg orally. Increase dose gradually in increments of 5–10 mg/week; individualize dose according to needs and response of the patient. Maximum dose: 60 mg/day. Titrate accordingly for extended release preparations.

Atomoxetine and the extended-release alpha-2 agonists guanfacine and clonidine remain the secondary alternative medications. Initial dose of atomoxetine is 0.5 mg/kg/day orally. Increase dose to 1.2 mg/kg/day after a minimum of 3 days at the initial dose. Maximum dose: 1.4 mg/kg/day or 100 mg/day, whichever is less.

The number of extended-release forms of stimulant medications has increased.

Educational interventions: This may include provision of tutoring or resource room support (either in a one-on-one setting or within the classroom), classroom modifications, accommodations, or behavioral interventions.

Combination therapy with medications and behavior/psychological therapy is superior to behavior/psychological therapy alone and necessary for restoration of function.

Re-evaluation of children with ADHD is essential in absence of response to appropriate intervention, whenever symptoms worsen or new symptoms emerge.

FURTHER READING

1. American Psychiatry Association. Diagnostic and Statistical Manual of Mental Disorders, 5th edition. Arlington, VA: American Psychiatric Association. 2009:59-65.
2. Brown T. A New Understanding of ADHD in Children and Adults: Executive Function Impairments. London, UK: Routledge; 2013.
3. Dalwai S, Unni J, Kalra V, Singhi P, Shrivastava L, C Nair MK. Consensus Statement of the Indian Academy of Pediatrics on Evaluation and Management of Attention Deficit Hyperactivity Disorder. Indian Pediatr. 2017;54(6):481-8.
4. Wolraich ML, Hagan JF Jr, Allan C, Chan E, Davison D, Earls M, et al. Clinical Practice Guideline for the Diagnosis, Evaluation, and Treatment of Attention-Deficit/Hyperactivity Disorder in Children and Adolescents. Pediatrics. 2019;144(4):e20192528.

Chapter 35

Disruptive Behavior Disorders

Leena Deshpande

"Anyone can become angry—that is easy, but to be angry with the right person at the right time, and for the right purpose and in the right way—that is not within everyone's power and that is not easy."
Aristotle

Disruptive behavior disorders are conditions, which are easy to recognize as these have patterns of externalizing behaviors which can be readily seen as temper tantrums, extreme anger, aggression, and excessive argumentativeness on part of the child. These children have difficulty in controlling their emotions and have strongly uncooperative, defiant, aggressive, and destructive behavior. As the name suggests, the lives of the people around are severely disrupted because of the child's behavior.

Disruptive behavior disorders include two disorders—oppositional defiant disorder (ODD) and conduct disorder (CD).

OPPOSITIONAL DEFIANT DISORDER

Introduction

There are times when even the best behaved child may be disobedient, defiant or argumentative toward parents, or other authoritative figures. But, if this behavior is frequent and persistent, the child may have oppositional defiant disorder (ODD). Symptoms may be seen commonly by 6-8 years of age though in some cases, they may be seen as early as 3 years of age. These issues can last through their teenage years and into adulthood.

Oppositional defiant disorder affects around 2-16% of school age children and is seen more commonly in boys than girls (postpuberty, seen equally in boys and girls).

The etiology is not known but is thought to be multifactorial due to a cumulative effect of genetic, social factors, and parenting technique.

Clinical Features

"My child just does not listen to me, keeps arguing! He is so irritable, demanding, and stubborn!"

It is quite common to hear these complaints from parents in pediatric practice. When such concerns are voiced by parents, the clinician needs to evaluate the child's behavior and parent's response to these behaviors. The purpose of this evaluation is to differentiate the developmental and normal toddler tantrums from the maladaptive behaviors (argumentative, defiant, vindictive, and angry) meeting criteria for ODD as well to determine if the parenting style is perpetuating the child's negative behavior.

Key questions to ask:
- What is the age of the child?
  Although there are no definitive cutoff for age-related behaviors, a 2-year-old child's normal toddler resistance needs to be differentiated from a 5-year-old's angry, argumentative, or vindictive behavior.
- How long does the negative behavior last?
  This will give clues regarding the intensity of the behavior with respect to the child's, age and cultural expectations.
- What triggers the negative behavior?
  Understanding the antecedents (sleepy, tired, and not giving into demands) leading to the behavioral pattern.
- What is done to calm the child?
  This will help understand the parenting style, e.g., does the parent use distractions or give in to the demand of the child.
- How often does this happen?
  It is very concerning if the difficult behaviors happen on a daily basis for under 5-year-olds or even once a week for children who are above 5 years of age.
- How long has this been going on?
  Difficult behaviors lasting >6 months may fulfil the diagnostic criteria for ODD.
- Are these behaviors seen only at home or also occur in other settings, like school?
  This helps determine the severity.
- Is his development, including academic achievement and social relations with peer group, progressing well?
  This helps to understand the impact of his behavior on everyday life.

Apart from these, the clinician needs to be aware of the child's medical [attention-deficit/hyperactivity disorder (ADHD) and mood disorders] and social (lower socioeconomic status, marital discord, alcoholism, and abuse) history, which may put the child at an increased risk of ODD.

Checklists (child behavior checklist) and rating scales (Vanderbilt Parent Rating Scales) are available which can help the clinician to quantify the difficult behaviors.

Oppositional defiant disorder is a clinical diagnosis.

Management

Early identification and treatment for ODD is imperative. The behavioral symptoms, if left untreated, will worsen and children are at an increased risk of CD, substance abuse, and depression.

Treatment options for ODD in children include:
- Cognitive behavioral therapy which teaches to control impulses or emotions
- Social skills group therapy where children can learn to improve their relationships with peers
- Family therapy helps parents find support and improve their interaction with their child and learn effective parenting techniques. Learning these skills will require routine practice and patience
- *Medications*: No specific medication to treat ODD itself, but can be used to manage co-occurring disorders like ADHD, anxiety, or depression
- Management of comorbid conditions (which are very common) like ADHD and learning disorder
- Teacher training is also vital to help them manage the child in classroom.

Though with early treatment some children will outgrow the disorder, at least 30% develop CD and 10% may eventually develop antisocial personality disorder.

CONDUCT DISORDER

"A child whose behavior pushes you away is a child who needs connection before anything else!"

Kelly Bartlet

Introduction

Most cases of CD are preceded by ODD and continue to display ODD symptoms. However, the disruptive behaviors seen in CD are more serious, even illegal as compared to ODD.

Approximately 6-16% of boys and 2-9% of girls meet the diagnostic criteria for CD. The incidence of CD increases from childhood to adolescence.

The etiology is same as ODD with interplay of genetic, familial, and social environmental factors. Untreated ODD will progress to CD.

Clinical Features

Many adolescents show defiance on occasions, some may show occasional risk taking behavior and experiment with alcohol or drugs. However, in children with CDs, the behaviors are more serious, persistent, and frequent.

Diagnostic and Statistical Manual of Mental Disorders, 5th edition (DSM 5) mentions infractions such as aggression toward people and animals, theft or deceitfulness, and serious violations of rules. After the act, these children show no remorse or empathy toward the person harmed by their actions.

The clinician must be aware of the social and the psychological risk factors which predispose to CD. Psychiatric disorders, antisocial behavior, and substance abuse in the family, poverty along with poor parenting are known to increase the risk of CD.

Two subtypes are commonly seen:
1. *Childhood onset*: Children show at least one symptom of CD prior to 10 years of age.
2. *Adolescent onset*: There are no symptoms of CD prior to 10 years of age.

To be diagnosed with CD, the symptoms must cause significant impairment in social, academic, or occupational functioning. The disorder is typically diagnosed prior to adulthood.

Conduct disorder is a clinical diagnosis and the diagnostic criteria are mentioned in detail in DSM 5.

Conduct disorder has varying degrees of severity. Childhood onset of symptoms is generally associated with severe problems.

Conduct disorder may mimic or coexist with various other mental health disorders including ADHD, ODD, mood disorders, substance abuse, and these will increase the severity of CD.

Management

Many children and adolescents with CD will require specialized mental health treatment. There is almost always a dysfunctional family background that will significantly affect the treatment efficacy. Family therapy can be most effective in improving behavior. Medications may be tried to help improve compliance during therapy. Stimulant medications and antidepressants may help manage comorbid conditions.

In new-onset CD, e.g., seen after a family stressor, behavior may remit if appropriate support is given.

Conduct disorder increases the risk of several public health problems, including violence, weapon use, teenage pregnancy, and substance abuse. Early identification and treatment may help minimize these long-term issues.

FURTHER READING

1. Diagnostic and Statistical Manual of Mental Disorders (DSM-5)—American Psychiatry Association, 2013.
2. Harstad EB, Barbaresi WJ. Disruptive behavior disorders. In: Voigt RG, Macias MM, Myers SM (Eds). Developmental and Behavioral Pediatrics. American Academy of Pediatrics; 2011. pp. 349-58.
3. Searight HR, Rottnek F, Abby SL. Conduct disorder: Diagnosis and treatment in primary care. Am Fam Physician. 2001;63(8):1579-89.

Chapter 36

Anxiety

Manoj Bhatawdekar

"Of all the troubles, great and small, the greatest are the ones that do not happen at all."
Thomas Carlyle

INTRODUCTION

Emotions add colors to human life. However, sometimes the colors can be dark and scary. There are some emotions we like and some we do not. Fear is one of the deepest emotions and is perceived to be negative. It is mostly normal to have fear of darkness, snakes, wild animals, etc. Fear has a protective role in that it helps one take appropriate precautionary measures, as necessary, e.g., crossing the road after checking both sides.

When there is a threat perceived from a real stimulus it is called fear. For instance, a real tiger chasing a person would make the person feel scared. However, if the person feels threatened by a chasing tiger even when there is none in reality, it is called anxiety. Thus, anxiety is a fearful anticipation of future in the absence of any real danger. It is a state of the body, which is caused by a rush of stress hormones such as adrenaline, and is characterized by autonomic arousal and hypervigilance.

Anxiety is normal to a certain extent and disappears on its own most of the times. However, at times, it can be intense, persistent, pervasive, and can interfere with daily functioning. In that case, it requires medical attention. Children and adolescents commonly perceive anxiety during different stages of their life and their presentation varies from stage to stage.

It is observed that anxious parents beget anxious children. It is always a complex interplay between genetic and environmental factors that is operative in this case. In addition to genetic predisposition, it is possible that a child learns from parents to give anxious responses to stimuli.

Very often, the seeds of future anxiety disorders in adulthood are sown in early childhood and adolescence. Therefore, it is important to diagnose anxiety disorders during childhood and manage them well.

CLINICAL FEATURES

Case 1

A 9-year-old girl was brought for treatment with history of refusal to go to school, excessive crying at the thought of going to school which would result in vomiting for the past 1 month. She would keep worrying that something might go wrong with her mother if she went to school. She would also refuse to sleep alone in her room away from her parents. She had started getting nightmares about being alone in a jungle. She would frequently complain of abdominal pain for which no apparent physical cause was found.

This type of anxiety disorder wherein there is excessive anxiety concerning separation from home or attachment figures is called separation anxiety disorder. There may be nightmares of wild animals, monsters, ghosts, of being kidnapped, and of accidents happening to themselves or parents. The child may be grossly attention seeking or demanding. This can result into a disharmony in the family. The prevalence varies from 0.9 to 1.9%. It is more common in females. There is often a genetic predisposition and there could be environmental triggers such as the loss of a member in the family or of a pet, change of school or place of residence, parental separation, etc.

This disorder, if not treated well, results into complications such as academic underachievement, suicidal behavior, and relationship crises in the family. It can persist even in later life affecting independent functioning.

Case 2

A 6-year-old boy was referred for evaluation, with presenting complaint of a severe fear of dogs. Whenever he saw a dog, he would almost freeze, start crying loudly, wanting to escape the situation, and would tremble in fear. He would cry irresistibly and end up vomiting. This resulted in severe restriction on his movements outside home. He would always be on the lookout for a dog wherever he went. He stopped going out to play with friends because a dog might chase him. He would avoid walking on the streets and insisted on being carried in arms because he would invariably spot a dog on the street. He would refuse to visit relatives who had pet dogs. He would otherwise be comfortable at home and at school.

This type of anxiety is associated with a fear of a specific stimulus and is called specific phobia. There is marked anxiety about a specific object or situation such as flying, heights, animals, receiving injections, or seeing blood. The anxiety response is immediate and results in avoiding the specific stimulus. The magnitude of anxiety is out of proportion to the actual threat posed by the stimulus. The clinical manifestations differ depending on the stimulus causing anxiety. For instance, there is a hyperadrenergic state (increased heart rate, sweating, dryness of mouth, etc.) in animal phobias whereas there is often increased heart rate initially which drops later giving a vasovagal syncope in case of blood or injury-related phobias. Highly neurotic temperament, parental overprotection, broken family situation, recurrent physical illnesses, and sexual abuse are some factors which increase the risk of phobias.

This disorder can result into moderately severe impairment in daily functioning especially if the phobic stimulus is a common one and difficult to avoid. Severe physical symptoms such as choking, fainting, and vomiting can lead to a vicious cycle of anxiety leading to further anxiety. A well-planned treatment, therefore, is essential and helps to improve the quality of life.

Case 3

A 10-year-old girl, a good dancer, presented with fearfulness related to performance on stage in school. She would tremble with fear, experience a choking sensation, and go blank on stage. She also started avoiding talking to strangers. She often expressed a fear that others may ridicule her and laugh at her. She was seen as a very shy, nervous girl who would not mix easily in her peer or adult groups. She was otherwise very comfortable with her own family and known circles.

This type of anxiety disorder is called social anxiety disorder. It is typical in social situations where the person is likely to be evaluated or judged. The person feels negatively evaluated by others and feels anxious. There are often thoughts that others may laugh or mock at him/her and may perceive him/her as stupid, crazy, or weird. There is a fear of rejection by others. Trembling, sweating, staring, crying, clinging, and avoiding social situations are common behaviors found among children with social anxiety. The anxiety is out of proportion to the actual likely negative consequences of the social situation.

The most common age of onset is between 8 and 15 years. It especially has severe negative impact on interpersonal relationships of adolescents. Adolescents with social anxiety disorder may be predisposed to alcohol abuse and drug abuse. There could be increased rate of school dropouts, lowered academic performance and work performance in later life, and generally accompanied by a low self-esteem. Hence, it is important to treat this disorder well.

Case 4

A 16-year-old girl, a junior college student, was referred from the ICCU with complaints of sudden onset of palpitations, sweating, choking sensation in the throat, constriction in the chest, breathing difficulty, dizziness, and a severe fear of dying. She has been getting these attacks quite frequently in the past 3 months. They appear out of the blue. She often feels as if she is going to lose control over herself and go crazy. This has incapacitated her so severely that she is scared to move out alone, unless accompanied by a close relative. She has missed her college.

The above attacks are called panic attacks and the disorder is called panic disorder. The attacks could be nocturnal or during day-time. These are always unexpected, without any precipitating factor. The attack typically has multiple physical symptoms. In addition to the above-mentioned symptoms there could be nausea, abdominal distress, tremors, hot or cold sensations, dryness of mouth, tingling and numbness, and derealization. The person may develop a fear of open spaces called agoraphobia. This is associated with a fear of being detected in a helpless state outside a comfort zone. Individuals with agoraphobia may avoid public transportation, crowded places, or enclosed spaces since they fear getting a panic attack.

Panic disorder can develop during adolescence and persist in later adulthood. It is usually associated with severe psychosocial impairment leading to a poor quality of life. Similarly, agoraphobia can also impair the quality of life. Individuals who are sensitive and prone to negativity are more likely to suffer from these disorders. Both these disorders have a genetic predisposition.

Case 5

A 17-year-old boy presented with complaints of a dull bitemporal headache, irritability, difficulty falling asleep, worrying excessively about his academic performance for the past 6 months. He often anticipates failure in exams, gets tired very easily, is unable to concentrate, experiences palpitations and dizziness intermittently, and has undergone multiple investigations for the same, all reports being normal.

The above type of anxiety disorder is called generalized anxiety disorder. As against panic disorder, generalized anxiety disorder has ongoing symptoms. There is often an admixture of psychological and physical symptoms. The prevalence among adolescents is 0.9%. Genetic predisposition and parental overprotection are important risk factors. The distress caused by this disorder can impair academic, interpersonal, and work life of the individual.

Among other anxiety disorders are medication-induced or substance-induced anxiety disorder and anxiety disorder due to other medical conditions.

MANAGEMENT

Anxiety disorders generally run a chronic course, if not intervened properly. These can impair schooling, academic performance, interpersonal relations, and thus the overall quality of life.

Many of these disorders can progress into adult life, causing psychosocial impairment. Therefore, early detection and proper evaluation followed by adequate treatment are essential.

A well-timed referral (as against a referral after multiple half-hearted trials of various drugs) to a psychiatrist is always recommended. Basic physical workup is needed only in order to consider primary or comorbid medical conditions. Unnecessary investigations just "to complete the list" or investigations which relieve the treating clinician's anxiety (!) only reinforce somatic symptoms in anxious patients and should be avoided. Appropriate psychological tests such as CAT/TAT might throw more light on psychopathology and are worth considering after a clinical assessment.

The line of treatment of anxiety disorders is a combination of pharmacotherapy, cognitive behavior therapy, and relaxation training. In children <12 years of age, small doses of tricyclic antidepressants such as imipramine and nortriptyline may be used. Selective serotonin reuptake inhibitors (SSRIs) such as sertraline, fluoxetine, and serotonin norepinephrine reuptake inhibitors (SNRIs) such as venlafaxine are useful in older children and adolescents. Parental counseling is an integral part of managing children and adolescents with anxiety. Very often, parents also have anxious personality predispositions or even a frank anxiety disorder which may warrant treatment.

"Anxiety is having to remind myself that being afraid of things going wrong is not the way to make things go right." —**Anonymous**

FURTHER READING

1. American Psychiatric Association. Diagnostic and Statistical Manual of Mental Disorders (DSM-5), 5th edition. Arlington, Virginia: American Psychiatric Publishing. 2013:193-234.
2. Bernstein BE. Pediatric social phobia and selective mutism. Medscape. 2018.
3. Bhatawdekar M. Modern Parenthood through the Eyes of a Psychiatrist. Mens Sana Monogr. 2015;13(1):125-33.
4. Forrest JS. Pediatric panic disorder. Medscape. 2018.

Chapter 37

Depressive Disorders

Kersi Chavda, Alka A Subramanyam

INTRODUCTION

The prevalence of depression is about 1-2% in prepubertal children, rises to 4-5% mid-teens, and then reaches an adult prevalence of 10-17%, with a preponderance in girls. Depression is slated to be the second leading cause of disability worldwide by 2020, which is why it is so important for medical professionals to be familiar with this disorder.

CLINICAL FEATURES

Depressive disorders include disruptive mood dysregulation disorder, major depressive disorder (MDD), persistent depressive disorder (previously called dysthymia), depressive disorder due to another medical condition, and other specified depressive disorder.

The common feature of all these is the presence of sad, empty or irritable mood, accompanied by somatic, and cognitive changes that significantly affect the individual's capacity to function.

The differences between them lie in duration, timing, and presumed etiology.

Major Depressive Disorder

- Five (or more) of the following have been present during the same 2-week period, represent a change from previous functioning: at least one symptom is either depressed mood or loss of interest or pleasure.
    - Depressed mood: Most of the day, nearly everyday
    - Diminished interest or pleasure in all, or almost all, activities, most of the day, and nearly everyday
    - Significant weight loss when not dieting or weight gain (>5% of body weight in a month), or increase/decrease in appetite nearly everyday
    - Insomnia/hypersomnia almost everyday

- Psychomotor agitation/retardation nearly everyday
- Fatigue/loss of energy nearly everyday
- Feelings of worthlessness/guilt
- Diminished ability to think or concentrate, or indecisiveness, nearly everyday
- Recurrent thoughts of death and suicidal ideation/plan/attempt.
• The symptoms cause clinically significant impairment in social, occupational, or other important areas of functioning.
• The episode is not attributable to the physiological effects of a substance or another medical condition.
There should never have been a manic or hypomanic episode.

Note: In children and adolescents, the mood may be irritable rather than sad. Some emphasize somatic symptoms (body aches and pains) rather than reporting feelings of sadness.

Chronicity of depressive symptoms substantially increases the likelihood of underlying personality disorders, anxiety and substance-use, and decreases the likelihood that treatment will be followed by full symptom resolution.

Recency of onset is a strong determinant of the likelihood of good recovery. Features associated with lower recovery rates, rather than current episode duration, include psychotic features, prominent anxiety, personality disorders, and symptom severity.

The risk of recurrence becomes progressively lower overtime as the duration of remission increases. The risk is higher in individuals whose preceding episode was severe, in younger individuals, and those who have already experienced multiple episodes. The persistence of mild depressive symptoms during remission is a powerful predictor of recurrence.

Differential Diagnosis

- Mood disorder due to another medical condition: Multiple sclerosis, hypothyroidism, etc.
- Substance/medication-induced depression, e.g., withdrawal from cocaine
- Attention deficit/hyperactive disorder: Mood is characterized by irritability rather than sadness or loss of interest
- Adjustment disorder with depressed mood—full criteria of major depressive disorder (MDD) are not met.

Persistent Depressive Disorder (Dysthymia)

Here the depressed mood is persistent for at least 2 years/in children, the mood must be irritable for at least 1 year. It might be preceded by MDD.

During this 2-year period, any symptom-free interval does not last longer than 2 months.

There are other disorders such as premenstrual dysphoric disorder, substance/medication-induced depressive disorder, depressive disorder due to another medical conditions, and other specified depressive disorders though these are more relevant to adults and not children per se.

Disruptive Mood Dysregulation Disorder

- Severe recurrent temper outbursts: Verbal/physical
- These are inappropriate with the developmental level
- They occur three or more times/week
- Mood between episodes is consistently irritable for most of the day, nearly everyday.

Above criteria present for at least a year, and in at least two out of three settings. Diagnosis made between 6 and 16 years.

Clinical Viewpoint

Usually, an alert clinician would watch out for increased irritability, changes in sleep (either increased or decreased quantity), excessive sensitivity to minor comments/criticism, and or excessive use of the internet/mobile/substance.

Adolescence being a period of rapid developmental growth, there is accelerated hormonal and neurochemical surge. This itself could confound the picture and make it difficult to differentiate between normal adolescent development and depression.

Proposed Etiology

Depression in an individual is a result of:
- *Genetics*: Genes, shape, brain structure, and function
- *Brain structure and function*: Abnormal connectivity between neurons, abnormal neurotransmitter connectivity between various brain regions lead to abnormal emotional processing
- Environmental situations can trigger off depression in an already compromised individual
- Genes are present in every cell of the body, so the effects are not limited to abnormal low mood and negative thoughts, but all body systems are affected
- Depression is also linked to immune-medicated changes and the inflammatory cascade. Which is why very often depression may present as medically-unexplained symptoms (MUS).

MANAGEMENT

It is falsely believed that children and adolescents need not receive medical treatment for depression but can manage by "easing out the stressful environment". While it is true that the child needs a supportive environment, recognition of depression as a treatable medical entity is of paramount importance.

The treatment of depression thus involves a multipronged approach for a child:
- Life skills modification
- Cognitive behavior therapy (CBT) or interpersonal therapy (IPT)
- Pharmacotherapy
- Support groups.

Life Skills Modifications

Life skills are acquired abilities imparted to children to develop adaptive behaviors, in order to deal with the stress of daily life. This assumes greater importance in childhood and adolescence which are tumultuous periods of development. These are *preventive strategies* for children to improve their coping skills.

A suitable program for life skills with five modules is as follows (Bharat et al., NIMHANS):
- Critical thinking and creative thinking
- Decision-making and problem-solving
- Communication skills and interpersonal relations
- Coping with emotions and stress
- Self-awareness and empathy.

Cognitive Behavior Therapy or Interpersonal Therapy

Cognitive behavior therapy is the process of changing one's behavior by altering the thought process or cognitive pattern. Patterns of predictive behavior and responses can thus be worked upon.

Interpersonal therapy, which is focused and time limited, involves the impact of life events, and interpersonal problems. Resolution of the same can affect mood and resolve depression.

Both CBT and IPT are recommended as first line management for children and adolescents with depression, and should be continued for at least 3 months.

Pharmacotherapy

The only recommended medications for this age group [United States Food and Drug Administration (US FDA) approved] are fluoxetine and escitalopram (above the age of 12 years). Medications should be initiated after (1) a failed trial of psychotherapy, (2) in case of moderate to severe symptoms and/or (3) suicidality. These should be continued for a period of at least 6 months.

Support Groups

Peer influences are very strong at this age. Hence, forming a strong support network through support groups (both virtual and real) help deal with the illness better.

Should the above not work, or if there is worsening of symptoms at any given point, the help of a mental health professional should be sought.

Depression in children and adolescents is thus very real and very treatable. It must be addressed early, diagnosed soon, and intervened timely to yield optimal results. Untreated depression may lead to school dropouts, substance use, and even suicide.

FURTHER READING

1. Clark MS, Jansen KL, Cloy JA. Treatment of childhood and adolescent depression. Am Fam Physician. 2012;86(5):442-8.
2. Maughan B, Collishaw S, Stringaris A. Depression in childhood and adolescence. J Can Acad Child Adolesc Psychiatry. 2013;22(1):35-40.
3. Srikala B, Kishore KK. Empowering adolescents with life skills education in schools—school mental health program: Does it work? Indian J Psychiatry. 2010;52(4):344-9.

Chapter 38

Tics

Kawaljit Singh Multani

"Nobody understood me and I got into trouble. It seemed like I was crying and screaming a lot. When I was in first grade it was awful. Nobody knew why I was so unhappy and why I would get so angry. I had three teachers that year. What really bugged me was that one of my teachers kept yelling at me. She would get mad at me because of stuff I did, like not being able to write out words and not finishing my math. I just wanted to kill myself, but not really."
"Hi! I am Adam" A child's book about Tourette syndrome

INTRODUCTION

Tic disorder is an inherited childhood onset movement disorder characterized by sudden repetitive nonrhythmic twitches/movements or sounds. The movements lasts for less than a second, tends to occur in bouts, which are paroxysmal in nature. Older children and adults often describe somatosensory phenomena preceding the tics, which are called "premonitory urges" which are relieved by the performance of tics. Tics can be suppressed partially. This suppression results in significant discomfort in the affected person and further enhances the tics severity.

Tourette syndrome is characterized by multiple motor tics and one or more vocal/phonic tics lasting more than a year, although not necessarily concurrently. The disorder affects 1–2% of the population and is much more common in males than females.

The etiology of the disorder is multifactorial with genetics, perinatal events, and autoimmune conditions each playing some role. Twin and family studies have shown a high rate of tics among monozygotic twins and those with positive family history though no single gene has been identified. Postinfectious conditions like PANDAS (pediatric autoimmune neuropsychiatric disorder associated with streptococcal infections) which present with tics like movement disorders and worsening of symptoms in patients during streptococcal infections makes a strong case for an autoimmune mechanism. Basal ganglia and corticostriatothalamocortical

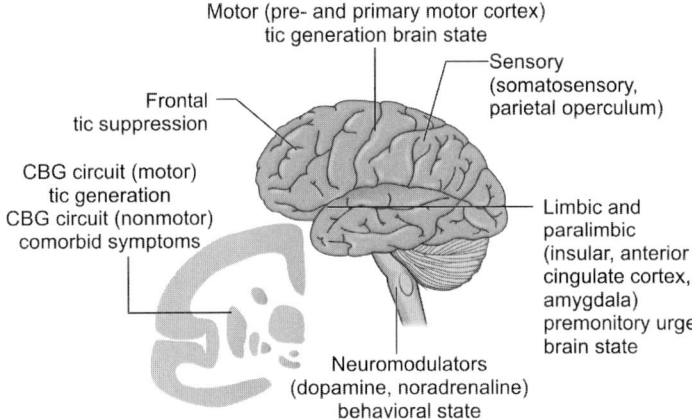

Fig. 1: Brain pathways involved in tic disorders.
Source: Yael D, Vinner E, Bar-Gad I. Pathophysiology of tic disorders. Mov Disord. 2015;30(9):1171-8.
(CBG: cortical-basal ganglia)

(CSTC) circuits play crucial role in sensorimotor integration and motor control **(Fig. 1)**. The dopaminergic system in these regions is altered in functional brain studies and this has led to improved understanding of the disease and the associated comorbid conditions as well as discovery of new treatment modalities like deep brain stimulation and transcranial magnetic stimulation.

CLINICAL FEATURES

The American Psychiatric Association's diagnostic and statistical manual of mental disorders, 5th edition (DSM-5) manual categorizes tic disorders into three types based on the duration and type of tics: provisional tic disorder (<1 year), persistent/chronic motor or vocal tic disorder, and Tourette's disorder **(Flowchart 1)**.

Most tics appear in the prepubertal period (usually between 3 and 8 years of age) with motor tics appearing early as compared to vocal tics. They usually follow a waxing and waning pattern of frequency, intensity, and severity with most showing a peak of symptoms in the second decade of life. Severity peaks around 10–12 years of age and many cases show a reduction in severity toward the end of the second decade. New-onset tics in older children and adults are uncommon and is commonly related to either drug use or a central nervous system (CNS) infection.

Common tics include eye blinking, grimacing, jaw, neck shoulder movements, sniffing, grunting, or throat clearing. Complex tics can appear purposeful, e.g., obscene gestures (coprolalia), repeating one's own words (palilalia), repeating the last-heard word (echolalia), mimicking someone

Flowchart 1: Classification of tic disorders.

```
                        Tics
                         │
            ┌────────────┴────────────┐
    Persistent tic              Transient tic
       disorder                    disorder
     (>12 months)                (<12 months)
            │
   ┌────────┼──────────────┐
Simple tics  Complex tics   Tic disorder-
   │              │          unspecified
┌──┴──┐       Tourette
Motor Vocal    syndrome
tics  tics
```

(echopraxia), and mouthing obscenities/slurs (coprolalia). Many cases especially those with complex tics and Tourette syndrome have significant comorbid conditions such as attention deficit hyperactivity disorder (ADHD), autism and obsessive compulsive disorder (OCD), depression, substance abuse, and bipolar disorder.

Patients with mild to moderate tics may be unaware of their symptoms while those with severe tics may have significant impairments in daily activities and/or social isolation, victimization, and reduced quality of life. Presence of a comorbid condition may worsen the situation further. Rarely, patients with complex tics and Tourette disorder may get physical injury due to tics.

Diagnosis is mainly clinical and requires four criteria to be fulfilled—(1) presence of motor or vocal tics, (2) duration of tic symptoms, (3) age at onset, and (4) absence of any known cause.

Tic disorders are diagnosed in a hierarchical order (highest Tourette's disorder and lowest unspecified tic disorder) and once a higher order diagnosis is made, a lower order diagnosis cannot be made.

Detailed clinical history including family history and examination is needed to rule out other movement disorders and illnesses causing similar symptoms. Laboratory tests, neuroimaging, and electroencephalogram studies are indicated in atypical cases (new-onset tics in older children and adults) and to look for Wilson disease/neuroacanthosis/Huntington's disease. Tics must be distinguished from other movement disorders such as athetosis, chorea, ballismus, dystonia, myoclonus, stereotypies, and seizures as well as stereotypic movements **(Table 1)**.

Yale Global Tic Severity Scale (YGTSS) and physician-rated Diagnostic Confidence Index are commonly utilized by clinicians for diagnosis and evaluating the extent of severity and impairments due to tics. YGTSS rates

Table 1: Comparing tics and stereotypies.

Feature	Tics	Stereotypy
Age at onset	5–7 years	<2 years
Pattern	Variable	Fixed
Rhythm	Quick and sudden	Rhythmic
Movement	Abrupt jerky movements	Repetitive arms or hand movements
Premonitory urge	Yes	No
Trigger	Stress and excitement	Excitement and stress
Suppressibility	Self-directed and short period associated with discomfort	By external distraction
Family history	Positive in many cases	Uncommon
Associated conditions	ADHD, OCD	OCD
Treatment	Behavior therapy + Medication	Not responsive to medication

(ADHD: attention deficit hyperactivity disorder; OCD: obsessive compulsive disorder)

the impairment due to tics as mild, moderate, marked, and severe. Parent/self-rating scales such as motor tic, obsessions and compulsions, vocal tics evaluation survey (MOVES) and premonitory urge for tics scale, etc., are also useful in assessment of tic disorders. It is important to carry out detailed evaluation to look for comorbid conditions such as ADHD, learning disabilities, anxiety/depression, OCD/obsessive compulsive behavior (OCB) as many of these coexist in patients with tics and their presence plays a vital role in formulation of management strategy and drug therapy.

MANAGEMENT

Patient education, family supportive measures, and psychotherapy form the mainstay of treatment while medication is mainly used for treatment of severe tics, Tourette syndrome, and comorbid conditions associated with tics like ADHD, OCD, etc. Education of teachers and classmates about the illness with advice and the child's condition goes a long way in improving school performance of these kids. A simple advice like ignoring the tic in the child by the teacher and classmates results in reduced stress on the child and may reduce tics.

Behavior therapies (habit reversal training and comprehensive behavioral intervention) are found to be effective and safe and all that is required in mild to moderate tics. Severe tics and Tourette disorder require medication in addition to behavior therapy.

Table 2: Medications in tic disorders.

Medication	Usual dose range (starting dose)	Age range	Remarks
Haloperidol	1–4 mg/d (0.25 mg/d)	≥18 years	FDA approval +
Pimozide	2–8 mg/d (0.5 mg/d)	≥12 years	FDA approval +
Risperidone	0.75–3 mg/d (0.125 mg/d)	≥18 years	Metabolic effects, raised prolactin
Ziprasidone	10–40 mg/d (5 mg/d)	≥18 years	Metabolic effects
Clonidine	0.1–0.4 mg/d (0.025 mg/d)	≥12 years	Use in ADHD + tics
Guanfacine	1–4 mg/d (0.5 mg/d)	≥12 years	Use in ADHD + tics
Fluoxetine	10–60 mg/d (5 mg/d)	≥7 years	Use in OCD + tics
Sertraline	50–250 mg/d (25 mg/d)	≥6 years	Use in OCD + tics
Atomoxetine	0.5–2 mg/d (0.5 mg/d)	≥6 years	Use in ADHD + tics
Topiramate	50–200 mg/d (25 mg/d)	≥6 years	Reduces tic severity

(ADHD: attention deficit hyperactivity disorder; FDA: Food and Drug Administration; OCD: obsessive compulsive disorder)

Most cases of tics with marked and severe impairment on YGTSS and those with comorbid conditions need medication. Dopamine receptor antagonists (Haloperidol, pimozide, etc.), atypical neuroleptics (risperidone, ziprasidone, etc.), and centrally acting α-2 agents like clonidine have been used. Motor tics show better response as compared to vocal tics **(Table 2)**. Sedation, dry mouth, and constipation are the common side effects seen with use of medication. The usual approach is "start low and go slow" with medication and keep, a close watch for side effects. Stimulant medications for ADHD can be used along with tics medication but needs careful monitoring and consultation with a pediatric neurologist. Newer therapies include use of botulinum toxin, deep brain stimulation, and repetitive transcranial magnetic stimulation have shown promise especially in resistant cases.

FURTHER READING

1. Greydanus DE. Tic disorders. Neurodevelopmental Disabilities. 2011;213-26.
2. Murphy TK, Lewin AB, Storch EA, Stock S. Practice parameter for the assessment and treatment of children and adolescents with tic disorders. J Am Acad Child Adolesc Psychiatry. 2013;52(12):1341-59.
3. Pringsheim T, Okun MS, Müller-Vahl K, Martino D, Jankovic J, Cavanna AE, et al. Practice guideline recommendations summary: The treatment of tics in people with Tourette syndrome and chronic tic disorders. Neurology. 2019;92(19):896-906.
4. Robertson MM. Tourette syndrome in children and adolescents: Aetiology, presentation and treatment. Br J Psych Advances. 2016;22:165-75.

Chapter 39

Hearing Abnormalities in Children: Assessments and Management

Abraham K Paul

"Blindness separates people from things, deafness separates people from people."

Helen Keller

INTRODUCTION

Hearing impairment is one of the most devastating sensory impairments with significant social and psychological implications, the extreme form labeled as deaf. Nearly half of these are due to environmental factors and the rest are due to genetic and other congenital causes.

Failure to detect children with congenital or acquired hearing loss may result in lifelong deficits in speech and language acquisition, poor academic performance, personal-social maladjustments, and emotional difficulties that can be prevented or ameliorated by early identification and appropriate intervention within the first 6 months of life.

The incidence of profound congenital hearing loss (PCHL) is 1 per 1,000 in well-baby nursery population and increases sharply to 2–4 per 100 in neonatal intensive care unit (NICU) population. While most children with congenital hearing impairment can be potentially identified by newborn and infant hearing screening, infectious diseases especially meningitis and otitis media, trauma, damaging noise levels, and ototoxic drugs can lead to acquired hearing loss later.

CLINICAL FEATURES

Risk factors associated with a higher incidence of PCHL include the following:
- Family history of hereditary childhood sensorineural hearing loss
- In utero infection such as cytomegalovirus inclusion disease, rubella, syphilis, herpes, and toxoplasmosis
- Craniofacial anomalies including those with morphological abnormalities of the pinna and ear canal

- Birth weight <1,500 g
- Hyperbilirubinemia at serum level requiring exchange transfusion
- Ototoxic medications
- Bacterial meningitis
- Apgar score 0–4 at 1 minute or 0–6 at 5 minutes
- Mechanical ventilation lasting 5 days or more
- Stigmata or other findings associated with a syndrome known to include sensorineural and/or conductive hearing loss.

Hearing impairment is classified depending on various types (as below) or the degree of impairment **(Fig. 1)**.

- Sensorineural hearing loss occurs in the inner ear (sensory) or auditory nerve/auditory pathway (neural) and is usually permanent.
- Conductive hearing loss occurs in the external and middle ear pathology. Many causes can be treated successfully with surgery.

Screening in the First Year of Life: Newborn Hearing Screening

American Academy of Pediatrics (AAP) Task Force on Newborn and Infant Hearing as well as Indian Academy of Pediatrics (IAP) recommends Universal Newborn Hearing Screening using otoacoustic emissions (OAEs) test by 1 month of age. If the OAE is abnormal, then a repeat OAE test is advised.

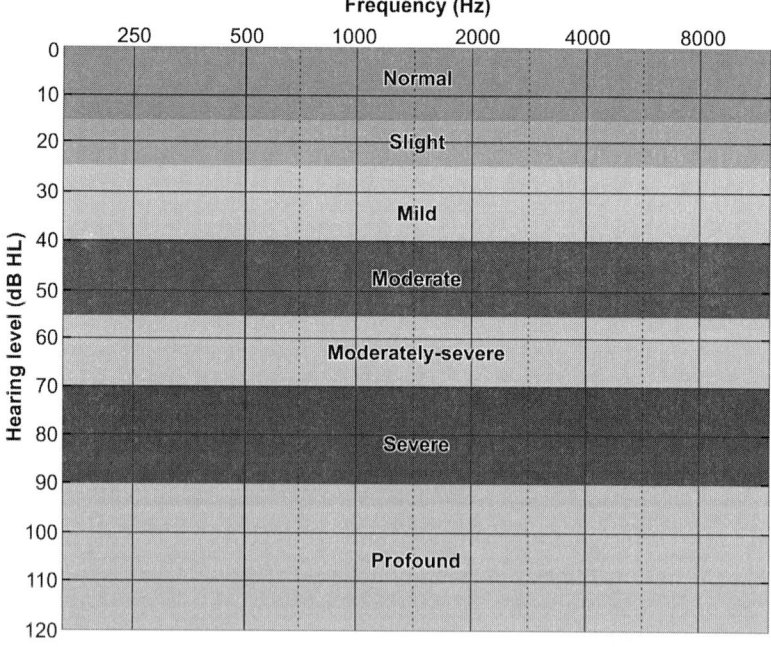

Fig. 1: Levels of deafness.

If OAE is abnormal on two occasions, auditory brainstem response (ABR) and full evaluation before 3 months of age and remediation before 6 months of age will get the best outcome in babies with hearing difficulties. All NICU babies should undergo ABR.

Hearing Assessment in Children

There are two types of assessments:
1. *Behavioral tests of hearing*: These are subjective assessments and some can be done from the first month of life.
2. *Auditory electroacoustic measures*: These are electrophysiologic recordings of response to sounds and are used for objective assessment of hearing.

Some of the tests commonly used to assess hearing in children have been summarized in **Table 1**.

MANAGEMENT

The fundamental goal of audiologic management is to limit the extent of any communication disorder that results from a hearing loss. To this end, the first step is to make use of the residual hearing by using the most suitable hearing aid. In some cases, other assistive technology may be used to supplement or substitute hearing aid use. In individuals with severe-to-profound hearing loss and those not benefitting from hearing aids, cochlear implant (CI) may be indicated.

Although the goal of audiologic management is relatively constant, the approach can vary significantly depending on patient's age, nature, and degree of the hearing impairment and the communication demand that patients have in their daily life.

Hearing Aids

Hearing aids vary from analog to digital with a wide variety of internal adjustments. The types of hearing aids, based on technology, include analog, analog programmable, digital, and digitally programmable hearing aids. Hearing aids based on placement includes body level (BL) hearing aids, behind the ear (BTE) hearing aids, in the ear (ITE) hearing aids, in the canal (ITC) hearing aids, completely in the canal (CIC) hearing aids, and postauricular canal (PAC) hearing aids. Hearing aids also vary based on features inside such as compression, noise cancelation, adaptive microphone, blue tooth technology, and data logging function.

Cochlear Implant

Candidates with severe-to-profound hearing loss and those not obtaining adequate speech perception after hearing aid use, are recommended

Table 1: Summary of audiological tests for children.

Developmental age of child	Audiological test	What does it measure?	Procedure	Advantages	Limitations
All ages	OAE (otoacoustic emissions)	Outer hair cell response in cochlea	Small probe is placed in the ear canal, click sounds delivered and response detected	Quick, ear-specific objective	Child must be quiet, does not measure level of hearing, subject to middle ear status
All ages	ABR (auditory brainstem response)	Electrophysiologic measurement of activity in auditory nerve and brainstem pathways	Electrodes placed on child's head detect response to sounds presented through earphones	Ear-specific gives level of hearing, objective, can be done in natural sleep in young infants	Child must remain still/asleep, may not always correlate with behavioral hearing levels (auditory neuropathy, neurological difficulties)
All ages	ASSR	Electrophysiologic response to sounds from brainstem/cortical pathways	Electrodes placed on child's head detect response to sounds presented through earphones	Estimates threshold in severe/profound hearing loss, can be used binaurally, objective threshold determination	Child must remain still/asleep, bone conduction data needed
All ages	Tympanometry	Middle ear function (i.e., diagnosis of glue ear)	Small probe is placed in the ear canal to pressurize it and movement of the ear drum is traced	Quick, ear-specific	Does not measure hearing

Contd...

Contd...

Developmental age of child	Audiological test	What does it measure?	Procedure	Advantages	Limitations
6/8 months to 2/2.5 years	Visual reinforcement Audiometry	Behavioral test, measures response of the child to frequency-specific stimuli	Child is conditioned to associate sound with a reinforcement stimulus, such as a lighted toy, response measured when head turns toward the sound	Versatile test, can be done using ear-specific inserts, bone conduction	Needs a soundproof room, depends on attention and cooperation of child
2.5–4 years	Play audiometry	Behavioral test, measures responses of the child to frequency-specific stimuli	Child is conditioned to put a peg in a peg board/similar game	Versatile test, can be done using ear-specific inserts, bone conduction	Needs a soundproof room, depends on attention and cooperation of child
4 years onward	Conventional pure tone audiometry	Behavioral test, measures responses of the child to frequency-specific stimuli	Child is instructed to raise his or her hand or press a button when a sound is heard	Versatile test, can be done using ear-specific inserts, bone conduction	Needs a soundproof room, depends on attention and cooperation of child

(ASSR: auditory steady-state response)

cochlear implantation. CI is a prosthetic replacement for the inner ear. The CI bypasses damaged parts of the inner ear and directly electronically stimulates the nerve of hearing. Part of the device is surgically implanted in the skull behind the ear and tiny electrodes are inserted into the cochlea. Microphone, speech processor, transmitter, receiver/stimulator, and electrodes are the major parts of CI.

Rehabilitation Process

Any child receiving a CI will require rehabilitation in order to maximize their listening potential. Auditory training activities form a major component of oral education. These help children who have hearing impairment to develop their ability to recognize speech using the auditory signal. Auditory-verbal and auditory-oral are two auditory training approaches used.

Auditory-Verbal Approach

Auditory-verbal philosophy encourages the maximum use of hearing in order to learn language and stresses listening rather than watching. This approach discourages lip reading and excludes the use of sign language. It views parents as the child's primary teacher.

Auditory-Oral Approach

In this method, children learn to use whatever hearing they have, in combination with lip reading and contextual cues (speech reading) to understand and use spoken language. Here, daily one-to-one instruction provides the needed intense early intervention.

Educational Considerations

Integrated education in regular school, especially preschool programs, is possible with early intervention and assistance from special teachers.

Segregated Education in a Special School

Children diagnosed late or those who have not developed adequate functional language are enrolled in special preschool programs. In special schools, special teachers help children build a strong foundation of language, which would ease out the formal education in primary and secondary school, again, either in an integrated setup or in a special school depending upon the child's achievements.

Assistive devices such as frequency modulation, induction loop, infrared, and induction loop systems can be used in school setup for better signal-to-noise ratio. The unoccupied classrooms should have <35 dB ambient noise levels and <0.4 seconds reverberation time for better speech perception. Usage of sound absorbing materials and classrooms away from recreational places will also help to increase signal-to-noise ratio.

In short, listening and speech skills do not emerge spontaneously. A concentrated, deliberate rehabilitation is a must. Child learns to utilize the electrical signal for the purpose of speech recognition and speech and language acquisition. Rehabilitation process must include participation by the parents, speech and hearing professionals, and educators.

FURTHER READING

1. American Speech and Hearing Association. (2007). Year 2007 Position Statement: Principles and Guidelines for Early Hearing Detection and Intervention Programs Joint Committee on Infant Hearing. Retrieved 2011, from Joint Committee on Infant Hearing. [online] Available from: http://www.asha.org/docs/html/PS2007-00281.html. [Last accessed February 2022].
2. From National Consultation Meeting for Developing IAP Guidelines on Neurodevelopmental Disorders under the aegis of IAP Childhood Disability Group and the Committee on Child Development and Neurodevelopmental Disorders; Paul A, Prasad C, Kamath SS, Dalwai S, Nair MKC, et al. Consensus Statement of the Indian Academy of Pediatrics on Newborn Hearing Screening. Indian Pediatr. 2017;54(8):647-51.
3. Paul AK. Centralized newborn hearing screening in Ernakulam, Kerala - experience on a decade. Indian Pediatr. 2016;53(1):15-7.
4. Reng D, Müller M, Smolders JW. Functional recovery of hearing following AMPA-induced reversible disruption of hair cell afferent synapses in the avian inner ear. Audiol Neurootol. 2001;6(2):66-78.
5. Stach BA. Clinical Audiology: An Introduction. Clifton Park: Delmar, Cengage Learning; 2010.

Chapter 40

Visual Impairment

Neepa Thacker Dave

INTRODUCTION

Children with developmental delay often have associated visual impairment. These children with special need are a unique subset who have multiple comorbidities including visual impairment and should be recognized as a special category requiring particular strategies of visual assessment, protocols for examination, and intervention (as compared to normal children).

Prematurity remains a major cause but other causes like cerebral palsy, congenital brain malformations, prenatal and cerebral infections, hypoxic ischemic encephalopathy, hydrocephalus, hypoglycemia at birth, traumatic brain injury, nonaccidental trauma, etc., can affect visual systems and functioning along with other system involvement.

The need for a multidisciplinary approach to such a child inclusive of visual system assessment cannot be overemphasized.

Common causes for visual impairment in children with developmental delay:
- *Cortical visual impairment*: Cortical visual impairment (CVI) is a decreased visual response due to a neurological problem affecting the visual part of the brain. Typically, a child with CVI has a normal eye exam or has an eye condition that cannot account for the abnormal visual behavior
- Optic atrophy
- Retinal disorders
- High refractive errors
- Strabismus
- Amblyopia (lazy eye)
- Visual field defects.

CLINICAL FEATURES

Ophthalmic examination of a child with visual impairment and developmental delay is often difficult. Expressive delay, varied responses, and cognitive impairment make interpretation of subjective responses difficult to interpret. Different responses on different days are possible.

Ophthalmic evaluation should be a part of the initial screening and ongoing evaluations.

The various routine tests done are:
- *Visual acuity measurements:* Vision charts include the standard alphabet (Snellen) and letter (HOTV). Pediatric vision charts with symbols and pictures like the Allen cards, Kay pictures, and Lea symbols are used for verbal children
- Preferential looking with contrast gratings cards or paddles is used for nonverbal children (picture of various vision charts used is attached)
- Look for nystagmus
- Presence of squint
- Eye movement disorders
- Assessment of refraction (retinoscopy)
- Assessment of pupils
- Anterior and posterior segment evaluation
- Visual fields
- Contrast sensitivity.

A concept of FUNCTIONAL vision assessment is followed for these children in addition to the standard visual acuity measurement. This includes visual alertness to surrounding environment, robustness of visual function, etc. Basically, it maps the child's visual response to the surroundings. It is valuable to program visual tasks, which will be taught to the child in the form of VISION THERAPY.

MANAGEMENT

Management of visual impairment in children includes:
- Correcting refractive errors
- Patching exercises for lazy eye and associated squints
- Squint correction is selected cases
- Vision therapy and rehabilitation. Training for visual tasks such as fixing, following, tracking, orientation, and moment of eyes and body like in looking down while walking, etc.

AUTISM AND VISUAL IMPAIRMENT

Children with autism can present a special challenge. Atypical visual behavior and visual inattention can mimic CVI. Various centers that have studied visual functions in autism show that vision is often normal, there is higher prevalence of squint and astigmatism, susceptibility for visuomotor deficits in stereoacuity, accommodation, convergence abnormalities, atypical pupillary response, and near vision difficulties. Some retinal structure and function may be compromised either related to zinc levels or genetic abnormalities.

Role of a pediatric ophthalmologist:
- Awareness and knowledge of these vision problems, appropriate diagnosis, intervention, and regular monitoring of the visual status.
- To work with other specialist looking after the child and aid in reaching the child's potential.
- To provide essential information and specific recommendations for medically necessary services or schools. To provide recommendations to placement of such children in regular schools (with special visual aids) or schools for visually impaired.
- To provide low visual aids, recommendations for font sizes, time for examinations, use of large screens, etc., to both individual children (families) and schools.

FURTHER READING

1. Little JA. Vision in children with autism spectrum disorder: A critical review. Clin Exp Optom. 2018;101(8):504-13.
2. Swaminathan M, Jayaraman D, Jacob N. Visual function assessment, ocular examination, and intervention in children with developmental delay: A systematic approach. Part 1. Indian J Ophthalmol. 2019;67(2):196-203.

Chapter 41

Balance Disorders and Dizziness in Children

Waheeda Pagarkar

INTRODUCTION

Balance disorders and dizziness are common in children, questionnaire studies worldwide estimating their prevalence between 5 and 18%. This may be an underestimate, as younger children may not have the language to report this symptom, and it often commands less medical attention than other somatic symptoms in a pediatric clinic.

Dizziness is a nonspecific term to denote a sense of unsteadiness or lightheadedness whereas vertigo is an "illusion of movement" in the rotational or translational plane. Vertigo can be described as "spinning or tilting or moving" sensation of surroundings or of self. Whereas dizziness can be caused by a number of systemic and vestibular causes, vertigo implies a deficit in the vestibular system.

Balance is a complex multisensory function which depends on sensory input from the visual, proprioceptive, and vestibular systems. These inputs are integrated in the central nervous system and help to maintain posture through neural pathways such as the vestibulospinal tracts. The connections of these sensory pathways with the cerebral cortex are responsible for our spatial perception of posture and movement and, in disease states, for the sensation of dizziness. Conflict between these sensory inputs can lead to motion sickness, a common condition in children and adults.

The vestibular system serves two main functions, i.e., development of motor milestones and balance (through vestibulospinal pathways) and stabilizing the eyes during head movements, (through the vestibulo-ocular reflex), e.g., during reading and walking. This reflex is the reason why we do not see the world wobble, when we move our head! Vestibular dysfunction is more common in children with hearing loss affecting 30–60% of these children.

CLINICAL DIAGNOSIS

Balance difficulties and dizziness in children can be due to vestibular, neurological, and other causes, which can vary from being innocuous (vasovagal) to being serious (intracranial tumors) **(Box 1)**. Children present to the pediatric clinic with delayed motor milestones, frequent falls, and clumsiness. Dizziness and vertigo can be described as "being on a merry-go-round", "walls falling", "being pushed", and "head feeling funny".

Box 1: Causes of balance disorders and dizziness in children.

- Vestibular migraine and benign paroxysmal vertigo (BPV; migraine variant)
- Neurological disorders:
  - Anatomical abnormalities: hydrocephalus, Arnold Chiari malformation
  - Space occupying lesions, e.g. medulloblastoma
  - Epilepsy causing "funny turns"
  - Neurodevelopmental disorders: Cerebral palsy and developmental coordination disorder
  - Neuromuscular diseases, e.g., Duchenne muscular dystrophy
  - Neurodegenerative disorders, e.g., Charcot Marie tooth, Friedrich's ataxia, mitochondrial disorders, and episodic ataxia
  - Genetic syndromes causing developmental delay: Down syndrome and 22q deletion
- Vestibular diseases:
  - Trauma: concussion, fracture temporal bone, fistula, and cochlear implant surgery
  - Ototoxicity: Gentamicin, streptomycin, and amikacin
  - Middle ear disease: Chronic suppurative otitis media, cholesteatoma, otitis media with effusion
  - Anatomical abnormality of vestibular organs: vestibular malformations, dilated vestibular aqueducts, and semicircular canal dehiscence
  - Infections/inflammation: Vestibular neuritis, labyrinthitis, bacterial meningitis, congenital CMV, and autoimmune inner ear disease
  - Vestibular hypofunction with deafness: Usher, Pendred, Alstron, auditory neuropathy, Jervell and Lange-Nielsen
  - Others: Meniere's disease, benign paroxysmal positional vertigo (BPPV; different from BPV), vestibular paroxysmia, motion sickness, autoimmune disorders, and Cogan's syndrome
- Cardiac:
  - Arrhythmias
  - Postural hypotension/postural tachycardia syndrome (POTS)
  - Vasovagal syncope
- Metabolic:
  - Anemia, vitamin D deficiency, diabetes, thyroid dysfunction, and electrolyte imbalance
- Ocular:
  - Squint and uncorrected refractive errors
- *Skeletal disease*: Mucopolysaccharidosis scoliosis and rheumatoid arthritis
- Psychogenic:
  - Anxiety disorders and nonorganic symptom

Migraine and benign paroxysmal vertigo (BPV) are the most common causes of vertigo in children and diagnosis is based on clinical history.

Vestibular Migraine

This is the most common cause of dizziness in children, accounting for 30–40%. It presents as sudden onset episodic dizziness lasting for hours, with or without headaches, photophobia, phonophobia, visual symptoms, nausea, and vomiting. There is often a trigger such as stress, infection, and diet (cheese, chocolate, and caffeine). A family history of migraine and motion sickness is often present.

Benign Positional Vertigo

This presents between 2 and 4 years of age, as sudden onset of paroxysmal, recurrent episodes of vertigo lasting for a few seconds to minutes, and rarely hours. The child appears frightened, sweaty, anxious, pale, imbalanced, or may stay immobile. Older children may complain of "spinning". Children may have nausea and vomiting; and spontaneous nystagmus may be seen. Differential diagnosis in this age group includes epilepsy and posterior fossa or cerebellopontine angle tumors. The diagnosis is clinical and one of exclusion and rests on the typical history and normal findings on examination. This is a migraine variant, which resolves as the child gets older, but may evolve into migraine headache.

Points to Remember

- Vestibular disorders are often overlooked in a general pediatric clinic and should be included in the differential diagnosis, particularly where hearing loss is present.
- Loss of consciousness should prompt neurological/cardiac investigations. It is not a feature of vestibular disease.
- Psychological causes are seen in children older than 7 years.
- Vestibular loss occurs in 40–80% of children with bacterial meningitis and is more common than deafness.

Key Points to Note in History

- Detailed milestones and evidence of regression
- Duration of vertigo, triggers, associated symptoms, relation to position
- Seizures, headaches, loss of consciousness, and focal neurological symptoms (neurological)
- Hearing and ear discharge (vestibular causes)
- Systemic symptoms: Palpitations and syncope (cardiac)

- Vision
- Psychological history.

Key Points in Clinical Examination

- *General examination*: Anemia and dysmorphism
- *Full neurological examination*: Focal/generalized weakness
- *Eye movement examination*: For squint, smooth pursuit, saccades, and nystagmus
- Skeletal system examination including spine, feet, and joints
- Cardiac examination and blood pressure in lying and standing positions
- Ears, nose, throat (ENT) examination
- *Examination of neonatal reflexes*: Moro reflex, head righting reflex, and parachute reflex are mediated by vestibular inputs and their presence in a floppy infant indicates presence of vestibular function
- *Examination of the vestibular system:*
  - *Posture and gait tests*: Romberg test, standing on one leg, standing on foam, tandem gait, and Unterberger test. Children with neurological conditions and vestibular hypofunction will have difficulty doing these tests.
  - *Vestibulo-ocular reflex tests*: These tests are specific for vestibular pathology:
    - *Head thrust test*: The child is asked to focus on the examiner's nose. A rapid sudden head rotation in the yaw plane (like saying "no") to the right or left of approximately 30° is made. A "catch-up" saccade indicates hypofunction of the lateral semicircular canal on the side of the head thrust. This is the single most useful test in detection of vestibular hypofunction.
    - *Head shaking nystagmus/vibration-induced nystagmus*: These tests serve to bring out vestibular asymmetry by use of head shaking and vibration.
    - *Dynamic visual acuity*: A simple test that can be done in the clinic with use of a visual acuity chart. The child is asked to read a vision chart from a distance of 1.5 m with the head steady to obtain their baseline visual acuity. The child's head is then rotated horizontally (like saying "no") at 1–2 Hz. A loss of three lines or more of visual acuity may indicate vestibular hypofunction.
  - *Other tests*: Dix-Hallpike test [diagnostic of benign paroxysmal positional vertigo (BPPV)] and Tullio test (for semicircular canal dehiscence).

Investigations

These are necessary only in selected children and are guided by history and examination. Blanket use of expensive tests is not useful.
- *Magnetic resonance imaging (MRI) scan*: Where hydrocephalus or a space occupying lesion is suspected, investigation of sensorineural hearing loss
- *Electroencephalography (EEG)*: For suspected seizures in "Funny turns"
- *Electrocardiogram (ECG)/Holter monitoring/cardiology referral*: If cardiac symptoms syncope
- *Blood tests*: Anemia, vitamin D, calcium
- *Microarray*: With undiagnosed dysmorphism
- *Relevant neurometabolic investigations*: With neuroregression.

Vestibular Function Tests

Their availability for children is limited, expensive, and involves a degree of cooperation that is not always forthcoming in children. They can be used for children with permanent hearing loss and suspected vestibular hypofunction and include:
- Video head impulse test
- Computerized rotational chair testing
- Bithermal caloric testing
- *Cervical/ocular vestibular evoked myogenic potentials (VEMPs)*: Can be done using special software on a brainstem evoked response audiometry (BERA) machine
- Computerized dynamic posturography
- Subjective visual vertical.

MANAGEMENT

This depends on management of the underlying cause. Migraine is amenable to prophylactic treatment with drugs such as propranolol, pizotifen and topiramate, if symptoms impact on quality of life. Management of otologic conditions with appropriate medication and surgery proves useful. Children with vestibular deficits often compensate using their residual vestibular function, visual, and proprioceptive information, due to the inherent plasticity of the nervous system, improving overtime. Children with bilateral vestibular hypofunction should use thin-soled shoes to optimize proprioception and well lit surroundings to provide visual input to maintain balance. They will need supervision during swimming as disorientation can occur when the head is underwater. Vestibular physiotherapists can advise on vestibular rehabilitation exercises to improve balance and vertigo in children with vestibular disorders.

FURTHER READING

1. Dasgupta S, Mandala M, Salerni L, Crunkhorn R, Ratnayake S. Dizziness and balance problems in children. Curr Treat Options Neurol. 2020;22(8).
2. International Classification of headache disorders: Diagnostic criteria of vestibular migraine. [online] Available from: https://ichd-3.org/appendix/a1-migraine/a1-6-episodic-syndromes-that-may-be-associated-with-migraine/a1-6-6-vestibular-migraine/ (Last accessed December, 2021).
3. Jahn K. Vertigo and dizziness in children. Handb Clin Neurol. 2016;137:353-63.
4. Luxon L, Pagarkar W. The dizzy child. In: Graham J, Scadding G, Bull P (Eds). Textbook of Pediatric ENT. Springer; 2007.
5. Wiener-Vacher SR, Quarez J, Priol AL. Epidemiology of vestibular impairments in a pediatric population. Semin Hear. 2018;39(3):229-42.

Chapter 42

Developmental Coordination Disorder

Leena Deshpande

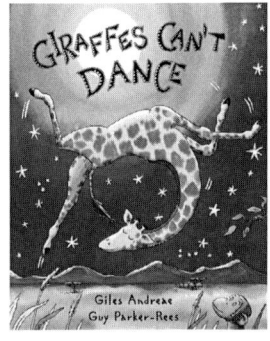

"Giraffes cannot dance" is a children's book where Gerald, the tall giraffe, is clumsy! When he tries to run, he buckles at his knees. When he tries to dance, he is awkward and uncoordinated. The book is about Gerald's triumphant journey where he learns to dance in his own way. The moral of the story is—"We all can dance if we find the music that we love."

For decades, clumsy movie characters from Hollywood like Mr Bean or Inspector Clouseau of "The Pink Panther" fame have delighted audiences across the world and have made for some hilarious film moments.

In reality, however, individuals who are clumsy are usually ridiculed. They struggle through childhood getting teased, isolated, and bullied.

INTRODUCTION

Developmental coordination disorder (DCD) is a childhood developmental disorder where otherwise healthy children have marked clumsiness. This condition makes it hard for children to learn how to plan, organize, perform, and modify their movements and hence has a significant impact on many aspects of life, mainly academic and activities of daily living.

This condition is prevalent in about 5% of school going children and is more common in boys. Though exact etiology is not known, it is seen more commonly in premature and intrauterine growth restriction (IUGR) babies and occurs commonly with other neurodevelopmental disorders such as attention-deficit/hyperactivity disorder (ADHD), learning disorders, and autism spectrum disorders. It also has a genetic predisposition.

CLINICAL FEATURES

Children with DCD may achieve basic motor milestones like sitting unsupported, walking independently at typical ages, or there may be slight delay, however, the child will then have ongoing difficulties in learning new skills which require gross motor coordination and balance (e.g., accessing stairs, throwing and catching a ball, riding a tri or a bicycle, balancing on one leg) and fine motor manipulation (such as feeding self, brushing teeth, unbuttoning and buttoning, tying laces, holding a crayon, and using scissors).

Some characteristic features:
- Children with DCD take significantly more time and require more practice to learn any new motor skills as compared to other children of their age. This results in the child having motor coordination below expectations of his chronological age.
- They have difficulties in generalization of learnt tasks, e.g., they may learn with difficulty to catch a large ball, but then will be unable to transfer the learnt skill to catch a smaller ball.
- Once they have learnt an activity, performing the same in a group situation with other children can be very challenging. This is because children with DCD are unable to process incoming information from a changing environment and then plan their response in a timely manner, thus making them appear extremely awkward.

Presenting features:
- Children with DCD will present in preschool age as being clumsy with frequent falls, bumping into and knocking down objects, tripping and spilling things.
- As they start schooling, they struggle with many tasks needed for learning in school. Writing and copying from board requires a lot of motor planning and will be a struggle resulting in slow and immature writing. Ongoing difficulties in dressing self will hamper independence.
- They have low muscle tone so may appear floppy with poor posture and balance and can get easily fatigued. Performing motor skill requires significant effort and the child will start avoiding tasks.
- They struggle with sports activities and tend to withdraw and avoid play with peers as they fear ridicule and bullying and tend to play with younger children.
- Developmental coordination disorder affects the child's self-care activities, academics, and sports activities on a daily basis and the child's self-confidence and motivation diminishes. They become introverted and secondary behavioral issues such as anxiety and depression may set in.

EVALUATION

- The Pediatrician has to ensure that the difficulties are not due to any systemic problems (e.g., vision problems), neurological disorders (such as cerebral palsy, muscular dystrophy, cerebellar problems, and global developmental delay) or connective tissue disorder. This can be done by a detailed history of perinatal events, progress (or any regression) of developmental milestones, and thorough medical and neurological examination.
- Pediatricians can use the DCD questionnaire, which is a brief parent questionnaire designed to screen for coordination disorders in children aged 5–15 years.
- Diagnostic and Statistical Manual of Mental Disorders, 5th edition (DSM-5) enlists the criteria needed to diagnose DCD.
- It is important to look for coexisting developmental and behavioral disorders such as ADHD, autism spectrum disorders, learning disorders, and intellectual disability as symptoms often overlap.
- Further assessment to identify and quantify deficient skills can be done by a trained occupational and physiotherapist using standardized tools.

MANAGEMENT

The focus of management is improving coordination, balance, and body awareness by trained occupational and physiotherapists. The activities need to be task oriented. Offering help with easier alternatives like Velcro instead of buttons and laces, computer typing instead of writing will increase child's participation. The child needs encouragement to participate alongside his peers without judgment or competition. Children with DCD will improve slowly with practice, so patience and ongoing counseling is important. Making the child aware of his strengths in language and cognition skills helps to maintain self-esteem.

Children with DCD do not outgrow the clumsiness and many adults struggle with coordination issues throughout life. The long-term outcome depends on severity, age of diagnosis, and intervention and associated comorbid conditions.

FURTHER READING

1. American Psychiatry Association. (2013). Diagnostic and Statistical Manual of Mental Disorders (DSM-5). [online] Available from: https://www.psychiatry.org/psychiatrists/practice/dsm.
2. Biotteau M, Danna J, Baudou É, Puyjarinet F, Velay JL, Albaret JM, et al. Developmental coordination disorder and dysgraphia: Signs and symptoms, diagnosis and rehabilitation. Neuropsychiatr Dis Treat. 2019;15:1873-85.

3. CanChild. Recognizing and referring children with developmental coordination disorder: The Role of the Physician. [online] Available from: https://www.canchild.ca/en/resources/120-recognizing-and-referring-children-with-developmental-coordination-disorder-the-role-of-the-physician (Last accessed December, 2021).
4. Harris SR, Mickelson ECR, Zwicker JG. Diagnosis and management of developmental coordination disorder. CMAJ. 2015;187(9):659-65.

Chapter 43

Sensory Processing Disorders: Developmental Aspects

Leena Deshpande

"The things that make me different are the things that make me ME!"
Piglet, Winnie, the Pooh

Sita and Gita are identical twins; most people can not tell them apart by just looking at them! But their personalities are very different. While Sita enjoys spicy food, Gita has a sweet tooth. Sita loves rollercoaster rides; Gita is scared of them. Sita loves playing in sand and mud; Gita would rather not have a speck of dirt on her hand.

This holds true for so many of us. These are called sensory preferences—while some like it hot, others like it cold! As long as these sensory preferences do not interfere with our life and do not cause day to day issues, it all becomes a part of our personality.

However, there are children who are so adversely affected by their sensory preferences, that it starts interfering with their normal, everyday functioning. These are the children who may have sensory processing disorder (SPD).

INTRODUCTION

Sensory processing disorders, also called sensory integration disorders, were first described by Dr A Jean Ayres, an occupational therapist in the early 1970s. Sensory integration is the process by which we register, modulate, and discriminate sensations received through the sensory systems to produce purposeful and adaptive behaviors in response to the environment. Effective integration of our five senses, i.e., vision, auditory, olfactory, gustatory, and tactile along with two more sensory inputs, i.e., vestibular and proprioceptive, helps in development of skills needed for smooth participation in everyday life. If this process is affected, the child will present with developmental and behavioral issues.

Though general prevalence is about 5%, SPD is significantly higher in children with autism spectrum disorder, learning disabilities, ADHD, cerebral palsy, syndromes such as fragile X, trisomy 21, and other neurodevelopmental diagnoses.

The exact cause is not known.

CLINICAL FEATURES (FLOWCHART 1)

Sensory modulation is the ability to regulate the degree, intensity, and nature of responses to sensory input. Most children with sensory modulation disorder (SMD) will over-react or under-react (or both) to one or more of the seven sensory modalities.

Children who are over responsive may show severe behavioral response to simple everyday situations—from brushing their teeth, eating food with different textures, simple hugs, everyday car or bus rides, noisy, or crowded places (like school or play area). This over reactive, over aroused child will quickly become disorganized and anxious and may show a fight (aggression, severe tantrums, and irritability) or a flight (running helter-skelter trying to escape from the situation) response.

Children who are under responsive will appear to be passive, lacking alertness, and attentiveness. These children will be difficult to engage and may seem lethargic.

Children who are sensory seeking crave sensory input and may self-rock, run purposelessly deliberately falling, and bumping into objects or chew on objects. These children will appear overexcited, impulsive, and disruptive.

Thus, children with SMD will have a very atypical behavioral response to simple everyday environmental and sensory stimuli. This will cause problems in peer relations, play and learning, and secondary effects will set in.

Clinical features of sensory-based motor disorders are discussed elsewhere.

Flowchart 1: Clinical classification of sensory processing disorder (SPD).

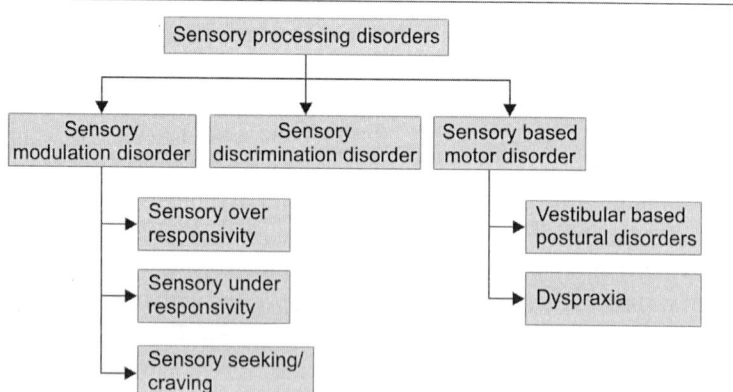

ASSESSMENT

A detailed history and examination will help understand the child's presenting behavioral and developmental issues.

Children with perinatal problems are at a high-risk to develop neurodevelopmental disorders including SPD. Early concerns of an infant who is irritable, a poor sleeper, and has feeding difficulties may be elicited. History to elicit an association between a particular sensory experience and the child's extreme behavior may help.

A detailed developmental and behavioral history will also help identify any other associated conditions. SPD may co-occur, mimic, or exacerbate neurodevelopmental disorders such as autism spectrum disorder and attention-deficit/hyperactivity disorder (ADHD).

Examination may reveal soft neurological signs such as dysdiadokokinesia, coordination problems, right-left discrimination problems, etc.

EVALUATION

Referral to a therapist experienced in SPD will be needed. Some standardized tools [Sensory Integration and Praxis Test (SIPT) and standardized questionnaire for parents] are available but there is no consensus regarding the best tool for diagnosis.

Caution: SPD is not recognized as a stand-alone diagnosis by Diagnostic and Statistical Manual of Mental Disorders, 5th edition (DSM-5) or International Statistical Classification of Diseases and Related Health Problems (ICD-10).

MANAGEMENT

The main intervention modality for SPD is sensory integration therapy provided by trained therapists. Sensory diet consists of individualized set of activities which help the child's arousal and attention throughout the day and includes deep pressure, rhythmic movement, weighted vests, etc., depending on the child's sensory needs.

Principles

- Educating the caregivers and the teachers about how the child's SPD is causing the behavioral and developmental issues
- Teaching the caregivers ways to accommodate to their children's sensory needs
- Introducing sensory diet appropriate to the child's needs which will fit into the child's daily routine
- Modifications in the classroom environment and routine to help accommodate child's sensory needs
- Teaching the child methods to compensate for their disorder so they can maintain optimal level of arousal and attentiveness (**Table 1**).

Table 1: Interview questions to screen for sensory processing problems (discuss the severity of symptoms and the environment they are associated with).

System	Questions
Auditory	• Does your child have trouble understanding what other people mean when they say something? • Is your child bothered by any household or ordinary sounds, such as the vacuum, hair dryer, or toilet flushing? • Does your child respond negatively to loud noises, as in running away, crying, or holding hands over ears? • Is your child distracted by sounds not usually noticed by other people? • Does your child seem overly sensitive to sounds?
Gustatory/olfactory	• Does your child gag, vomit, or complain of nausea when smelling odors such as soap, perfume, or cleaning products? • Does your child like to taste nonfood items such as glue or paint? • Does your child gag when presented with certain foods?
Proprioception	• Does your child sometimes grasp objects so tightly that they break? • Does your child grind his or her teeth? • Does your child seem driven to seek activities such as pushing, pulling, dragging, lifting, and jumping? • Does your child seem to exert too much pressure for a task, such as slamming doors or pressing too hard when using pencils or crayons? • Does your child have difficulty positioning himself or herself in a chair? • Does your child bump or push other children?
Tactile	• Does your child pull away from being touched lightly? • Does your child seem to lack the normal awareness of being touched? • Does your child react negatively to the feel of new clothes? • Does your child show an unusual dislike for having his or her hair combed, brushed, or styled? • Does it bother your child to have his or her face touched or washed? • Does your child avoid foods of certain textures?
Vestibular	• Is your child excessively fearful of movement, such as going up and down stairs, or riding swings, slides, or other playground equipment? • Does your child exhibit distress when he or she is riding on moving equipment? • Does your child have poor balance? • Does your child spin and whirl his or her body more than other children? • Does your child rock himself or herself when stressed?

Source: Adapted from Parham LD, Ecker C. Clinical observations of neuromotor performance, evaluation of sensory processing and touch inventory for elementary school children. In: Bundy A, Lane S, Murray E (Eds.). Sensory Integration Therapy and Practice. Philadelphia, FA Davis; 2002.

FURTHER READING

1. Ayres AJ. Sensory Integration and Praxis Tests (SIPT): Manual. Los Angeles: Western Psychological Services; 1989.
2. Ayres AJ, Robbins J. Sensory Integration and the Child: Understanding Hidden Sensory Challenges. Los Angeles: Western Psychological Services; 2005.
3. Diagnostic Classification of Mental Health and Developmental Disorders in Infancy and Early Childhood (DC: 0-3R). Washington, DC: Zero to Three Press; 2005.
4. Miller LJ, Anzalone ME, Lane SJ, Cermak SA, Osten ET. Concept evolution in sensory integration: A proposed nosology for diagnosis. Am J Occup Ther. 2007;61(2):135-40.
5. William Carey, Allen Crocker et al. Other Sensory Problems. Developmental-Behavioral Pediatrics. 4th edition. 2009;730-36.

Chapter 44

Language and Speech Disorders

Patricia Osbourn

INTRODUCTION

Language and speech disorders are a broad category of developmental communication disorders. The diagnostic and statistical manual of mental disorders, fifth edition (DSM-5) has identified the following four communication disorders:
1. Language disorders
2. Social (Pragmatic) communication disorders
3. Speech sound disorders
4. Childhood onset of fluency disorder (stuttering).

These disorders are developmental in nature and appear in early childhood. The pediatrician may be the first professional to identify communication disorders, therefore, it is important that pediatricians recognize the symptoms and understand how to best guide parents of these children. Developmental language and speech disorders are not an uncommon developmental issue; Western literature finds prevalence rates from 2.63 to 16%. Two population studies conducted in India place prevalence rates from 6.2 to 13.7% of children under the age of 6 years.

CLINICAL FEATURES

Language disorders broadly refer to difficulties in the ability to communicate one's needs, desires, and emotions with expected proficiency based upon one's age. Language disorders may be evidenced in a child's inability to communicate freely with family and/or peers or in an inability to comprehend the language spoken to him. Thus, language disorders have both an expressive and receptive realm; both areas will be considered when assessment for language disorders occurs. While there are certainly developmental differences among children, general language acquisition milestones are helpful in determining the possible presence of a language disorder.

Clinically, the child may have minimal verbal communication or few words. His/her parents may describe a child who does not seem to know many words or a child who resorts to tantrums in order to get needs met. The child may be unable to follow simple commands or point to common nouns such as body parts, colors, shapes, and the like. The child may be unable to respond to simple who, what, or where questions when another child of his age could easily do so.

Pragmatics refers to the social use of language for communication. Children with social communication disorders may exhibit challenges in using the language in a social context with another person. Greetings, understanding and using conversational norms, and changing communication style to accommodate one's listener all are characteristics of social communication disorders. These may be present both in verbal and nonverbal communication.

Speech sounds are phonemes, which are conventionally combined to form words of one's language. Children with speech sound disorders may be difficult to understand or unintelligible to the listener. Speech sound disorders may be characterized by omissions, deletions, or substitutions of one speech sound for another. Children may labor to produce sounds or have no awareness that their speech production is outside of the norm.

Fluency disorders involve the timing and patterning of speech sounds. Children with fluency disorders may exhibit repetition or prolongation of sounds and/or syllables. Audible or silent blocks may also occur. Frequently, this is accompanied by physical symptoms such as facial grimacing, or obvious tension in the mouth, lips, or tongue. These difficulties frequently lead to anxiety about speaking.

Specific diagnostic criteria can be referred from the DSM-5 (2013).

MANAGEMENT

Management of language and speech disorders ideally is an interdisciplinary effort, however, the pediatrician may be the first professional to acknowledge parental concerns. While screening for other developmental issues, pediatricians identify potential delays in language, and speech. Delayed identification and treatment may contribute to increased maladaptive behaviors as children are unable to get needs met, increased challenges with socialization, and decreased academic functioning. We know that early identification and intervention provides children with the greatest opportunities for successful outcomes. Pediatricians then are involved in identification, referral, and rule out of other possible contributing medical conditions. Pediatricians become critically important in counseling parents regarding their child's potential disorder and in assisting parents with next steps.

All children suspected of language and speech disorders should be referred for a current audiological assessment to rule out hearing impairments if this has not already occurred. A thorough history of developmental milestones is indicated to rule out global or developmental delay as well as to identify motor deficits that may be present.

Regardless of co-occurring medical conditions, children with suspected language and speech disorders that significantly interfere with everyday functioning should be seen by a qualified speech-language pathologist. The speech-language pathologist will provide assessments that are both culturally and age appropriate for the child. The speech-language pathologist will also take into account a child's bilingual or multilingualism. This assessment will not only seek to ascertain whether or not a significant disorder exists but will provide parents with an accurate look at their child's functioning level in terms of language and speech and will point to initial intervention goals. Intervention goals will consider parental priorities for their child. Evidence-based practices are selected based upon clinical and research results as well as family desires. The speech-language pathologist may enlist other team members such as special education teachers, occupational therapists, or others as appropriate to encourage language and/or speech production.

All children have a basic right to communication. The goal of speech and language intervention is to ensure that the individual child has a useful and effective communication system that supports his/her socialization and academic functioning. Speech and language therapy is effective; children can and do learn to communicate in more functional ways given proper identification and intervention. The pediatrician is an important link in the interdisciplinary management of the child with language and speech disorder.

FURTHER READING

1. American Psychiatric Association. Diagnostic and Statistical Manual of Mental Disorders, 5th edition (DSM-5). 2013. pp. 40-8.
2. Binu A, Sunil R, Babaraj S, Mohandas M. Sociodemographic profile of speech and language delay up to six years of age in Indian children. Int J Med Res Health Sci. 2014;3(1):98-103.
3. Law J, Boyle J, Harris F, Harkness A, Nye C. Prevalence and natural history of primary speech and language delay: Findings from a systematic review of the literature. Int J Lang Commun Disord. 2000;35(2):165-88.
4. Nair MKC, Prasad C, Unni J, Bhattacharya A, Kamath SS, Dalwai S. Consensus statement of the Indian Academy of Pediatrics on evaluation and management of learning disability. Indian Pediatr. 2017;54(7):574-80.
5. Orellana CI, Wada R, Gillam RB. The use of dynamic assessment for the diagnosis of language disorders in bilingual children: A meta-Analysis. Am J Speech Lang Pathol. 2019;28(3):1298-317.
6. Sidhu M, Malhi P, Jerath J. Early language development in Indian children: A population-based pilot study. Ann Indian Acad Neurol. 2013;16(3):371-5.
7. Verdon S, McLeod S, Wong S. Reconceptualizing practice with multilingual children with speech sound disorders: People, practicalities and policy. Int J Lang Commun Disord. 2015;50(1):48-62.

Chapter 45

Selective Mutism

Samir H Dalwai

"Kaise keh doon ke mulakaat nahin hoti hai, Roz miltein hain magar baat nahin hoti hai."

Shakeel Badayuni

"I was a prisoner inside my own body. I felt desperate, angry, stupid, confused, ashamed, hopeless, and absolutely alone... and that this was of my own making. I could speak at home, how come I could not outside it? I have never been able to find the right words to describe what it was like." Carl Sutton, Selective mutism (SM) in our Own Words: Experiences in Childhood and Adulthood.

INTRODUCTION

Selective mutism is one of the seven anxiety disorders seen in children. Though considered as a differential diagnosis with autism spectrum disorders, it is completely different in that it is caused due to social anxiety, whereas autism spectrum disorder (ASD) is due to a deviancy in social communication development, which is pervasive in all situations.

Thus, children with SM would show inability to speak in certain social settings like school or day care, despite speaking normally in usually more familiar settings like home and with family. Whereas, children with ASD would have similar deficits in all settings. 90% of children with SM also have social phobia (social anxiety disorder); thus selective mutism is a disturbance that affects the child's daily functioning. Onset is usually before 5 years and may come to attention when entering the preschool setting or becoming a part of the community systems.

Not surprisingly, SM is seen more commonly in first degree relatives of those with social phobia, which ascribes a genetic basis to the condition, and less commonly in those with speech and language disorders.

The prevalence of SM is <1% in the general population, twice as common in girls than boys and lasts at least for a month (excluding the first month of school entry). Bi- or multilingualism may lead to a child unfamiliar or uncomfortable with the new environment to refuse to speak with strangers—this must not be misdiagnosed as SM.

CLINICAL DIAGNOSIS (BOX 1)

The essential feature is to be sure that the child talks well at home but not outside in community settings.

This requires a good clinical history from the parents that the child is very chatty at home (home videos on mobile phones are easily captured by parents and can be shared with the clinician).

Behavioral observations in the clinic correlates with history from the school setting. Typically, the child would show withdrawal, poor eye contact and social interaction, blank facial expression, rigid body language, and clinging to parents. They may resort to gesturing, nodding, pointing, or whispering.

Key questions to ask:
- How was your child's social interaction as an infant and a toddler?
- When did your child begin using meaningful words?
- How is the behavior and speech at home?
- How is the behavior and speech at school and other community and social settings?

Besides evaluations for anxiety, the selective mutism questionnaire is helpful in clinical as well as research settings.

Differential diagnoses include the oppositional and defiant strong-willed child who refuses to speak as opposed to a child with selective mutism who

---

Box 1: Diagnostic criteria for selective mutism.

- The child shows consistent failure to speak in specific social situations in which there is an expectation for speaking (e.g., at school), despite speaking in other situations
- The disturbance interferes with educational or occupational achievement or with social communication
- The duration of the disturbance is at least 1 month (not limited to the first month of school)
- The failure to speak is not attributable to a lack of knowledge of, or comfort with, the spoken language required in the social situation
- The disturbance is not better explained by a communication disorder (e.g., child-onset fluency disorder) and does not occur exclusively during the course of autism spectrum disorder, schizophrenia, or another psychotic disorder

Source: American Psychiatry Association. (2013). Diagnostic and Statistical Manual of Mental Disorders (DSM-5). [online] Available from: https://www.psychiatry.org/psychiatrists/practice/dsm (Last accessed December, 2021).

is truly afraid of speaking in social settings. This misconception had been strengthened by the earlier name "elective mutism".

Selective mutism is distinguished from speech disorders such as developmental language disorder, which is seen in all settings; and from dysarthria and fluency disorders in terms of the morphology as well as the developmental history.

Tests include audiogram, which is the mandatory test for any speech and language disorder and a detailed speech and language evaluation considering that 20–30% children with SM also have some speech and language delay. Evaluation for anxiety is equally important.

MANAGEMENT

"I have packed myself into silence so deeply and for so long that I can never unpack myself using words. When I speak, I only pack myself a little differently."

Herta Müller, The Hunger Angel

It is a misconception to believe that children with always outgrow their selective mutism; many may gradually speak a little more with time. However, with an increased "expectation" to speak, the anxiety may actual worsen the performance. Social situations where the child is expected to "perform" by speaking prelearned poetry or prose in social gatherings of family or friends to demonstrate scholarship can worsen the anxiety and the fear of speaking. Encouragement, positive reinforcement, reducing pressure to speak, and nurturing supportive relationships go a long way in reducing anxiety and increasing self-esteem. The clinician's role includes winning the confidence of the family and the cooperation from the school authorities. Techniques of cognitive behavior therapy like contingency and stimulus fading, gradual desensitization and extinction help.

Relaxation and breathing techniques, group therapy sessions, and social skill groups can all help. In difficult to resolve cases, selective serotonin uptake inhibitors (SSRIs) in low doses over 9–12 months have been shown to help lower the anxiety threshold in combination with the above interventions.

FURTHER READING

1. Bergman RL, Keller ML, Piacentini J, Bergman AJ. The development and psychometric properties of the selective mutism questionnaire. J Clin Child Adolesc Psychol. 2008;37(2):456-64.
2. Diagnostic and Statistical Manual of Mental Disorders, 5th edition (DSM-5). (2013). American Psychiatry Association. [online] Available from: https://dsm.psychiatryonline.org/doi/book/10.1176/appi.books.9780890425596 (Last accessed December, 2021).
3. https://www.rekhta.org/ghazals/kaise-kah-duun-kii-mulaaqaat-nahiin-hotii-hai-shakeel-badayuni-3-ghazals

4. Müller H, Boehm P. The Hunger Angel. [online] Available from: https://www.goodreads.com/book/show/13165142-the-hunger-angel?from_choice=false&from_home_module=false (Last accessed December, 2021).
5. Naomi S. Selective mustism. In: The Zuckermann Parker Handbook of Developmental and Behavioural Pediatrics for Primary Care; 3rd edition. Wolters Kluwer. 2011. pp. 327-8.
6. Sutton C, Forrester C, Williams D. Selective Mutism in Our Own Words: Experiences in Childhood and Adulthood. Jessica Kingsley Publishers. 2015.

Chapter 46

Medical Comorbidities in Autism Spectrum Disorder

Yamini Jagannath Howe, Ann M Neumeyer

INTRODUCTION

Autism spectrum disorder (ASD) is a lifelong neurodevelopmental condition characterized by impairments in social communication and ongoing repetitive and restricted pattern of interests and behaviors. ASD is a heterogeneous condition with varying etiology with both environmental and genetic factors thought to be involved. Worldwide prevalence of ASD is generally increasing, largely due to increased recognition, more widely available treatments, and decreasing stigma related to the disorder, with recent estimates ranging from 1 out of 100 children diagnosed with ASD under the age of 10 in India and one in 58 children diagnosed with ASD in the United States (US).

The diagnosis of ASD can be made as early as 14 months of age in some individuals though in milder cases symptoms would not become apparent until school age or whenever social demands exceed their capabilities. Some individuals with ASD will present with regression in language or social communication skills, typically between the ages of 1 and 3 years. The diagnosis is a clinical one based on expert clinical examination using published criteria, ideally consulting with a multidisciplinary team and using standardized testing. As of yet, there are no biomarkers to aid in diagnosis. Risk factors include family history of ASD, advanced parental age, pregnancy and birth complications, and with folic acid likely having a protective effect.

Medical comorbidities are common in ASD, likely related to the underlying neurobiological etiology of the disorder, as well as secondary to symptoms of ASD. Due to advances in medical technology, it is increasingly possible to identify genetic causes of ASD for more individuals. ASD is a common neurodevelopmental presentation in some genetic conditions (such as fragile X, Rett syndrome, tuberous sclerosis, Phelan–McDermid syndrome, PTEN hamartoma tumor syndrome, and Prader–Willi and Angelman syndrome) or can be a co-occurring condition in others (such as Down syndrome). Medical care should proceed as is recommended for the child with an identifiable genetic syndrome. In children who have ASD that are not associated with a known genetic condition, certain medical conditions are still more common than in the general population of children. These include sleep disorders, feeding disorders, constipation, and seizure disorders. Psychiatric comorbidity is also common, most commonly, attention deficit/hyperactivity disorder (ADHD) and anxiety disorders.

CLINICAL DIAGNOSIS

In general, assessing medical concerns in children with ASD are not different from that of the general population of children, except that communication challenges make it difficult for children to express pain and sensory processing differences may lead to hyper- or hyporesponsiveness to pain. Behavioral presentations for medical symptoms are common.

Sleep disorders in particular are very common in children with ASD and can present early in life. Collecting a detailed sleep history is important with every patient with ASD as identification and treatment of sleep disorders can significantly improve quality of life for the child and family. As with sleep disorders in general, it is important to rule-out medical causes for insomnia such as iron deficiency, gastroesophageal reflux, obstructive sleep apnea, and restless leg syndrome. Children with ASD can have difficulty falling asleep, maintaining sleep, or waking too early in the morning and often seem to require less sleep (have a shortened sleep duration) as compared with typically-developing peers.

Feeding problems are also very common among children with ASD and can be seen even in infancy. Children with ASD often refuse new foods and have difficulty transitioning to eating solid foods. Sensory-mediated feeding difficulties are common, as well as selective eating patterns. Some may have oral motor dysphagia related to hypotonia and difficulty with oral motor coordination. Multidisciplinary evaluation is helpful, including gastroenterologists, nutritionists, as well as speech-language pathologists, and occupational therapists.

Constipation is common in children with ASD. As with other children, this can be related to the child's self-restricted diet or due to stool with-holding behaviors during potty training. As mentioned previously, symptoms of chronic constipation may present different in children with ASD, due to communication impairments and possibly related to differences in processing of abdominal pain. Some patients may present with worsening behaviors in general, or self-injurious behaviors targeted at the abdomen. Some may present with gastroesophageal reflux symptoms such as increased drooling or chewing/mouthing behaviors or sleep disruption.

Seizure disorders are common in ASD occurring in about 6–27% of people with ASD with rates varying depending on genetic etiology, sex, age, and presence of intellectual disability. For example, seizures are very common in tuberous sclerosis, more common in girls with ASD, and intellectual disability and there are two peaks of onset, one in early childhood and the other in adolescence. Children are more likely to have a higher rate of electroencephalogram (EEG) abnormalities without clinical seizures and may often have seizure like events with no epileptic EEG correlate. Therefore, routine EEG testing of children with autism is not recommended without clinical reports of seizure like behavior.

Many children with ASD can have behaviors that look like seizures including staring spells and repetitive behaviors. They are often less responsive to their name being called (less verbally attentive) or can hyper focus on a stimulus making it difficult to judge if the child is having a seizure. The caretaker is advised to touch the child when staring off to see if they alert better with touch than with voice. The family is encouraged to take a video of the event to show the doctor. A child who has incontinence or drooling or loss of tone during a spell is also more likely to have a seizure.

The physical examination of children with suspected epilepsy should focus on identification of neurologic injury or neurogenetic disorders, which present with epilepsy such as looking for the hypomelanotic macules of tuberous sclerosis with a UV light or Wood's lamp. Marked hypotonia is also often associated with genetic disorders such as Angelman syndrome (UBE3A deletion), 5q11.2-13.1 duplication (Dup15) and Phelan McDermid syndrome (22q13.1 deletion). The microcephaly of Rett syndrome and facial characteristics of fragile X syndrome should also be sought.

MANAGEMENT

Treatment of sleep disorders in children with ASD should proceed similarly to the general population of children, however, underlying sleep disorders requiring medication management is more common. The initial treatment of sleep problems should focus on counseling parents on healthy sleep development and sleep hygiene. Caregivers should be counseled on establishing clear and consistent bedtime routines as well as establishing safe and comfortable sleeping environments. Parents should consider what environmental factors may be present at the time of sleep onset. Children can develop sleep onset associations, such that whatever is present when the child is falling asleep (i.e., a parent cuddling or rocking the child) are the same conditions needed when the child awakens at night. If addressing sleep hygiene practices are inadequate to address the sleep problem, then medications can be considered. Melatonin is safe and relatively well-tolerated medication that can be used for the treatment of sleep-onset difficulties in children with ASD.

Feeding problems in ASD are generally best treated with feeding therapy, once contributing medical conditions (i.e., gastroesophageal reflux disease and food allergies) have been assessed and treated. Feeding therapy is generally guided by an occupational therapist, behavioral therapist, or speech-language pathologist, to address sensory, behavioral, and/or motor challenges that might be affecting the child's willingness or ability to eat healthy foods.

Constipation for children with ASD is treated the same was for other children, however, it is generally more difficult for children with ASD to tolerate oral medications and supplements and parents need more support around recognizing signs and symptoms of constipation and monitoring response to treatment.

Treatment of seizures will be determined by the seizure type as well as the identification of an underlying genetic etiology. The diagnosis of ASD should not affect antiepileptic medication choice.

FURTHER READING

1. American Psychiatric Association. Diagnostic and statistical manual of mental disorders (DSM-5), 5th edition. Washington, D.C: American Psychiatric Association; 2013. p. 947.
2. Autism Speaks. Autism Statistics and Facts. [online] Available from: https://www.autismspeaks.org/autism-facts-and-figures (Last accessed December, 2021).
3. Global Autism Prevalence Map by Spectrum. [online] Available from: https://prevalence.spectrumnews.org/ (Last accessed December, 2021).
4. Hyman SL, Levy SE, Myers SM. Identification, evaluation, and management of children with autism spectrum disorder. Pediatrics. 2020;145(1):e20193447.
5. Jeste SS, Tuchman R. Autism spectrum disorder and epilepsy: Two sides of the same coin? J Child Neurol. 2015;30(14):1963-71.
6. Malow BA, Byars K, Johnson K, Weiss S, Bernal P, Goldman SE, et al. A practice pathway for the identification, evaluation, and management of insomnia in children and adolescents with autism spectrum disorders. Pediatrics. 2012;130(Suppl 2):S106-24.

Chapter 47

Autism Spectrum Disorder

Samir H Dalwai

"I know of nobody who is purely autistic, or purely neurotypical. Even God has some autistic moments, which is why the planets spin."

Jerry Newport
Your Life is Not a Label

INTRODUCTION

Autism spectrum disorder (ASD) is a biologically-based neurodevelopmental disorder characterized by impairments in two major domains of development: (1) social communication and social interaction and (2) restricted, repetitive patterns of behavior, interests, or activities, with severity based on impairments and symptoms presenting when social demands exceed limited capacities. The term includes disorders previously known as autistic disorder (classic autism, early infantile autism, childhood autism, or Kanner's autism); childhood disintegrative disorder; pervasive developmental disorder-not otherwise specified (PDD NOS) and Asperger disorder (syndrome).

The term "spectrum" in ASD indicates that each individual is affected in different ways, with mild to severe symptoms. The manner in which ASD affect a person's functioning, depends on the severity and combination of symptoms, the presence or absence of associated conditions (e.g., intellectual impairment, language impairment, etc.) and the quality of intervention received.

Prevalence ranges from one in 68 children [Centers for Disease Control and Prevention (CDC), United States of America (USA)] to one in 65 (INCLEN, India). ASD has a genetic etiology, which alters brain development, affecting social and communication development. Children, who have a sibling with ASD, have increased risk (3–20%) of developing the condition. Epidemiologic evidence does not support an association between immunizations and ASD.

CLINICAL DIAGNOSIS

Earliest symptoms are absence of normal behavior (rather than the presence of abnormal ones), i.e., the baby resists cuddling, avoids eye contact, or fails to spread her arms in anticipation of being picked up, or to and fro babbling and jargoning; similarly, a "very good" baby, i.e., quiet and undemanding.

Symptoms of ASD may not be apparent until later, i.e., when social demands (age appropriate-expected behavior and speech) exceed limited capacities. Parents commonly notice these in the second year of life, when there is a delay in speaking meaningful words and sentences as well as in following oral instructions **(Flowchart 1)**.

Children with ASD often lack joint attention and protodeclarative pointing (may point toward an object but not necessarily to draw someone's attention to it), but not protoimperative pointing. Some children with ASD achieve early language milestones, but have regression of language, communication, and/or social skills between 15 and 24 months of age.

As they grow, children fail to develop and maintain peer relationships, prefer solitary play, involving others in activities only as tools or "mechanical" aids. Older children may lack understanding of what behavior is appropriate in a particular situation, nor the needs and emotions of others.

Stereotyped behaviors may be seen in the form of motor mannerisms or complex whole-body movements (e.g., hand or finger flapping or twisting, toe walking, rocking, and swaying) or behaviors like lining up toys in the same manner in a stereotyped ritual without apparent understanding of what the toys represent. Other repetitive behaviors may be seen like echolalia and memorized phrases (nursery rhymes and audio jingles). Inflexible adherence to specific, nonfunctional routines, or rituals are characteristic of ASD, leading to anxiety and distress at small changes in routines and difficulty with change. Some show restricted interests (preoccupation or focused interests only on certain objects or part of an object to the exclusion of all else). Restricted interests in younger children may center on peculiar sensory stimuli. Restricted and repetitive interests of older children (higher functioning) may

Flowchart 1: Clinical features of autism spectrum disorder (ASD).

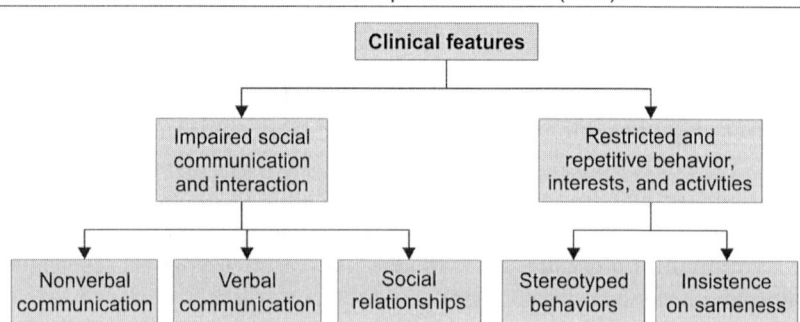

Table 1: Tools (scales) for assessment of autism.

Screening tools	Diagnostic tools
1. M-Chat-R	Autism diagnostic interview revised (ADI-R)
2. Social Communications Questionnaire (SCQ)	Autism Diagnostic Observation Schedule (ADOS)
3. Gilliam Autism Rating Scale (GARS)	
4. Childhood Autism Rating Scale (CARS)	

include phone numbers, dates, schedules, license plates, popular animation characters, or subtypes of any groups (e.g., cars, dinosaurs, and planes). Heightened comfort or choice with certain sensory stimuli may present as preference to particular tactile, vestibular, proprioceptive, auditory, olfactory and visual stimuli, and resistance to others.

Associated conditions to be assessed for all children with ASD include intellectual disability, medical disorders (e.g., seizures; genetic disorders; and lead poisoning in children with pica), language impairment, developmental and mental health comorbidities (e.g., hyperactivity, anxiety, depression, and behavioral regulation), sleep problems, feeding, and nutrition problems (e.g., constipation and restricted diet), delays in acquisition of activities of daily living (ADL), or self-help skills (e.g., toileting, dressing, and hygiene).

The tools for assessment of autism spectrum disorders are given in **Table 1**.

DIAGNOSIS

The diagnosis of ASD is clinical, based upon the history, examination, and observations of behavior. Accurate and appropriate diagnosis requires a team led by a developmental pediatrician, neurologist, or psychiatrist who is experienced in the diagnosis and treatment of ASD. The diagnostic evaluation should include documentation of whether the child's symptoms meet the DSM-5 criteria for ASD or the International Classification of Diseases (ICD)-10.

DIFFERENTIAL DIAGNOSIS

- Global developmental delay/intellectual disability
- Hearing impairment
- Developmental language disorder/language-based learning disability
- Landau–Kleffner syndrome
- Rett disorder (MECP2)
- Severe early deprivation/reactive attachment disorder
- Anxiety disorder
- Obsessive-compulsive disorder.

A comprehensive history is the best tool for distinguishing these disorders from ASD, although sometimes ancillary tests are necessary. Additional evaluation in patients with comorbid global developmental delay/intellectual disability and seizures may reveal associated conditions like tuberous sclerosis complex, fragile X syndrome, and Angelman syndrome to name a few. Evaluation for genetic testing and metabolic testing, neuroimaging, and/or electroencephalography (EEG) may be considered, only if the history and clinical presentation indicate associated conditions.

Key questions to ask:
- How was your child's social interaction as an infant and a toddler?
- How is the child's behavior and speech at home?
- Does your child use nonverbal language meaningfully?
- When did your child begin using meaningful words?
- How is the behavior and speech at school and other community and social settings?

MANAGEMENT

General principles of management of ASD include:
- Intervention should begin as early as possible. A definitive diagnosis is not necessary for commencing intervention.
- Management of ASD should target core features of autism, i.e., deficits in social communication and interaction and restricted repetitive patterns of behavior, activities, and interests.
- Pharmacologic interventions may be used to address comorbidities or provide symptom control but do not treat the core deficits.
- Intervention should be specific, evidence-based, and structured.
- Management of children should be provided through interdisciplinary teams, coordinated by the developmental pediatrician. This team should include pediatrician, child neurologist, psychiatrist, clinical psychologist, occupational therapist, speech and language therapist, special educator, nutritionist, and social worker.

The domains of management have been summarized in **Flowchart 2**.

The following interventional models are being used for ASD with limited outcomes:
- Behavioral [e.g., Applied Behavior Analysis (ABA)]
- Structured teaching [e.g., The Treatment and Education of Autistic and Related Communication—handicapped Children (TEACCH)]
- Integrative programs that use a combination of strategies within the treatment program [e.g. Social Communication, Emotional Regulation, Transactional Support (SCERTS)]
- Developmental/relationship-based (e.g., "Floor time")
- Early start Denver model

Flowchart 2: Domains of management of autism.

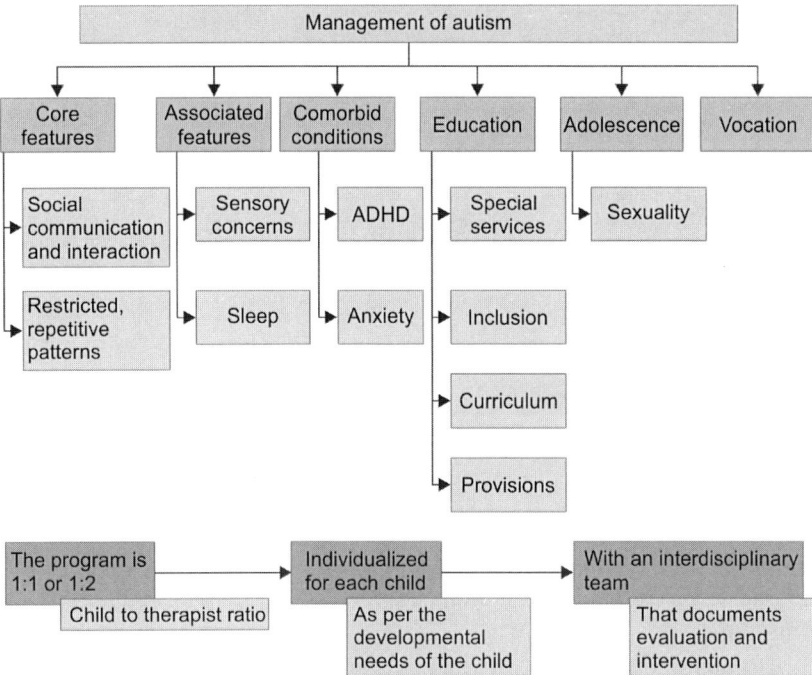

Fig. 1: Components of an ideal intervention program for autism.

- Cognitive behavioral therapy may work for anxiety and anger management in high functioning children
- An eclectic approach using elements of different therapies as well as parent and community-based programs.

A good Autism Intervention Program is based on the child's chronological age and developmental level, specific strengths and weaknesses, and the goals and needs as per the child's family. Involving the child's family is of paramount importance in intervention and outcomes **(Fig. 1)**.

Educational management of children with ASD should consider the following components:
- *Inclusion:* Meaningful inclusion is the goal of educational management.
- *Curriculum:* Educational plan should reflect an accurate assessment of the child's strengths and weaknesses leading to academic skills. Modified or special curricula must be adapted and provided to meet optimum education needs of the child.
- *Special services:* Appropriate individualized educational plan (IEP) is central in providing effective service.
- *Provisions:* Various boards provide for certification with special provisions for children with autism.

Table 2: Psychopharmacologic intervention.		
Symptoms	Drug	Option
Inattention and hyperactivity	Methylphenidate (S/E: sleep disturbances, decreased appetite, irritability, tics, and dullness)	Atomoxetine
Maladaptive behaviors including aggression and self-injury	Risperidone	Stimulants (SSRIs)
Repetitive behaviors	Fluoxetine (or another SSRI)	
Anxiety	Fluoxetine (or another SSRI)	
Dysregulated mood	Risperidone or SSRI	
Depressive symptoms	SSRI or serotonin norepinephrine reuptake inhibitor	

(SSRI: selective serotonin reuptake inhibitors)

Psychopharmacologic intervention: Psychopharmacologic interventions should be used in conjunction with appropriate behavioral and environmental interventions. **Table 2** mentions the medications to be given for specific symptoms.

Though complementary therapies have no evidence to support their use, they should be discussed with parents and explained.

AUTISM: AN ALTERNATE HYPOTHESIS

With observation of diagnosis, management, and outcomes in children at New Horizons Child Development Centre and Research Foundation across two decades, we hereby propose a novel hypothesis that has helped us understand how the symptoms develop, as well as identify children with autism more easily, as well as achieve better outcomes. We have proposed this as the "theory of social interaction of autism" with the "social communication sequence" and an acronym "interactive, meaningful, and purposeful (IMP)".

A common error is to construe early echolalia as words. We believe the history of "the child was speaking at 1 year and then regressed" needs to be examined in detail. We propose that three elements need to be looked into carefully. For a sound to be considered a word and not echolalia, it needs to be qualified by checking whether it is "interactive, meaningful and purposeful". We have proposed an acronym "IMP" for the same. If a child is reported to have achieved the milestone of saying a word at a particular age, we need to examine in detail whether it was done interactively, meaningfully, and purposefully; if not, it is doubtful if it can be considered as a true milestone; rather, is more likely to be echolalia.

Table 3: Social communication milestones as per the theory of social interaction of autism.

Normal social communication	Autism spectrum disorders
Normal social communication begins at birth, as the child learns that its needs are met by living beings in the environment. This helps it to differentiate between living (human) and the nonliving (object) world; it can interact with the former for its needs—meaningfully and purposefully, as against the latter	The child who lacks the ability to interact, fails to engage—meaningfully and purposefully—with humans for its needs
This interaction drives the child to observe, learn, and then master meaningful and purposive (1) Social interaction, (2) Social behavior, (3) Nonverbal communication, and (4) Verbal communication in a sequential manner (The "Social Communication Sequence")	This prevents the child from observing, learning, and (especially) mastering meaningful and purposive (1) Social interaction (2) Nonverbal communication, and (3) Verbal communication
Finding profit in the above, the child gravitates toward learning the nuances of human social behavior and communication, a sly smile, a happy face and angry word, a heated conversation; and comparatively ignores the nonhuman (object) world	With the overwhelming presence of objects in the environment, the child gravitates toward learning the patterns of object "behavior" rather than the nuances of human social behavior and communication. Thus, a child with autism can master the use of a mobile gadget or patterns of movement or alphabets and numbers or musical melodies or the façade of a building to recreate it in a painting, but fails to understand a sly smile, a happy face, and angry word or a warm conversation

Autism is not the presence of a disease but it is absence of normal social communication milestones **(Table 3)**. In autism, the child fails to learn interaction, meaningfulness, and the purpose of human behaviors as well as communication (i.e., the meaning of symbols—nonverbal as well as verbal). This concept helps in early suspicion as well as pediatrician-guided intervention by parents.

FURTHER READING

1. American Psychiatric Association. Diagnostic and statistical manual of mental disorders (DSM-5), 4th edition. Washington, DC: American Psychiatric Association; 2000.
2. Community Report from the Autism and Developmental Disabilities Monitoring (ADDM) Network. (2014). Centers for Disease Control and Prevention. [online]

Available from: http://www.cdc.gov/ncbddd/autism/states/comm_report_autism_2014.pdf (Last accessed December, 2021).
3. Dalwai S. Autism spectrum disorders. In: Gowrishankar NC, Nedunchelian K, Ramachandran P, et al. (Eds). Differential Diagnosis in Pediatrics. New Delhi: Jaypee Brothers Medical Publishers; 2020. pp. 35-8.
4. INCLEN survey findings. [online] Available from: http://indiatoday.intoday.in/story/autism-autisitic-mind-western-syndrome-myths-about-autism-autistic-children/1/322242.html (Last accessed December, 2021).

Chapter 48

Scholastic Backwardness

SS Kamath, Kawaljit Singh Multani

"If children cannot learn the way we teach, may be, we should teach the way they learn."

Ignacio Estrada

"Lazy. Unmotivated. Not living up to his potential. Daydreams. Needs to work harder. Does not try his best." Year after year, my grades slipped. Instead of developing my strengths, I tried to fit into the expectations of the school. I was not able to access learning the way it was presented and I felt like a failure."
Biography of a struggling student: My story

Seth Perler

INTRODUCTION

All children learn as they grow, though, the rate and pattern of learning may differ. Once children enter school, we expect them to learn at the same pace as their peers. This comparison between children leads to trouble when they are performing poorly in school as it not only affects the child's self-esteem leading to issues such as anxiety, depression, school absenteeism, etc. but also results in stress in the family, if unresolved.

There is no standard definition of scholastic backwardness (SB). SB can be considered as a condition wherein a child is failing in one or more subjects, or when a child's marks are below the 10th percentile in a class, or a teacher finds a child "difficult to teach". SB is seen in 15–50% of school-going children in India in different studies and is a major cause of school dropouts during adolescence when the academic pressure on the child increases manifold.

The causes of SB are multifactorial and include individual causes, family causes and school-related causes. Individual causes include prematurity, low birth weight, genetic conditions (e.g., fragile X, Klinefelter syndrome, etc.), autism, attention-deficit/hyperactivity disorder (ADHD), specific learning disability (LD), vision/hearing issues, head injury, poor motivation, substance abuse, child abuse, and chronic illnesses. Family factors include poor socioeconomic status, low maternal education, marital discord/divorce, domestic violence, and high parental expectations. School factors include frequent school changes, bullying, change in language at school (e.g., shift from Hindi to English medium), overcrowding in classes, and poor teaching methodology. One or more of these factors may be present in a child and a thorough history and clinical examination is needed to correctly diagnose the condition/s and also identify the strengths of the child which can help design an individualized plan for every child as one size does not fit all. In a study conducted at a tertiary care center in Kerala, common causes among children referred with SB were detected to be slow learners [intelligence quotient (IQ) 70–90] 35%, intellectual disability (IQ < 70) 28%, specific LD 12%, other neurodevelopment disorders (autism/ADHD, etc.) 15%, and no specific diagnosis in 10% of cases. Males are affected more commonly as compared to females. Children from rural areas are affected more than urban areas and this may be related to poor education and medical infrastructure in rural areas.

CLINICAL FEATURES

Scholastic backwardness may present as poor grades in school, or as a medical or psychiatric condition. The majority of students with SB are identified during middle school or high school when their performance falls sharply, or when other features like school refusal or behavioral issues manifest. The "no detention policy" for children up to class eighth has further compounded the issue and children who could have been picked up earlier in school are now being diagnosed rather late. These children lose critical time during early formative years of school which is most crucial for early effective remediation methods.

Screening can be carried out by teacher's feedback using Rutter's child behavior questionnaire. Intelligence testing can be done using standard tests of intelligence, e.g., Binet–Kamat Scale of Intelligence or Malin Intelligence Scale for Indian children. Specific LD can be tested using curriculum-based assessment or National Institute of Mental Health and Neuro-Sciences (NIMHANS) specific learning disability (SLD) battery. Autism and ADHD screening can be carried out using standard tests.

Based on the different assessments, children with SB without any specific underlying condition can be divided into two types: (1) deprived cases: those with significant familial/environmental factors, (2) poor learners—those with poor learning habits/styles. This differentiation is important as it will decide which interventions will benefit the child more.

MANAGEMENT

Early recognition is the single most important factor in management which requires a team effort of an interdisciplinary team comprising of a pediatrician, developmental behavioral pediatrician, psychologist, special educator, counselor as well as highly-motivated parents supportive to the child. A detailed vision and hearing assessment should be carried out in all children to rule out any underlying pathology. HEEADSSS (home, education, eating habits, activities, depression, substance use, sexuality, and safety) is an essential tool for eliciting psychosocial history and find the strengths and weaknesses of a child. Routine hemogram to look for underlying anemia and thyroid function tests to look for hypothyroidism are needed in all cases. Intelligence testing should be carried out, especially to find the cases with borderline IQ. Electroencephalography (EEG), neuroimaging, and genetic testing should be carried out for clinical indications (dysmorphism, positive family history, history of seizures, etc.) **(Flowchart 1)**. Child's strengths and weaknesses should be identified and individualized education plans (IEPs) should ideally be prepared for every case consisting of academic curriculum as well as extracurricular activities using the help of a special educator. Both parents and the child should be kept informed of the plan and regular follow up should be carried out by the pediatrician. They should be made aware of the various provisions by the Central Board of Secondary Education (CBSE). Management of specific LD is discussed in a separate chapter. The aim of management is "inclusive education" and the child should be kept in the mainstream school. Children with borderline IQ who find the mainstream

Flowchart 1: Algorithmic approach to scholastic backwardness.

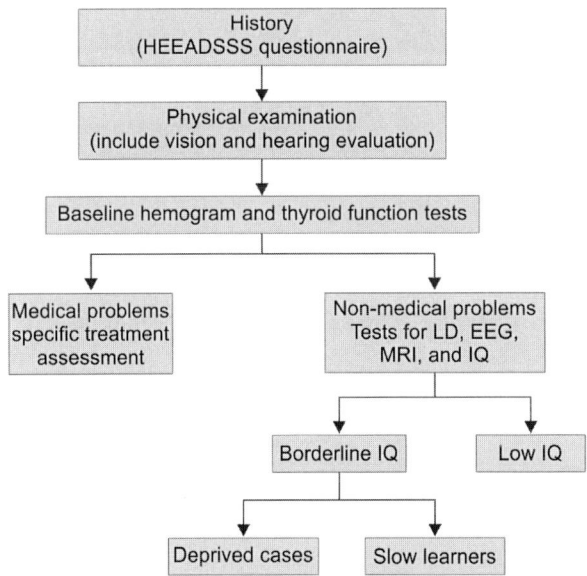

(EEG: electroencephalography; HEEADSSS: home, education, eating habits, activities, depression, substance use, sexuality, and safety; IQ: intelligence quotient; LD: learning disability; MRI: magnetic resonance imaging)

school education too difficult or stressful should be given the option of National Institute of Open Schooling (NIOS). Only very rarely should the child be referred to a special school.

Medications have little role in the management of poor scholastic performance. Iron supplements, thyroxine, antiepileptics, or stimulant medications for cases with ADHD may be used in diagnosed cases. One should look for features of anxiety and depression in these children as these may require referral to a child psychiatrist. Children with chronic medical/surgical conditions need condition specific enhancements in the classroom environment for better performance.

To summarize, early recognition and remediation of SB are essential as delays can result in a negative lifelong impact on the child and family. Pediatricians should look for SB in children presenting with vague, recurrent symptoms in the absence of any significant physical findings. Judicious use of the accommodations to the child that are offered by the CBSE/state boards, vocational training, and innovative ways of teaching using technology and multisensory methods will go a long way in helping the child with SB perform better.

"Tell me and I forget. Teach me and I remember. Involve me and I learn."
Benjamin Franklin

FURTHER READING

1. Baker R, Matulich E, Papp R. Teach me in the way I learn: Education and the internet generation. J Coll Teach Learn. 2007;4(4):27-32.
2. Galgali PM, Luiz N. Poor school performance in adolescence. Ind J Pract Pediatr. 2015;17(2):116-21.
3. Karande S, Kulkarni M. Poor school performance. Indian J Pediatr. 2005;72(11):961-7.
4. Nair MKC, Paul MK, Padmamohan J. Scholastic performance of adolescents. Indian J Pediatr. 2003;70(8):629-31.
5. Ramadas S, Vijayan VV. Profile of students referred for the assessment of scholastic backwardness at a tertiary care center. Indian J Psychiatry. 2019;61(5):439-43.
6. Unni J. Poor scholastic performance module. India: IAP Action Plan; 2011.

Chapter 49

Developmental Behavioral Disorders in Adolescence

Dilip R Patel, Swati Y Bhave

INTRODUCTION

Most neurodevelopmental and neurobehavioral disorders have their onset during early childhood and most persist through adolescence and adult years. A wide spectrum of developmental and behavioral disorders has been described during adolescence that range from predominant motor disability on one end to subtle learning and cognitive deficits at the other end of the spectrum. Major categories of developmental and behavioral disorders include intellectual disability, learning disabilities, communication disorders (including speech, language, and disorders of voice), neurogenetic disorders, neurometabolic disorders, movement disorders, cerebral palsy, sensory impairments, traumatic brain injuries, vision impairment, autism spectrum disorder, attention deficit hyperactivity disorder (ADHD), and aggressive and oppositional behaviors. In addition to the well characterized disorders, a range of behavioral issues is an important consideration within the adolescent cognitive and psychosocial developmental contexts, such as adolescent parenting issues, adolescent risk taking behaviors, motivation to change behavior, exposure and impact of violence, dating violence, tobacco and other substance use, and impact of increasing use of social media.

The incidence and prevalence of various developmental-behavioral disorders in adolescence vary depending upon the specific disorder and the population studied, as there may be geographical confounding factors and variations in ascertainment of population-based data. Epidemiological surveys indicate prevalence of intellectual disability at 6 per 1,000 population. The prevalence of autism spectrum disorder is 1%, ADHD is 5%, and learning disabilities are between 5 and 15% of the adolescents. Developmental disabilities or neurodevelopmental disorders comprise a diverse group of conditions that first manifest during early childhood and persist through adolescence and adult life.

Conceptually, development and behavior are linked from infancy through childhood through adolescence; however, the associated manifest behaviors evolve and change over time with neurocognitive and psychosocial development from childhood through adolescence. Most of the generally recognized behavioral disorders as categorized in the American Psychiatric Association Diagnostic and Statistical Manual of Mental Disorders and the International Classification of Disorders are well characterized by cluster of behavioral symptom criteria. More toward the disability spectrum of disorders with behavioral symptoms, it is important to understand the interplay of disability, function, and behavior.

The World Health Organization International Classification of Function, Disability, and Health (ICF), consists of three key components—body function and structure, activity, and participation. This concept provides a framework for delineating disabilities based on normal function or lack of normal function as follows:

Normal function:
- *Body function:* The physiological functions of the body
- *Body structure:* Anatomic parts of the body
- *Activity:* The execution of a task or action by an individual
- *Participation:* Involvement in a life situation
- *Functioning:* A global term used to encompass body function, body structure, activities, and participation.

Lack of normal function:
- *Impairment in function or structure:* Problems in the body function as a significant deviation or loss
- *Activity limitation:* Difficulties as individual may have in executing activities
- *Participation restrictions:* Problems an individual may have an involvement in life situation
- *Disability:* A global term used to encompass problems with body functions, body structures, activity limitations, and participation restrictions.

Intellectual functioning may range from normal to various degrees of subnormal in different developmental and behavioral disorders. It is important to also understand the concept of intellectual disability. According to the American Association of Intellectual and Developmental Disabilities (AAIDD), intellectual disability "is a disability characterized by significant limitations both in intellectual functioning and in adaptive behavior as expressed in conceptual, social, and practical adaptive skills." The determination of intellectual functioning and adaptive behaviors must take into consideration the expectations based on an individual's age and cultural context. The cognitive and adaptive functioning should be measured by individually administered standardized tests. The influence on cognitive assessment of sensory, motor, communication, or behavioral factors should be considered in the administration and interpretation of standardized tests.

The term learning disorders or disabilities describe a group of conditions with difficulties in specific areas of learning that have direct relation to scholastic performance. The failure to succeed academically in adolescents who have learning disabilities occurs in the context of age appropriate instructions and learning experiences and not necessarily a reflection of underlying cognitive deficits or sociocultural factors.

Various communication disorders have direct behavioral implications and manifest as behavioral symptom during adolescence. Language based disorders manifest various deficits in receptive or expressive language. The main underlying causes of language disorders are autism spectrum disorder, intellectual disability, and specific or developmental language disorder.

CLINICAL FEATURES

Clinical features of developmental-behavioral disorders in adolescents vary depending upon specific disorder. The diagnostic criteria for behavioral disorders such as ADHD, autism spectrum disorder, tic disorders, stereotypical movement disorder, intellectual developmental disorder, speech disorders, and developmental coordination disorder are well-characterized and described in the American Psychiatric Association Diagnostic and Statistical Manual of Mental Disorders.

The most important consideration during adolescence in terms of developmental-behavioral disorder is academic or scholastic difficulties. In addition to specific signs associated with learning disorders, these adolescents may present with behavioral problems. The differential diagnoses should also include anxiety disorders, ADHD, disruptive behavior disorders and substance abuse, and depressive disorders.

Developmental learning disorder is diagnosed when the adolescent's scores on an individually administered standardized achievement test (in reading, mathematics, or written expression) are substantially below that expected based on his or her age, education, and level of intelligence (on individually administered standardized tests). Reading disorder may not be apparent until fourth grade, especially, if mild and in children and adolescents with high intelligent quotient. Some of the clinical features of reading disorder include delayed language, problems with rhyming words or words that sound alike, difficulty learning letters of the alphabet, spelling errors, difficulty reading (decoding) unfamiliar or nonsense words or single words, and slow reading. Adolescents with mathematics disorder will demonstrate problems with skills in arithmetic. Some of the features include difficulties understanding or naming mathematical terms, operations, or concepts; difficulties decoding or recognizing mathematical symbols or signs; difficulties copying numbers or figures, following sequences of mathematical steps, counting, or multiplication tables.

Disorder of written expression is apparent by the end of the fifth grade and manifests problems with writing skills, which include grammatical errors, punctuation errors, poor paragraph organization, spelling errors, and very poor handwriting. Nonverbal learning disability demonstrates difficulties with problem solving, visual-spatial, and visual-perceptual deficits, while the language-based skills and intelligence are normal.

In addition to the neurobehavioral and neurodevelopmental disorders that is generally well-described in the standard biomedical literature, a range of behaviors are important to consider within the context of adolescent development. These disorders present clinically to the physician as parent adolescent conflicts, various forms of adolescent risk taking behaviors, lack of motivation to change from negative to positive health behaviors, impact of exposure to various forms of aggression and violence, the adolescent anger-hostility-aggression syndrome, dating violence, use of tobacco and other forms of recreational substances, and exposure and use of social media, and internet addiction.

MANAGEMENT

The management of the diverse group of developmental-behavioral disorders seen in adolescents vary depending upon the specific disorder; however, a set of general principles in management of these disorders in adolescent age group should guide the overall management. These include:
- It is important to delineate the underlying disorder and comorbid conditions by thorough assessment before starting treatment. Such diagnostic evaluations should include medical as well as behavioral assessment.
- Recognize that environmental accommodations and support systems play a vital role in the success or failure of any treatment approach, such as the home and family context, the school system, and access to community-based resources.
- The treatment of developmental behavioral disorders requires application of the multidisciplinary or interdisciplinary team care approach. The team members will include as appropriate to the given condition, physician, behavioral counselor, psychologist, medical social worker, physiotherapist, occupational therapist, speech-language pathologist, and audiologist.
- Pharmacotherapy is supported, based on evidence of effectiveness for specific conditions, e.g., stimulants for ADHD. On the other hand, pharmacotherapy can be used for alleviating specific target symptoms.
- Various forms of behavioral treatment approaches are applicable depending upon specific target symptoms or specific conditions—parent skills training for aggression and disruptive behaviors.

- In the learning environment, certain accommodations can be made to allow for compensation of deficits in skills for learning.

A wide range of therapeutic techniques are available to help manage parent adolescent conflicts, various forms of adolescent risk taking behaviors, lack of motivation to change from negative to positive health behaviors, impact of exposure to various forms of aggression and violence, the adolescent anger-hostility-aggression syndrome, dating violence, use of tobacco and other forms of recreational substances, exposure and use of social media, and internet addiction. These include parent skills training, cognitive-behavior therapy, motivational interviewing techniques, aggression replacement therapy, anger control training, relaxation exercises, yoga, meditation techniques, family life education programs in school systems, positive discipline, application of transactional analysis, and various forms of counseling—family, individual, and vedantic.

FURTHER READING

1. American Psychiatric Association. Diagnostic and Statistical Manual of Mental Disorders: Neurodevelopmental disorders, 5th edition. Washington DC: American Psychiatric Press; 2013. pp. 31-86.
2. Greydanus DE, Patel DR, Pratt HD, Calles JL Jr, Nazeer A, Merrick J. Behavioral Pediatrics, 4th edition. New York: Nova Science Publishers; 2015.
3. Parthasarathy A, Bhave SY, Nair MKC, Menon PSN, Greydanus DE. Bhave's Textbook of Adolescent Medicine. New Delhi: Jaypee Brothers Medical Publishers; 2006. pp. 875-949.
4. Patel DR, Greydanus DE, Calles JL Jr, Pratt HD. Developmental disabilities across the lifespan. Dis Mon. 2010;56(6):304-97.
5. Patel DR, Merrick J. Neurodevelopmental disabilities: Introduction and epidemiology. In: Patel DR, Greydanus DE, Omar HA, et al. (Eds). Neurodevelopmental Disabilities: Clinical Care for Children and Young Adults. New York: Springer Medical; 2011.
6. Patel DR. Principles of developmental diagnosis. In: Greydanus DE, Feinberg A, Patel DR, et al. (Eds). The Pediatric Diagnostic Examination. New York: McGraw Hill Professional; 2008. pp. 629-44.
7. Rubin IL, Merrick J, Greydanus DE, Patel DR. Rubin and Crocker Health Care for People with Intellectual and Developmental Disabilities Across the Lifespan, 3rd edition. Switzerland: Springer International; 2016.

Chapter 50

Specific Learning Disability

Samir H Dalwai, Hilla Sukhadwala

INTRODUCTION

Learning disabilities (LDs) are a heterogeneous group of neurodevelopmental disorders where the individual unexpectedly fails to competently acquire, retrieve and use information, resulting in profound academic, and psychosocial consequences. Unexpectedly so, because the child's overall intelligence seems far superior to the academic performance. The terms LD, specific LD, and specific LD [Diagnostic and Statistical Manual of Mental Disorders, 5th edition (DSM-5)] are often used synonymously. In some countries, LD refers to the intellectual disability.

Learning disabilities are caused by inborn or acquired abnormalities in the brain structure and function and have a multifactorial etiology (including genetic influences). LD is frequently (but not invariably) preceded in preschool years by motor, attention, and language delays, which may persist and co-occur with learning. LD can only be diagnosed after formal education starts, but can be diagnosed at any point afterward in children, adolescents, or adults provided there is evidence of onset during the years of formal schooling.

Risk factors include a family history of LD; prematurity; neurologic conditions (e.g., seizure disorders, neurofibromatosis, tuberous sclerosis complex, and Tourette syndrome); chromosomal disorders (e.g., fragile X syndrome, Turner syndrome, and Klinefelter syndrome); chronic medical conditions [e.g., type-1 diabetes mellitus and human immunodeficiency virus (HIV) infection], and history of central nervous system infection, irradiation, or traumatic brain injury.

CLINICAL DIAGNOSIS

In India, prevalence rates between 5 and 10% have been reported. Clinical features are associated with difficulties learning and using academic skills that have persisted for at least 6 months, as follows: (1) Inaccurate or slow and effortful word reading, (2) difficulty understanding the meaning of what is read, (3) difficulties in spelling, (4) difficulties in written expression, (5) difficulties mastering sense of number, number facts, or calculation, and (6) difficulties in mathematical reasoning.

Disabilities in reading, language, and mathematics frequently co-occur, and coexist with or may lead to deficits in social skills, and emotional or behavioral disorders.

Even mild deficits, if not intervened early are likely to snowball into significant academic underachievement as the child goes to higher grades **(Fig. 1)**.

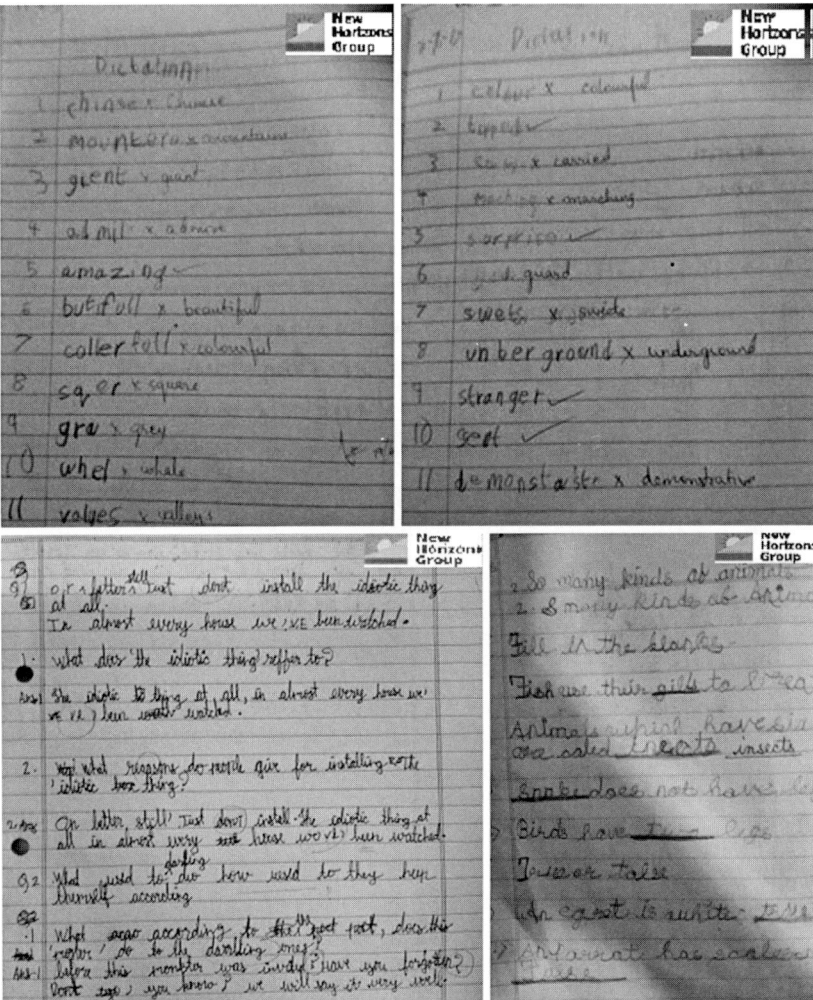

Fig. 1: Handwriting samples of a children presenting with academic concerns.
Source: ©New Horizons Child Development Center, Mumbai.

Functional consequences of LD include lower academic attainment; higher rates of high school dropouts; high level of psychological distress; poor mental health with a higher risk for adverse mental health outcomes including suicidal tendencies.

Specific types of LDs: Dyslexia or reading disability presents initially with problems in letter-sound relationships (i.e., connecting the sound to the alphabet) thus leading to a difficulty in (1) decoding alphabets, (2) words, and (3) reading fluently in kindergarten or grade one and later, problems in (4) reading comprehension. This can be identified by low overall reading achievement as compared to peers, or by low reading ability as compared to the child's overall intelligence.

Dysgraphia or writing disabilities are caused by a range of neurodevelopmental weaknesses like problems with handwriting (fine motor concerns and/or graphomotor concerns—correctly producing the alphabet on the paper) and visual-spatial perception (e.g., being able to correctly judge the space available in which to write). Children present with difficulties in copying efficiently from the board; may show excessive grammar and punctuation errors; formulating, expressing, and organizing ideas in writing and/or produce disorganized text that is difficult to follow.

Dyscalculia or math disabilities are marked by inability to correctly read and interpret math symbols and numbers. Students may reverse numbers or make errors while reading them aloud. Students with reading disability and dyscalculia have greater difficulty in solving word problems, because they do not understand the meanings of sentences as well.

Comorbid conditions include attention-deficit/hyperactivity disorder (ADHD), autism spectrum disorder (ASD), communication disorders, and developmental coordination disorders.

DIAGNOSIS

The diagnosis of LD is made primarily by educational history; psychometric tests help to confirm the presence of LD, and identify targets for intervention. Vision and audiology examination is mandatory.

The diagnosis cannot be LD, if learning difficulties are better explained by intellectual disabilities, uncorrected visual or auditory acuity, other mental or neurological disorders, psychosocial adversity, lack of proficiency in the language of academic instruction, or inadequate educational instruction.

Differential diagnosis includes the comorbid conditions as well as normal variations in academic achievement due to lack of educational opportunity, frequent school absenteeism, learning in a second language, or unrealistic expectations.

Assessments for LDs: If suspected, the pediatrician can review the features of LD described in DSM-5 and refer the child for a comprehensive developmental evaluation.

Recommended psychoeducational tests include: (1) Intellectual assessment: Wechsler Adult Intelligence Scale, 3rd edition (WAIS III); (2) Academic achievement: Woodcock Johnson Psycho-166 Educational Battery-Revised; (3) Cognitive processing abilities: Woodcock Johnson Psychoeducational Battery Revised, Raven-Colored Progressive Matrices, Bender Visual Motor Gestalt Test, and NIMHANS (National Institute of Mental Health and Neurosciences) Index.

MANAGEMENT

Delays in identification and intervention, as well as children with extreme reading deficits, make intervention more challenging with lower rates of success. These children are also at greater risk of acquiring severe social-behavioral deficits. LD with ADHD needs superior and better-planned intervention. An interdisciplinary approach toward intervention led by a developmental pediatrician (DP) is warranted to cover all aspects of the problem. A basic intervention approach should focus on (1) interpretation of specific skills that may be delayed (e.g., phoneme awareness and phonics; reading comprehension; spelling; number sense, and organizational skills); (2) identification of comorbidities, and (3) well-planned interdisciplinary and skill-based approach to each child **(Flowchart 1)**.

The DP has to judiciously select among various interventions (remedial education, occupational therapy, and counseling) to formulate a goal-oriented individual education program (IEP) for each child. The DP monitors the child's progress and updates the IEP accordingly.

The remedial educator is assigned assessments for strengths and weaknesses in academic skills and intervention sessions (i.e., twice or thrice weekly) to work on building the child's skills such as (1) reading—phoneme awareness, (2) reading—phonics, (3) writing skills—basic principles; and (4) Math—basic principles.

Due to inadequate awareness about LD, parents undergo immense stress in coping with their child's academic difficulties, and even in accepting the diagnosis. The pediatrician plays a crucial role in ensuring that parental and student stress is effectively minimized by (1) explaining them the nature of the disability, (2) explanation of the rationale of evaluations and provisions for children with LD, (3) gradual preparation of parents to accept that LD is a lifelong condition, (4) empowerment of parents to guide their child in selecting an appropriate career, and (5) effective peer sensitization.

Flowchart 1: Management of learning disability (LD).

```
                    Presenting concerns
                    for the three types of LD
         ┌──────────────────┼──────────────────┐
         ▼                  ▼                  ▼
  Academic concerns   Behavioral concerns   Emotional concerns:
  in areas of reading, of impulsivity, inattention, Poor confidence and
  writing, and Math   demotivation for academics  self-esteem, and anxiety
         │
         ▼
  Evaluations to        History and evaluation: To
  establish diagnosis   identify comorbid conditions, and
                        to rule out differential diagnosis
    ┌────────┼─────────────┐
    ▼        ▼             ▼
History (birth,  Physical        Standardized tools to
developmental,   examination:    assess IQ and LD:
and              Vision and hearing, DSM-5 screening,
educational)     CNS examination  MISIC, BKT,
                 (tone, power,    NIMHANS index,
                 reflexes, and visual- WJ III-achievement
                 motor index), and tests and GLAD
                 blood tests
                          │
                          ▼
                 Intervention (team approach)
                 • Remedial education
                 • Parental and child counseling
                 • Occupational therapy
                 • Career counseling
```

(BKT: Binetkamat Test for Intelligence; CNS: central nervous system; DSM-V: Diagnostic and Statistical Manual of Mental Disorders, 5th edition; IQ: intelligence quotient; MISIC: Malin's Intelligence Scale for Indian Children; NIMHANS: National Institute of Mental Health and Neurosciences)

Provisions and Advocacy

Concessions for students with LD include: (1) Extra time in examinations; (2) No mark deduction for grammar and spelling mistakes; (3) Use of calculator in Maths exam; (4) Exemption from writing one language exam; (5) Use of scribe or typing answers on a computer; and (6) Grace marks.

FURTHER READING

1. American Psychiatry Association. Diagnostic and Statistical Manual of Mental Disorders, 5th edition. Arlington, Virginia: American Psychiatric Association; 2009. pp. 59-65.
2. Levine M. A Mind at a Time. New York, NY: Simon and Schuster; 2002.
3. Nair MKC, Prasad C, Unni J, Bhattacharya A, Kamath SS, Dalwai S. Consensus statement of the Indian Academy of Pediatrics on evaluation and management of learning disability. Indian Pediatr. 2017;54:574-80.

Chapter 51

Child Abuse

Shabina Ahmed

INTRODUCTION

Child abuse or child maltreatment is defined by World Health Organization (WHO) as all forms of physical or emotional ill treatment, sexual abuse, neglect or negligent treatments, commercial or other exploitations resulting in actual or potential harm to the child's health, survival, development, or dignity. It is now recognized as a continuum of family violence, partner violence, abuse of animals, and the elderly.

INCIDENCE

As per WHO 2017 report, 1 billion minors between 2 and 7 years, experience violence annually of which 115 million children are engaged in extremely harmful form of work [International Labor Office (ILO) 2010] while 150 million girls and 73 million boys are subject to sexual violence (WHO 2000).

These figures, however, do not represent the true extent of the phenomenon as one out of third do not report violence.

India is home to one-fifth of the child population and incidence of abuse as reported by Ministry of Women and Child Development (MWCD) (2007) is one in every 10 children are sexually abused at any given time.

There is a great deal of knowledge about the causes of violence and protective factors for prevention. However, the above figures indicate that it is an ongoing process and is considered a human rights crisis. Traditional responses are failing, and we need to consider urgently this as a public health issue.

TYPES OF ABUSE AND NEGLECT

- *Physical abuse* is the use of physical force, body posture or gesture, or body movement that inflicts pain on a client. Examples being slapping, kicking, pushing, shouting, choking, hair pulling, biting, and use of corporal punishment. The rate of abuse in boys is higher than in girls.

- *Neglect* is failure of adequate care by a service provider or a person in care of children.

Types of neglect:
- *Physical neglect*—Denial or inadequacy of food, shelter, clothing, protection, medical, and dental care.
- *Passive neglect* is withholding or failure to provide the necessities of life.
- *Willful deprivation* is willfully depriving support, and thereby exposing to risk of physical, mental, and emotional harm.
- *Emotional neglect* is restricting social, intellectual and emotional growth, and verbal abuse; namely calling names and bring out inadequate comparisons with others.
- *Sexual abuse*—Any contact or interactions between child and an older person or with a more knowledgeable child, or adult, or a stronger sibling or person, in position of authority such as parent or a caretaker who uses the child as an object of gratification for the older child's or adult's sexual needs constitutes sexual abuse. These contacts or interactions are carried out against the child, using force, tricking, bribes, threats, or pressure.

RISK FACTORS FOR CHILD ABUSE

It is a highly complex phenomenon where the parent, child characteristics, and environmental characteristics play a part. Majority of abuse occurs at home, school, or the neighborhood. Research has revealed that parents that have low self-esteem, poor impulse control, substance, and alcohol abuse as well as young parents with low knowledge of child development and child behavior have great chances of abusing children. Research has shown that their personal experiences as a child affect parenting style. Risk of abuse is also high where parental support system is poor, namely social isolation, single parents, poverty, and partner violence.

Children with disabilities are 3–4 times more vulnerable to abuse, as well as those who have emotional, behavioral difficulties, and chronic illness.

IMPACT OF ABUSE IN CHILDREN

Adverse experiences in childhood are thought to produce effect on health by influencing biological adaptations, to response to stress, neuromaturation, and function of immune system, leading to impacts on psychosocial health. These have short and long-term consequences.

Early adverse experiences are associated with poor health and alters developmental trajectory of psychological development leading to internalizing and externalizing behavioral problems, as well as long-term chronic health issues such as chronic asthma, cardiovascular disorder, diabetes, and often may lead to suicidal tendencies.

ROLE OF PEDIATRICIANS

- Pediatricians are in a unique relationship with families and are well placed to enhance their ability to protect children and address issues that may put children at increased risk
- To recognize and respond to ongoing maltreatment
- Routine healthcare visits, provide ample opportunities to access, and give anticipatory guidance on child development
- Obtain a thorough social history initially and periodically
- Guide parents in providing effective discipline
- Talk to parents about sexual development and how to prevent abuse
- Understand the legislations that protect children and be aware of the support system available in the community.

LEGISLATIONS

1. The Protection of Children from Sexual Offences (POCSO ACT 2012) has been drafted to strengthen legal provisions of children from sexual abuse and exploitation. The national response to child maltreatment is mandatory reporting.
2. United Nations Convention on the Rights of the Child (UNCRC)—The UNCRC under international law, protects children from all kinds of maltreatment and is incumbent on all nations, to use appropriate measures to protect children. India is a signatory of the law since 1992.

FURTHER READING

1. Appleton JV, Sidebotham P. Safeguard children and young people is everyone's responsibility. Child Abus Rev. 2018;27(6):423-8.
2. Camp C, Thorogood W. The association of child protection professionals: Moving forward with a new identity. Child Abus Rev. 2019;28:11-2.
3. Christian CW; Committee on Child Abuse and Neglect, American Academy of Pediatrics. The evaluation of suspected child physical abuse. Pediatrics. 2015;135(5):e1337-54.
4. Committee on Child Abuse and Neglect. Policy Statement—protecting children from sexual abuse by health care providers. Committee on Child Abuse and Neglect. Pediatrics. 2011;128(2):407.
5. Flaherty EG, Stirling J Jr; American Academy of Pediatrics. Committee on Child Abuse and Neglect. Clinical Report—the pediatrician's role in child maltreatment prevention. Pediatrics. 2010;126(4):833-41.

Chapter 52

Role of Evaluation in Developmental Behavioral Pediatrics

Anjan Bhattacharya

"A medical evaluation is a comprehensive assessment of a patient's overall medical history and current condition for the purpose of identifying health problems and planning treatment."

"He just looked at my child and told my child has autism. Please tell me doctor, how can one just look and tell? We are here to be sure. Is there a test?"

Parent

INTRODUCTION

Evaluation in neurodevelopmental conditions starts at the initial contact. Since, the evaluation schema of a child with special needs involves various aspects and initial contact triggers assessments that are listed in **Table 1**.

CLINICAL EVALUATION

Key questions to ask:
- Is the child showing normal, delayed, or deviant development?
- When did the child's problem begin?
- How is the behavior and functionality at home?
- How is the behavior and functionality at school and other community and social settings?
- How is my clinical evaluation going to add value to what is offered currently?

Evaluations should also aim at:
- Ruling out mimics
- Considering differential diagnoses
- Detecting complications
- Detecting comorbidities
- Measuring baseline for pre-postintervention
- Benefiting clinical as well as research settings
- Management planning
   A systematic approach toward physical examination should help.

Table 1: Evaluation of neurodevelopmental conditions.

Evaluation schema	Child	Family/Caregiver	Society
Observation	Limping, hyperactive, poor-eye-contact, wheelchair, stature, etc.	Kempt, caring, affect Keen, qualified, expectant, etc.	Joint family, gated-society, slum-dweller, urban, semiurban, etc.
History	Antenatal/perinatal Presenting complaints Relevant complaints Past history, diet, and sleep Family history Drug/vaccine history	Composition, working family, businessman, primary caregiver, home help, family support, earnings, siblings, and elderly	Looked-after child, fund-rising, disability access—locally, to healthcare or educational facility, supportive, or discriminatory
Physical evaluation	General survey, anthropometry, condition-based-checks, and evaluation of gadgets	Family health Midparental height Genetic examination Dysmorphology search	Institutional health and health promotional practices of the community
Tests	Screening Investigations	Genetic testing Dysmorphology database search	Means testing Educational placement suitability testing

TESTS

Evaluation also involves screening and confirmatory tests, including laboratory tests.

The following schema shown in **Table 2**, could be quite helpful, albeit not comprehensive.

There is plenty of room for cross usage as well. The need for further evaluation, depending on needs, can hardly be overemphasized. This is where the need for a well-experienced developmental pediatrician can be acutely felt. For example, International Classification of Functioning, Disability and Health (ICF) can be used in all of the above and ICF core sets can be used in the ones available, e.g., cerebral palsy (CP), autism spectrum disorder (ASD), and attention-deficit–hyperactivity disorder (ADHD).

Moreover, there are many other validated and peer-reviewed tests, which can be adopted by specialists conversant with their usage. Due to the complex nature of neurodevelopmental disabilities, it is important to ensure that no child is denied access to good quality evaluation. The pediatrician can guide parents regarding the pros and cons of these.

Table 2: Different tests for evaluation of neurodevelopmental conditions.

Presenting types	Screening	Confirmatory tests	Laboratory tests
Cerebral palsy	GM (Prechtl's) assessment	GMFM ICF/ICF core set	Brain imaging metabolic/genetic
Autism spectrum	M-CHAT R/F CARS	• ISAA • ADI-R • ADOS • 3Di	• Audiometry • Visual tests • Thyroid
Attention deficit	Pediatric symptom checklist (PSC)	Connors Vanderbilt (teacher/parent)	• Audiometry • Visual tests • Thyroid
Behavioral difficulties	Pediatric symptom checklist (PSC)	CBCL (Child behavior checklist)	Sensory profiling SIPT/SPM
Learning difficulties/developmental delay	• Denver developmental screening test • Pediatric symptom checklist (PSC) • Trivandrum development screening chart	• Griffiths • Bayleys • DASII	• Audiometry • Visual tests • Thyroid • Metabolic/Genetic
Epilepsy	Clinical (semiology)	EEG and brain imaging	Do
Dysmorphic/genetic	Clinical (dysmorphology)	Genetic counseling	Genetic tests

(ADOS: Autism Diagnostic Observation Schedule; ADI-R: Autism Diagnostic Interview-Revised; CARS: Childhood Autism Rating Scale; EEG: electroencephalography; GMFM: gross motor function measure; ICF: International Classification of Functioning, Disability and Health; ISAA: Indian Scale for Assessment of Autism; M-CHAT R/F: Modified Checklist for Autism in Toddlers, Revised with Follow-up; SIPT: Sensory Integration and Praxis Tests; SPM: sensory processing measure; 3Di: Developmental, Dimensional, and Diagnostic Interview)

MANAGEMENT

Management will vary according to the findings, since even within a diagnosis, complexities, complications, and comorbidities will vary. Based on the diagnoses or the probable list of possible diagnoses, the following axial schema given in **Flowchart 1**, can be easily followed based on ICF by the World Health Organization.

A well-published example may be as follows:

The rehabilitation problem-solving form (RPS-Form) as presented by Steiner et al. (2002) is given in **Table 3**.

The numbers used in **Table 3** are ICF codes, where every disability can be coded in their current form of functionality.

Flowchart 1: Diagnostic approach to the neurodevelopmental conditions.

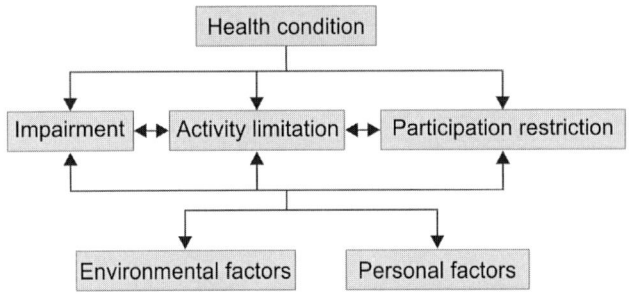

Table 3: Rehabilitation problem-solving form.			
Child name: Age: 7 years/Sex: Male	Disorder/disease: Cerebral Palsy (ataxic)		Therapist: Rehab-goal: walking
Patient/family perception of problems and disabilities	• Deformity of the feet • Weakness of both hand and leg • Poor body balance • Speech difficulties	Difficulties in walking without support	• Child has little contact to children from the neighborhood • Child cannot go somewhere independently without helper
Functions/ Structures	⟵⎯⎯⟶ Activities	⟵⎯⎯⟶	Participation
Health professional identification of mediators relevant to target problems	• Pronated foot (both) (pes planus valgus with abducted forefoot)-s75021.373 • Tonal abnormality-hypotonic (b735.2) • Low muscle power in both lower limb (b7303.2) • Low muscle power of trunk (b7305.2) • Impaired coordination (b7603.3) • Poor vestibular function b235.2 • Voice and speech functions (articulation functions-b320.3)	• Walking short distance (d4500.3) • Walking around different surface (d4502.3) • Walking around obstacles (d4503.3)	• Difficulties engaging in leisure activity and sports (d920.3) • Over-protection from the mother (e310)

Contd...

Contd...

Personal factors			Environmental factors
Cooperative nature—attitude toward health professional and other health professional (e450+4 and e455+4)			• Immediate family (good support and cooperation) (e310+4) • Less space for moving at home (e1558.2)

Pediatricians can offer guidance to parents/families by familiarizing themselves with these through various educational portals, thus remaining updated and relevant to current pediatrics and recent advances.

FURTHER READING

1. Diagnostic and Statistical Manual of Mental Disorders (DSM-5). American Psychiatry Association. 2013.
2. Einspieler C, Prechtl HF. Prechtl's assessment of general movements: A diagnostic tool for the functional assessment of the young nervous system. Ment Retard Dev Disabil Res Rev. 2005;11(1):61-7.
3. Medical Evaluation. (2020). [online] Available from: https://www.workplacetesting.com/definition/1468/medical-evaluation (Last accessed December, 2021).
4. Novak I, Morgan C, Adde L, Blackman J, Boyd RN, Brunstrom-Hernandez J, et al. Early, accurate diagnosis and early intervention in cerebral palsy: Advances in diagnosis and treatment. JAMA Pediatr. 2017;171(9):897-907.
5. Schiariti V, Selb M, Cieza A, O'Donnell M. International Classification of Functioning, Disability and Health Core Sets for children and youth with cerebral palsy: A consensus meeting. Dev Med Child Neurol. 2015;57(2):149-58.
6. World Health Organization. (2001). International Classification of Functioning (ICF). [online] Available from: http://apps.who.int/iris/bitstream/handle/10665/42407/9241545429.pdf;jsessionid=D73D040956A983CA927B916B8C699BB1?sequence=1 (Last accessed December, 2021).

Chapter 53

Early Intervention

Zafar Mahmood Meenai

"Shubhasye Shighram"
Earliest, the Auspicious!

A recent meta-analysis (Ferreira et al., 2020) vindicates this ancient Indian teaching as it shows a positive impact of early intervention (EI) focused on the family on cognitive outcomes of children born premature and/or at social risk.

INTRODUCTION

Nature and nurture contribute equally toward recovery in neurodevelopmental disorders in children.

Early intervention services can optimize the development of children from birth to 3 years of age, who have or are at risk of having developmental delay or deviancies. The term "EI" encompasses a wide variety of medical, educational, and psychological treatments for at-risk babies as well as socioeconomically-disadvantaged children. The goals of EI are to empower the families, facilitate service provision, and coordination by developmental/pediatrician and, when required, to provide direct services by therapists. The target is to be family centered and individualized to meet the specific needs of each infant covering gross motor, fine motor, language, social, and self-help skills. The emphasis is on the initial 3 years of life, which is the critical period of brain development, as this is the period of effective synaptogenesis. This is also supported by an important UNICEF report 2001 (role of critical period 0–3 year).

CLINICAL FEATURES

Identifying the at-risk or red flags or absent building blocks of a particular milestone is the first step in planning EI services **(Boxes 1 and 2)**. This requires detailed family, antenatal, perinatal history as well as developmental history covering all domains of development. This is followed by detailed screening and assessment in relevant areas.

A collaborative perinatal project of National Institutes of Health (NIH) has suggested, simple Neuro-Behavior Scoring in the Neonatal Intensive Care Unit (NICU) can alert us to be vigilant as:
- Abnormal tone, weak suck, and lethargy for >24 hours indicate a 12–15 fold-increased risk of developmental delay.
- Decreased spontaneous movements for 24 hours increase the risk of 19-fold.
- Poor response to touch, poor cry for >24 hours indicates a 21-fold increased risk of developmental delay.

Vision screening **(Box 3)**—Fundoscopy for screening retinopathy of prematurity (ROP), retinoscopy and visual-evoked potential (VEP) (for details please refer Chapter 40).

Hearing screening **(Box 3)**—Universal hearing screening by oto acoustic emission (OAE) and brainstem-evoked response audiometry (BERA) (for details please refer Chapter 39).

Box 1: Red flag signs at 9 months.

Inability to:
- Sit well with support
- Motor symmetry without established handedness
- Should be able to grasp objects
- Transfer objects from hand to hand
- Roll over to both sides

Source: publications.aap.org

Box 2: Red flag signs at 18 months.

Inability to:
- Stand and walk independently
- Should grasp and manipulate small objects
- Any sign of regression in GM/FM skills
- Drooling

Source: publications.aap.org

Box 3: Community-based screening and identification can be carried out by the use of the direct observation card.

Confirm that child can see and hear:	
2 months old infant	Social smile
4 months old infant	Head holding
8 months old infant	Sitting independently
12 months old infant	Standing without support
15 months toddler	Should speak Mama and Papa (specific) in his native language
18 months	Follow one line command with no regression in communication, social, or play
If any of them is not achieved, EI should be provided to the child	

Source: publications.aap.org

The International Classification of Functioning (ICF) is developed by the World Health Organization (WHO). The ICF recognizes that functional abilities are a combination of the child's medical condition, activity limitations, and personal and environmental factors.

Red Flags for Communication, Behavior, and Socialization

Individualized direct services should be started if by 2 years of age:
- The mother is not satisfied with the child speech or if there is regression in speech
- The mother is not satisfied with the child behavior, he looks lost in his own world
- The child is not following 2 step commands, is hyperactive
- The child is having sensory issues such as hyperacusis, chewing difficulties and difficulty holding crayons.

As the ability to diagnose children with autism spectrum disorder (ASD) during the infant and toddler years increases, children with ASD will be a growing population for EI. Children diagnosed with ASD at 30 months or younger and provided EI were more likely to have a change in classification from ASD to non-ASD than children diagnosed with an ASD at 31 months or older (Wiggins et al., 2012).

Beside the above, the Denver Developmental Screening Tool (DDST), Gross Motor Function Classification (GMFC), Manual Ability Classification System (MACS), the Communication Function Classification System (CFCS), and the Eating and Drinking Ability Classification System (EDACS) can be used to identify the delay in specific domains.

Regardless of the scale used, it is important to identify the problems in developmental domains and to address each individually at the earliest rather than waiting for a final diagnosis.

Direct or definite services include speech and language therapy, occupational therapy, physical therapy, special instruction, and family education and behavioral counseling, although other services, such as assistive technology and nutrition may be required.

MANAGEMENT

Preventive strategies should focus on adolescent girls, maternal nutrition, and management of anemia, iron, folate, iodine, zinc, infection prevention, rubella vaccine, treating chronic medical illnesses, gynecological issues, and better obstetric care. Antenatal steroids should be administered in premature deliveries. Proper in utero and neonatal transport services should be available. Intrauterine growth restriction (IUGR) and girl child should be provided better neonatal care, literacy, and life skills.

Early intervention strategies should start as early as NICU:
- Unnecessary noises of alarms should be reduced (1 hour noise free period).
- Promote bonding through the kangaroo method.
- Passive exercises of the joints and gentle massage should be given to neonate.
- Individual lighting units should be dimmed at night to simulate cycles of day and night.
- Recording of mother's voice or music (hum) can be recorded and played near the baby but not constantly.

Early intervention for head control:
- Carry the child in upright position.
- Slowly lift the child from lying down position holding axilla, to sitting position, and then slowly put him back to lying position thereby stimulating to lift and hold head (5 minutes × 4 times/day).
- If the child does not lift his head, gently stroke downward over the neck muscle.

Early intervention for sitting:
- Make the child come to sitting position, hold her in this position and then make her lie down (5 minutes × 4 times a day).
- Make the child sit across his mother's knee, just tilt the child forward and sideways, so that he outstretches the hand. This helps in development of righting reflex.
- Make the child sit, provide support and toys, then slowly reduce support.

Early intervention for standing:
- Help him in coming to sitting position on his own.
- Make him come to standing position holding a stool and put toys.
- Help him to balance on an inclined surface.
- Help him to walk with support holding both hands and later with one.
- Outdoor playing with children will help holistic development.

Early intervention for vision and socialization:
- Hang brightly colored objects 12–15 inches above the crib.
- Hang black and white strip cloth across the crib.
- The mother while maintaining eye to eye contact performs singing or talking keeping face 6–8 inch away.
- Bright colored balls and balloons, etc., to be hung for providing visual stimulation.
- To promote visual following, use multicolored small bulb series, this is to be hung on the wall at the foot end of the child.
- Promote symbolization—it can be done by pointing and naming common objects when in front of the child's eyes.
- To promote joint attention, by to and fro sharing of something interesting; and something which is far, by pointing it to the child.

Early intervention in speech and communication:
- No electronic gadgets before 2 years of life.
- Quality communication between infant and family members and use single language.
- Speak clearly and with eye-to-eye contact with the child, do not use motherese.
- Talk to child whenever possible and encourage him to ask questions.
- Make the child listen to different sounds and do repetitions of what you say.
- Encourage him to share his experiences and to tell stories.

Early intervention for hand function:
- For opening of hand, pull the thumb or fingers from base.
- Place an object in his hand and bend his fingers around it to promote hand grasp.
- Apply dough or colored clay on thumb and index finger to promote pincer grasp.

One important benefit of EI is in helping families be hopeful about their child's future (NEILS 2014). Developmental trajectories can potentially be changed during the early years and the development of secondary disabilities can be prevented by the provision of services when the child is very young. We need to incorporate EI services in our daily practice which should be family-centered, individualized for the child, and culturally appropriate with prompt direct services as and when indicated.

FURTHER READING

1. CanChild. Gross Motor Function Classification system. [online] Available from: https://www.canchild.ca/system/tenon/assets/attachments/000/000/058/original/GMFCS-ER_English.pdf (Last accessed December, 2021).
2. Ferreira RDC, Alves CRL, Guimarães MAP, de Menezes KKP, Magalhães LDC. Effect of early intervention focused on the family in the development of children preterm and or at social risk: A meta-analysis. J Pediatr (Rio J). 2020;96(1):20-38.
3. Hadders-Algra M. Early diagnosis and intervention in cerebral palsy. Front Neurol. 2014;24(5):185.
4. Hebbeler K, Spiker D. National Early Intervention Longitudinal study (NEILS), the Study Overview, Context, and Purpose. Ency Spec Educ. 2014.
5. Nair MKC. Neuro-developmental follow up module on early stimulation & intervention. IAP President action plan.
6. Wiggins LD, Baio J, Schieve L, Lee LC, Nicholas J, Rice CE. Retention of autism spectrum diagnoses by community professionals: Findings from the autism and developmental disabilities monitoring network, 2000 and 2006. J Dev Behav Pediatr. 2012;33(5):387-95.
7. World Health Organization. International Classification of Functioning, Disability and Health (ICF). [online] Available from: https://www.who.int/standards/classifications/international-classification-of-functioning-disability-and-health (Last accessed December, 2021).

Chapter 54

Therapies and Interventions

Lata Bhat

INTRODUCTION

There are various interventions and therapies that are used for children with neurodevelopmental and behavioral problems. However, not all of them are evidence based or effective. The most effective treatment for all children with neurodevelopmental disorders is an appropriate educational training program that is tailored to the child's specific needs as even within the diagnostic checks, each child has unique behavioral patterns and causality. The intermingling interventions have to be planned according to each dimension of the individual needs of the child. A multidisciplinary team with inter- and intradisciplinary specialties and functioning that works under the care of a Developmental Behavioral Pediatrician who plans the overall program and outcomes should be involved in planning the interventions in the ideal setting.

BEHAVIORAL INTERVENTIONS

Behavioral interventions are now considered an established treatment for children with autism spectrum disorder (ASD), although they should not be expected to lead to normal functioning (National Autism Center, 2009; Spreckley and Boyd). They may help the child to substantially improve in their speech and communication along with bringing about a reduction in problem behaviors. Different learning techniques are used based on the principles of behavior modification depending on the individual child's problem.

Behavior modification is also very effective for children with attention-deficit/hyperactivity disorder (ADHD) and yields good results, especially when used along with medication.

Applied behavior analysis (ABA): Ivar Lovaas and colleagues pioneered ABA in the 1960s (Lovaas and Simmons, 1969). Programs based on ABA are currently one of the most popular interventions for autism. The theory behind using ABA is that children with autism have difficulty in learning through imitation and listening as their normal peers do. ASD individuals need a highly structured format with direct instructions and as such appropriate behaviors are taught by breaking down the tasks into small discrete steps along with training in a systematic and precise way. These include social, communication, and adaptive living skills such as various motor skills, both gross and fine, along with academics, and so on. Desired behaviors are rewarded by giving a preferred object as a consequence for a predecided span of time. Once, the desired behavior is achieved, the reinforcement can be delayed and blended into natural sources of reinforcement. Skills are broken down to smallest level as per the individual's level to make them successful and then, gradually, endurance is built. For example, in a child who is unable to sit at a place, we have to start with a target of sitting for 5 seconds and gradually build it up. Thus, the therapist has to reinforce desirable behaviors and decrease undesirable ones, teach new skills, and generalize them to different situations through repeated reward-based trials.

Each child needs attention and hence it necessitates a low student-to-therapist ratio along with very intensive intervention (25–40 hours a week). Child psychologists, special educators, and pediatric occupational therapists can acquire training in ABA.

Pivotal response training: It is a naturalistic intervention model derived from the principles of ABA to focus on "pivotal behaviors" such as motivation and self-management, rather than targeting individual behaviors at a time.

Floor time: This technique is used in children with autism. It encourages parents to engage with their children literally at their level by getting on the floor to play. Overall, floor time aims to help children reach the developmental milestones crucial for emotional and intellectual growth. A certified floor time specialist can assist the child and parents in this intervention.

TEACH (Treatment and Education of Autistic and Communication-related Handicapped children): This is a structured developmental teaching program. It aims to maximize educational attainment/life skills in children requiring structured teaching. This approach makes use of several techniques in various combinations and includes a focus on the person with autism, understanding autism, adopting appropriate adaptations, and the development of a program building on existing skills, emerging capabilities, and the individual person's unique needs. Addressing behavioral antecedents by organizing the physical environment, developing schedules and work systems, making expectations clear, explicit, and visual have been the effective ways of developing skills and allowing people with autism to use these skills independently.

Play therapy: Play therapy can supplement almost any existing autism intervention program. Children with autism not only need appropriate toys to play with, but also need to be taught how to play. A child psychologist who has experience in using play therapy techniques for autism or a qualified play therapist may be appropriate to use play therapy.

Occupational therapy (OT): The American Occupational Therapy Association defines OT as a "skilled treatment that helps individuals achieve independence in all facets of their lives. OT assists people in developing the "skills for the job of living" necessary for independent and satisfying lives" [American Occupational Therapy Association (AOTA) 2008].

Occupational therapy in children addresses the following issues:
- Helps to improve focus in children with inattention
- Helps to reduce hyperactivity and improve sitting tolerance
- Addresses the fine motor skills to improve the grasp, release, and handwriting skills
- Hand-eye coordination activities, help to improve play and concentration (hitting a ball with the bat, throwing at a target, copying from blackboard/book, etc.)
- Evaluates the need for specialized equipment, such as communication aids, wheelchairs, splints, bathing equipment, dressing devices, etc.

Sensory integration (SI): SI is about how our brain receives and processes sensory information so that we can do the things we need to do in our everyday life. Sensory issues may affect the social functioning, learning, and may aggravate feeding issues in children. SI may be customized for the hypo- or hyper-responsiveness of the child to sensory stimuli depending on the baseline sensory profile of the child. Repetitive behaviors have also been associated to the sensory modulation problems in children with developmental disorders. Sensory profile assessment and sensory integration therapy are given by occupational therapists (details in Chapter 43).

Physiotherapy versus OT: Physiotherapy deals with pain relief, strength, joint range of motion, endurance, and gross motor functioning. OT deals more with fine motor skills, visual-perceptual skills, cognitive skills, and sensory-processing deficits.

Social skills training is a promising intervention. Social stories, sociodramatic play, role modeling, and peer-mediated plans can be used for goals in social communication and behaviors in children with ASD, ADHD, and social communication disorder.

Role of special educator: Special educators carry out assessments for specific learning disorder and create an Individual Education Plan (IEP) for the child. They are also trained to deal with children with ASD and help them in achieving communication skills as well create an IEP to teach them academics. In children with ADHD, they can help with learning difficulties.

Special educators are specialized in different disabilities including intellectual disability, hearing impairment, ASD, cerebral palsy (CP), learning disability (LD), etc. They provide wholesome learning environment for every level.

Individual education plan: An IEP should be made under the guidance of a developmental pediatrician and a team of professionals should work on the goals. Different professionals working with the child include a special educator, a clinical psychologist, school teachers, and other allied professionals, if needed, such as an occupational therapist, language therapist and, of course, the parents. Response to intervention should be reviewed and documented at regular intervals. Outcomes should be measured and gaps examined.

Speech and language therapy: A sleep and language therapist works with children with ASD to address the following:
- Helping the child to understand communication
- Understanding of spoken language
- Stimulating the child to talk
- Stimulating the child (give means and reason) to communicate.

Speech and language therapists work with the child and the family to facilitate effective communication between them so that there is overall development. They also work on the child's cognition, understanding abilities, verbal repertoire, functional communication, and echolalia. During the early years, the neuroplasticity of the brain can be utilized to achieve better results. In a nonverbal child, both speech therapists and behavior therapists (clinical psychologists or special educators) can use alternative and augmentative communication such as keyboards, assistive devices, picture cards, and sign language. Picture Exchange Communication System (PECS) is also widely used. For children with fluent speech, focus should be on pragmatic language skills training.

COMBINED INTERVENTIONS

They include more than one interventional model, but are mainly based on a specific approach.
- *Social Communication, Emotional Regulation, Transactional Support (SCERTS)* program is a developmentally-based model (Wetherby and Prizant, 2000).
- *The Early Start Denver Model (ESDM)* uses a mixture of a clear behavioral approach with a relationship-based model, and it uses the parents as therapists (Dawson et al., 2010).
- *Learning Experiences* is an Alternative Program (LEAP) for preschoolers and parents.

THERAPEUTIC APPROACHES FOR CP

- *Neurodevelopmental therapy (Bobath) (NDT):* This rehabilitation intervention concept for CP was developed in the 1940s by Dr Karel and Berta Bobath. The concept aims to improve the gross motor function and postural control by facilitating muscle activity through key points of control assisted by the therapist. The technique has evolved and changed over years.
- Key elements in NDT are: Facilitation (using sensory inputs to improve motor performance), management of compensatory motor behavior, and an overall management strategy (a 24-hour interdisciplinary management approach) (Graham 2009; Veličković 2005). According to Kollen 2009, in NDT, "the patient must be active while the therapist assists him. The therapist assists the patient to move using key points of control such as the head, shoulders, and pelvis, and guides the movement of the whole body."
- *Sensory motor approach:* Modify muscle tone and activate voluntary movement by using cutaneous sensory stimulation.
- *Sensory integration therapy*: To improve efficiency of neural processing and organize adaptive responses. Vestibular and kinesthetic stimulation are given to develop adaptive purposeful response.
- *Proprioceptive neuromuscular facilitation (PNF)*: In this multisensory approach, facilitation techniques are used through therapist's manual contacts, verbal commands, and visual cues.
- *Constraint-induced movement (CIMT)*: Restrains the sound limb in hemiparesis to increase the use of affected limb. Currently modified CIMT is also used.
- *Traditional therapy*: Positioning, range of motion (ROM) exercises, strengthening of weak muscles, stretching of spastic muscles, compensatory techniques, and endurance training.
- Motor relearning approach.
- Task-oriented training.
- Hand arm bimanual intensive training (HABIT).

CONCLUSION

Interventions should be as intensive (25–40 hours/week) as possible. Every child needs an individualized plans with a target-based approach. Quarterly reports should be documented.

Follow-up assessments of skills achieved is necessary. An interdisciplinary team should be involved with a developmental pediatrician as the team leader with the involvement of parents/caregivers. Parental education is very important. Parents need to be kept in the loop with realistic expectations.

FURTHER READING

1. American Occupational Therapy Association. (2008). What is occupational therapy? Retrieved March 25, 2008, from: http://www.aota.org/Consumers/WhatisOT.aspx
2. Bobath K, Bobath B. The neurodevelopmental treatment. In: Scrutton D (Ed). Management of the Motor Disorders of Children with Cerebral Palsy. London: Spastics International Medical Publications; 1984. pp. 6-18.
3. Grazziotin Dos Santos C, Pagnussat AS, Simon AS, Py R, Pinho AS, Wagner MB. Humeral external rotation handling by using the Bobath concept approach affects trunk extensor muscles electromyography in children with cerebral palsy. Res Dev Disabil. 2015;36C:134-41.
4. Hoare BJ, Wasiak J, Imms C, Carey L. Constraint-induced movement therapy in the treatment of the upper limb in children with hemiplegic cerebral palsy. Cochrane Database Syst Rev. 2007;(2):CD004149.
5. Neurodevelopmental treatment approaches for children with cerebral palsy. Cochrane Systematic Review - Intervention - Protocol Version published: 05 November 2015.
6. Ortega JV. Applied behaviour analytic interventions for autism in early childhood: Meta-analysis, meta-regression and dose-response meta-analysis of multiple outcomes. Clin Psychol Rev. 2010;30(4):387-99.
7. Veličković TD, Perat MV. Basic Principles of the Neurodevelopmental Treatment. Rijeka: Croatian Medical Association. Cochrane Library. 2005.
8. Wendy Harron. Occupational Therapy. Children Health from Nemours.

Chapter 55

Principles of Pharmacotherapy in Developmental and Behavioral Pediatrics

Jeeson C Unni

INTRODUCTION

Management of neurodevelopmental and behavioral disorders in children is largely driven via multidisciplinary interventional programs, with early diagnosis and well-tailored early intervention being a key to a better outcome. However, there are certain conditions where medications have an important role in improving outcome. Appropriate medications can improve the child's functioning and the ability to participate in behavioral interventions.

GENERAL PRINCIPLES BEFORE STARTING MEDICATIONS IN CHILDREN WITH SPECIAL NEEDS

Create an individualized treatment plan, a long-term plan for treatment, which includes:
- Setting goals for improvements in behavior
- Programs envisaged for stimulating the baby neurodevelopmentally
- A timeline for monitoring progress
- Adolescent, parent, family, and other caregivers counseling and education
- Formulating the multidisciplinary team including doctors, parents, teachers, caregivers, and other healthcare professionals
- Cognitive behavior therapy wherever required
- Appropriate pharmacotherapy.

Pharmacotherapy may be needed for the following conditions (specific medications have been mentioned in the respective chapters):
- Attention deficit hyperactivity disorder (ADHD)
- Anxiety/obsessive-compulsive disorder (OCD)
- Depression
- Disruptive behavior and aggressive disorder
- Convulsive disorder
- Elimination disorders—encopresis/enuresis

- Schizophrenias
- Autism spectrum disorders (ASDs)
- Psychotropic management of cognitive-adaptive disability
- Sleep disturbances
- Tic disorders
- Substance abuse
- Self-injury.

Considerations before initiating drugs for children with neurodevelopmental and behavioral disorders are as follows:
- The child/adolescent and family must be informed about the purpose/goals of administering medications for the child.
- They must be made aware that medications are not being used to fully remedy or cure the problems of the given child.
- Start the medication after the patient's and family's approval for a trial of the intended pharmacotherapy and solicit final approval after that period of "trial."
- Emphasize the importance and the greater role of nonpharmacological interventions such as behavior therapy, psychotherapy, speech therapy, occupational therapy, and physiotherapy.
- Use of standardized behavioral rating scales will help quantify baseline problem areas and their severity. This can help guide the dosage and monitor the effectiveness of medications.
- Remember that starting with a low-dose and gradually increasing the dose, till expected effect or maximum dose is achieved or first signs of toxicity are manifested, is the best way of reducing side effects of medications in these children.
- Ensure regular follow-ups; knowledge of "what to look for" at every visit is mandatory; and an understanding that different doses and altogether different medications may be required at various stages of development from childhood to adulthood in differently abled children is essential.
- Increased renal clearance, lower body fat, efficient hepatic metabolism, and/or idiosyncratic metabolism of the drug would need consideration when treating adolescents as they would therefore need to be treated with higher doses than that recommended for adults.
- Responsibilities of every stakeholder, the child/adolescent, the family, school, the multidisciplinary medical and paramedical team, the society at large, the government health services, legislation, etc., in the care of the child should be detailed at the outset and reviewed periodically.

COMMON SIDE EFFECTS

Medications used to treat neurobehavioral disorders may exhibit a variety of side effects. Some are observed immediately after starting medications, e.g., lack of appetite with stimulants, while others are seen after long-term chronic treatment, e.g., weight gain with antipsychotics. Some are dose dependent, while some are seen on drug discontinuation, e.g., dyskinesia after stopping antipsychotics.

While prescribing, benefits of the medication have to be weighed against its side effects. One also needs to consider the problems and risks faced by child and the family if left untreated.

POLYPHARMACY

This is the practice of prescribing two or more medications for one or more diagnosed disorders. The concern arises due to increase in adverse events with polypharmacy, and hence extreme caution and regular monitoring is crucial. In children with multiple diagnosis or if symptoms are not responding to monotherapy, polypharmacy may be needed.

Most neurobehavioral disorders have significant comorbidities which sometimes necessitates the use of more than one drug, e.g., children with ASD with ADHD may need a combination of antipsychotics and stimulants.

It is natural that parents will be apprehensive about starting long-term medications in their child; however, there is scientific evidence to show that when used appropriately medications will improve behavior and subsequent learning in children with neurodevelopmental and behavioral disorders. Hence, it is crucial for the pediatricians to consider the same, and, in some cases, requisition the services of a developmental pediatrician or pediatric neurologist to understand if the child will benefit from medications.

FURTHER READING

1. Abbruzzese G. The medical management of spasticity. Eur J Neurol. 2002;9 Suppl 1:30-4.
2. Awaad Y, Rizk T, Siddiqui I, Roosen N, McIntosh K, Waines GM. Complications of intrathecal baclofen pump: Prevention and cure. ISRN Neurol. 2012;2012: 575168.
3. Chou R, Peterson K, Helfand M. Comparative efficacy and safety of skeletal muscle relaxants for spasticity and musculoskeletal conditions: A systematic review. J Pain Symptom Manage. 2004;28(2):140-75.
4. Dressler D, Eleopra R. Clinical use of non-A botulinum toxins: Botulinum toxin type B. Neurotox Res. 2006;9(2-3):121-5.
5. Keenan E. Spasticity management, part 2: Choosing the right medication to suit the individual. Br J Neurosci Nurs. 2009;5(9):419-24.
6. Kheder A, Nair KP. Spasticity: Pathophysiology, evaluation and management. Pract Neurol. 2012;12(5):289-98.
7. Kischka U. Neurological rehabilitation and management of spasticity. Medicine. 2008;36:616-9.

8. Kolaski K, Logan LR. A review of the complications of intrathecal baclofen in patients with cerebral palsy. NeuroRehabilitation. 2007;22(5):383-95.
9. Lapeyre E, Kuks JBM, Meijler WJ. Spasticity: Revisiting the role and the individual value of several pharmacological treatments. NeuroRehabilitation. 2010;27(2):193-200.
10. Milla PJ, Jackson AD. A controlled trial of baclofen in children with cerebral palsy. J Int Med Res. 1977;5(6):398-404.
11. Simon O, Yelnik AP. Managing spasticity with drugs. Eur J Phys Rehabil Med. 2010;46(3):401-10.
12. Tilton A, Vargus-Adams J, Delgado MR. Pharmacologic treatment of spasticity in children. Semin Pediatr Neurol. 2010;17(4):261-7.
13. Unni JC, Joseph RB, Sreerekha KB. Pharmacotherapy in attention deficit hyperactivity disorder. IJPP. 2017;19:56-62.
14. Unni JC, Joseph RB, Zachariah SM, Jafna F. Pharmacotherapy in autism. IJPP. 2018;20:206-11.
15. Vitiello B. IACAPAP Textbook of Child and Adolescent Mental Health. Principles in using psychotropic medication in children and adolescents. [online] Available from: https://drmsimullick.com/wp-content/uploads/2020/07/A.7-PSYCHOPHARMACOLOGY-072012.pdf. [Last accessed March 2022].
16. Zonfrillo MR, Penn JV, Leonard HL. Pediatric psychotropic polypharmacy. Psychiatry (Edgmont). 2005;2(8):14-19.

Chapter 56

Counseling

Leena Deshpande, Lavanya Iyer

The journey from "*I am low*" to "*I am motivated*", the change of attitude from "*I am unable to manage the behavior of my child*" to "*My child is doing very well*", the change of mindset from *looking at things negatively* to *having a positive outlook toward life*, from having *low self-esteem* to *being a confident person* and from the practice of *doing things for others* to *learning to love oneself*; all these positive transformations demonstrate the power of counseling.

Lavanya Iyer

INTRODUCTION

Counseling comes from the Latin word "consilium" which means "advice". It is a therapeutic process that allows individuals to share their feelings, outlook, mindset, and issues openly in order to deal with a situation in an effective manner.

Parents are the best advisers to guide their children. While generally they will do everything feasible for the health and happiness of their child, since they are emotionally invested in the situation as a parent, they may be unable to address certain problems or issues. In such situations, counseling will help. Depending on the problem area, developmental age, and maturity of the child, one may work directly with the child or indirectly through parental and/or family therapy. Parents play a vital role in child counseling to help make the child comfortable and build trust with the counselor.

CLINICAL COUNSELING

Counseling is a dynamic process of guiding and helping the child and family by identifying the core concerns, formulating goals, planning strategies, and advising specific ways to cope with or avoid a specific set of problems.

Counseling entails listening attentively, understanding the issue, and trying to find the root cause of the issue and give appropriate feedback.

Counseling needs to help develop insight to the problem, build emotional resilience, and help the child and the family to cope better.

Good counseling aims to identify the thought pattern, feelings, and behavior that shape up the person's life.

Counseling needs to be empathetic and follow professional and ethical guidelines of counseling and carried out in a warm, patient, responsible, respectful, nonjudgmental, and supportive manner.

Counseling can help overcome emotional and behavioral issues that plague the child and the family. However, results may take time and the child and the family have to invest their time and energy into proactively involving themselves in this process. The attitude and involvement of family and the individual, socioeconomic and educational level of parents, and family support also determines the success of counseling. For instance, while dealing with a child with anxiety, if the counselor realizes that the parent also has anxiety problems which in turn are affecting the child, this will also need to be considered and addressed.

Counseling sessions are custom made according to the needs of the child and family.

The counseling is designed in a way where the issue is considered and a time span is discussed at the outset. Over time, with regular follow-up, one must achieve short-term goals of the sessions. The sessions will eventually taper down from where it starts off once some goals are achieved. Homework is given to the child and family after each session, which will help them to apply and practice skills learnt in sessions in their daily life.

BEHAVIOR THERAPY (BT)

It is used to modify maladaptive behaviors and replace them with desirable ones by using various techniques of reinforcement and rewards for positive behaviors and consequences for negative behaviors.

The ABC model can be used as behavioral strategy. The process involves functional analysis of the problematic behavior, i.e., analyzing what the problematic behavior is achieving. For this purpose, the antecedent event (A), the behavior of the child (B), and the consequence of the child's behavior (C) are noted down in detail and analyzed.

Illustration: The mother took the mobile away from the child's hand (A), the child starts crying and hitting (B), and the mother gives the mobile back to the child to stop him from crying (C). Herein, the child has learnt that if he behaves in a certain way, the consequence will be that he will get whatever he desires. BT will work here by making parents understand this A-B-C principle of behavior, identifying the antecedents in their daily life which triggers the problematic behavior, and altering the consequences.

Different parenting styles in the family and inconsistent responses by family members exacerbate behavioral issues; this is part of counseling. It is vital to get all family members to implement the corrective techniques consistently. BT techniques are generally based on conditioning like classical conditioning and operant conditioning. Various techniques like time-out, token economy, shaping, and contingency contract can be used with children to modify their behavior.

Behavior therapy helps parents learn aspects of positive communication, positive reinforcement and bring about discipline in children. Children with attention deficit hyperactivity disorder (ADHD), autism spectrum disorders, and other behavioral issues benefit considerably from BT. Other techniques like aversion therapy are used for addictions while systematic desensitization is used for fears and phobias.

COGNITIVE BEHAVIOR THERAPY

"Your emotions are the slaves to your thoughts and you are the slave to your emotions."—Eat, Pray, Love.

Elizabeth Gilbert

Cognitive behavior therapy (CBT) is commonly used in counseling and works on the notion that human behavior and emotions are a result of ideas, beliefs, attitudes, and thinking related to events and never due to the events themselves. The main principle is that we are all guided by our thoughts, which will eventually create emotions and emotions will reinforce our behavior. So, if we change our thoughts, it will lead to a change in feelings and our behavior.

Illustration: A 15-year-old teenager is not invited to his classmate's birthday party. This becomes an activating event which then triggers negative thoughts in the child, whereby he feels rejected and unwanted. The emotion arising from this will be sadness and lead to anxiety and may make him withdraw from others which in turn will continue the vicious cycle of negative thoughts.

Cognitive behavior therapy is a focused therapy that works on modifying the initial thought process, replacing negative thoughts with positive ones which in turn will help the negative emotions. CBT works very well for clinical issues such as anxiety, depression, and panic attacks. It can also be used for personal counseling, anger management, and addictions.

Cognitive behavior therapy also helps us understand the cognitive distortions like polarized thinking, filtering, overgeneralization, jumping to conclusion, catastrophizing, personalization, control fallacies, emotional reasoning, and so on. Thoughts will revolve around these distortions and will eventually have to be identified and modified for any change to happen.

Illustration: A 12-year-old boy who is excellent in his academics and extracurricular activities has been facing anxiety issues and is constantly worried about his performance.

It was understood that fear of failure, disappointing his parents, and teachers was the root cause of his anxiety. He was disregarding his success and strengths and focusing on his perceived weakness.

Counseling helped the boy identify his negative thought processes and correcting them by replacing them with positive words and statements. The anxiety of his performance was challenged by relating to his consistent achievement over the years. Techniques like challenging irrational beliefs, restructuring, exposure, and positive self-talk were used. Parents were also counseled about the same and were asked to motivate him using positive words.

RATIONAL EMOTIVE BEHAVIOR THERAPY (REBT)

It is a therapy that works on ABC model where A is activating event, B is belief, and C is consequence. It coincides with CBT in a variety of ways but differs in its philosophic basis of emotional disturbances. It also highlights the significance of secondary disturbance, e.g., worrying about worrying. It teaches unconditional self-acceptance, e.g., if a child fails at an exam, he should rate his "performance" as poor but never overgeneralize and rate "himself" as a failure or being worthless. It focuses on the present and addresses attitudes, emotions, and behaviors. It is used to remodel the beliefs to more realistic ones by disputing them. Acceptance is a major component in this therapy to be worked on—whether it is toward self, others, or towards life.

Illustration: A 10-year-old girl has been refusing to go to school.

After detailed interview, it was understood that one incident of bullying by her friend in her classroom has led to this refusal.

Activating event—bullying by her friend.

Beliefs—she will be bullied everytime she goes to school and as a friend did this she cannot trust her friends. She also blames herself for being weak and allowing herself to be bullied.

Consequences—refusing to go to school and developing mistrusts, and poor self-esteem.

Disputing thoughts—she will not be bullied everytime and not all friends are evil, she can always ask for help from her other friends or complain about the same to the teachers and higher authorities. She was also counseled in self-acceptance to improve her confidence.

New thought—she needs to learn strategies to deal with such situations. Avoiding school will worsen the situation.

GESTALT THERAPY

It is the therapy that focuses on finding solutions in the present instead of focusing on the past. This therapy focuses on person taking accountability rather than blaming. Self-awareness and one's perception are keys factors in this therapy. It is used to work on various issues such as depression, anxiety, confidence issues, and relationship issues. Some common techniques used in this therapy are empty chair technique, role-play, words and language, exaggeration, etc. Gestalt is combined with various other techniques like art therapy. This therapy aims at making one more aware of what they are doing and what triggers them to bring about the change.

For instance, if an adolescent is struggling with how to be assertive with a bully in school, in Gestalt therapy's "empty chair technique", the child is asked to imagine that the bully is sitting in an empty chair across him and the counselor encourages dialogue with the empty chair and the child in order to engage the child's thoughts, emotions, and behavior and help child become mindful of the whole situation.

ECLECTIC THERAPY

It is an integrative method of using the above techniques together rather than using just one single therapy. The counselor needs to be choose the right technique for the presenting concern. This therapy can yield results for all short-term goals eventually leading to long-term results.

We all have imperfections and flaws; however, it is important to understand whether they are affecting our thought process, our daily life, and our relationships. Acknowledging, accepting, and working toward these issues will help us lead happy fulfilling lives. Counseling sessions can guide and help the individual and their families in overcoming their problems. But as good as the therapy techniques may be, counseling succeeds only if the individual and the family desire a change, are ready to accept advice and are proactive in the process. Hence, patience and empathy are essential in initiating the individual and family into the counseling process.

FURTHER READING

1. A Yuvaveer Initiative – Published by Central Chinmaya Mission Trust – Two volumes – Drop-Its Easy
2. Bratton SC, Landreth GL, Kellam T, Blackard SR. Child Parent Relationship Therapy (CPRT) Treatment Manual: A 10-Session Filial Therapy Model for Training Parents. Taylor & Francis; 2006.
3. Capuzzi D, Gross DR. Counseling and Psychotherapy: Theories and Interventions, 5th Edition. John Wiley & Sons, Inc.; 2014.
4. Miltenberger RG. Behavior Modification: Principles and Procedures, 6th edition. Cengage Learning; 2015.
5. Morgan CT, King RA, Schopler J, Weisz JR, Morgan M, Weiss JR. Introduction to Psychology, 7th edition. Mcgraw-Hill; 1986.

Chapter 57

Electronic Media and Gadgets

Samir H Dalwai, Barkha Chawla

"We are living in a gadget driven world and kids want their own gadgets. It makes them feel like they're part of the whole culture."
Chris Byrne

INTRODUCTION

Electronic media and gadgets have become a part of daily life particularly for children and adolescents. Its use is getting increasingly pervasive even in infants and toddlers. Caregivers often wax eloquent over the child's expertise with gadgets. Exposure to electronic media and gadgets is perceived by caregivers to be more beneficial than harmful; its utility in managing children during a busy day full of chores for caregivers easily tips the balance in favor of overuse. Consequently, its use is reported up to 7 hours of the day or more. With formal education coming online, this is only expected to worsen.

Screen time can be described as the time spent viewing of TV/video, computer, electronic games, hand-held devices, or other visual devices. There have been growing concerns about the impact of screens on children and young people's (CYP) health.

Language development in young children is directly related to the amount of time parents spend speaking to them. Human-to-human interaction has a strong influence on a child's social communication development. Infants learn social human behavior and language best by social interaction with other humans, and social feedback is important for the quantity and quality of infant social behavior and communication. Excessive television or excessive screen time interferes with a child's language and social development because children spend less time interacting with parents and may internalize what is seen on the screen.

Addictive behaviors are defined by the person's progressive exclusion of other activities, causing physical, mental, and social harm, while attempting to control one's dysphoric feelings. Addiction presents as abuse without control, alterations in mood, tolerance (the need for more), abstinence (ability to avoid), and personal harm or conflicts in the environment (family, peers, and school), as well as a tendency to relapse.

The internet, videogames, and cell phones constitute the highest form of behavioral addictions to their global use or to specific interactive addictive contents and activities (such as gaming, gambling, and social media).

Five broad forms of addictive behavior on the internet have been described:
1. The machine, i.e., the computer itself
2. Searching for information
3. Interaction compulsions, including contact with the web through online games, shopping, etc.
4. Cybersexuality, and
5. Cybercontacts

The smart phone, with its spectrum of applications and uses, driving excessive attention, and uncontrolled dedication to one's cell phone offers greater opportunity for abuse than regular cell phones or gadgets. Thus, cell-phone addiction is one of the greatest addictions of this century inspiring new terminologies, such as "FOMO" (fear of missing out), "nomophobia" (no-mobile-phobia), "textiety"—the anxiety of receiving and responding immediately to text messages.

CLINICAL FEATURES

Factors associated with high television and mobile screen viewing:
- *Child*:
  - Younger children watch more of television whereas older children are more likely to use mobile screen devices.
  - Higher number of media devices at home; gadgets allowed in the child's bedroom.
  - Younger age of possession of one's first cell phone.
  - Keeping cell phones switched on at night (vigilance behavior).
- *Caregiver*:
  - Higher parental use of mobile screen media.
  - Decreased parental control; poor or unstructured media use rules.

Children's exposure to screen time are similar for parents across all age groups and incomes.

Clinical features associated with high levels of screen time:
- Developmental delay—early exposure to screens and gadgets can lead to delay and/or deviance in the development of speech and language.
- Sleep—exposure to light and stimulating content from screens can delay or disrupt sleep. Teens with high number of calls and messages and on social networks are at greater risk for anxiety and insomnia.

- Obesity—decreased mobility due to activity displacement in favor of screen time for long parts of the day, along with increase in energy intake, may lead to obesity.
- Behavioral problems—irritability, inattention, emotional, and psychological issues including auditory and tactile illusions (heard a ring or felt a vibration).
- Poor academic performance.
- Physical problems—muscular rigidity and pain.
- Ophthalmological—screen time reduces blinking rates by half and causes dry eyes along with fatigue, blurry vision, irritation, or ocular redness.
- Risk taking behaviors—higher risk of addiction and earlier initiation of substance use, self-injury, or eating disorders. Sexting (sending nude or seminude images and sexually explicit text messages using a cell phone) is increasingly reported. Exploitation may lead to further behavioral emotional concerns. Cyberbullying leads to social, academic, and health issues.

Key Questions

- How much combined time does your child spend on the screen (television, smartphone, tablet, etc.) daily?
- Does your child have access to television or mobile screen device in the bedroom?
- Who decides how much and what to use screen time for? Is there a policy?
- Does taking away the gadget trigger a meltdown or tantrum that is difficult to control?
- Are activities of daily living (such as sleep or eating) supplemented with screen time?
- Does gadget use interfere in academic and social domains for adolescents?

Red flags needing professional intervention:
- Excessive use, frequent checking of phone; dependence and craving, feelings of unease when unable to use it; associated with insomnia and sleep disturbances
- Need to respond immediately to messages, preferring the cell phone to personal contact
- Urgency, need to be connected; anxiety, irritability, if cell phone is not accessible
- *Tolerance*: Increased use to achieve satisfaction or relaxation or to balance a low mood
- Sexting, bullying, or posting self-harm images
- Frequent family and conflicts; loss of interest in other activities.

Addiction and dependence may signify underlying emotional disturbances such as impulsivity and sensation seeking, poor conflict resolution, and low self-esteem.

MANAGEMENT

Health workers need to educate and guide caretakers about the potential of addiction and abuse of electronic media and gadgets and counsel them about expert recommendations. This should be a part of routine consultation.

World Health Organization has recommended maximum screen time of 1 hour/day for children below 5 years; infants <1 year old should not be exposed to electronic screens at all. Infants under one should interact in floor-based play and avoid all screens (**Box 1**).

Dos

- Set limits. Make your own family media use plan. Designate time and place for media activities. Limit digital media for the youngest family members. Limit your own media use. Teach and role model good manners online. Create tech-free zones. Banish media use from mealtimes, sleep times, and playtimes.
- Encourage playtime. Physical unstructured interactive play is essential on a daily basis.
- Sleep. Remove all devices from the child's bedrooms, including televisions (TVs), computers, and smartphones. Avoid screen time for 1 hour before going to bed.
- Exercise. Children age 6 years and older should get at least 60 minutes of physical activity each day [American Academy of Pediatrics (AAP)].
- Eye care. Follow the 20/20/20 rule: look away from the screen every 20 minutes, focus on an object at least 20 feet away, for at least 20 seconds

---

Box 1: American Academy of Pediatrics: Recommendations for children's media use (2016).

- For children younger than 18 months, avoid use of screen media other than video-chatting
- Parents of children 18–24 months of age who want to introduce digital media should choose high-quality programming, and watch it with their children to help them understand what they are seeing
- For children ages 2–5 years, limit screen use to 1 hour/day of high-quality programs. Parents should co-view media with children to help them understand what they are seeing and apply it to the world around them
- For children ages 6 years and older, place consistent limits on the time spent using media, and the types of media, and make sure media docs not take the place of adequate sleep, physical activity, and other behaviors essential to health
- Designate media-free times together, such as dinner or driving, as well as media-free locations at home, such as bedrooms
- Have ongoing communication about online citizenship and safety, including treating others with respect online and offline

(American Optometric Association). Take frequent breaks from the screen—at least 10 minutes every hour. Remember to blink. Encourage your child to try to blink extra, especially when they take breaks. Use moisturizing eye drops or a room humidifier, if indicated. Screen positioning. Make sure the screen is slightly below eye level. Some experts suggest positioning device screens based on the 1/2/10 rule: mobile phones ideally at one foot, desktop devices and laptops at two feet, and roughly 10 feet for TV screens. Increase the font size. Ambient lighting. Prevent light from windows and overhead light fixtures shining directly on screens. Decrease the brightness of the screen to a comfortable level for viewing. Get regular ophthalmological screening done.
- Children should be counseled about the dangers of privacy settings, predators, and sexting. Caregivers are encouraged to know your children's friends, both online and off, and what platforms, software, and apps they are using, the sites they visit what they are doing online.
- Children will make mistakes. Be kind, empathetic, and guide them to learn from mistakes.

Donts

- Screen time should not always be alone time. As far as possible, co-view, co-play, and co-engage with children when they are using screens.
- Do not use technology as an emotional pacifier. Children need to be taught how to identify and express strong emotions, manage their boredom with activities, or self-sooth.

Myths

- Which is the best app for my child? >80,000 apps are labeled as educational, but little research has demonstrated their actual quality. In his clinical practice, the author has counseled caregivers whose children as young as 3–6 months of age were shown apps and nursery rhymes on devices with a belief that this would increase their cognitive and communication abilities or simply to help them consume more nutrition or to sooth them. The author has counseled parents about the need to increase social interaction with their child and that "their lap is the best app for infants and toddlers". Infants and toddlers learn best through two-way communication. Children learn more by a "face-to-face" "back-and-forth conversation" direct-animated interaction, with hugging and playing, rather than with "passive" listening or one-way interaction with a screen. In his service evaluation, the author recounts the significant number of children with social communication concerns whose parents had reported compelling amount of screen time and who anecdotally reported significant improvement on eliminating screen time.

FURTHER READING

1. De-Sola Gutiérrez J, Rodríguez de Fonseca F, Rubio G. Cell-phone addiction: A review. Front Psychiatry. 2016;7:175.
2. Hill D, Ameenuddin N, Chassiakos YR, Cross C, Hutchinson J, Levine A, et al. Media and young minds. Pediatrics. 2016;138(5):e20162591.
3. Madigan S, Browne D, Racine N, Mori C, Tough S. Association between screen time and children's performance on a developmental screening test. JAMA Pediatr. 2019;173(3):244-50.

Chapter 58

Technology in Practice

Kawaljit Singh Multani

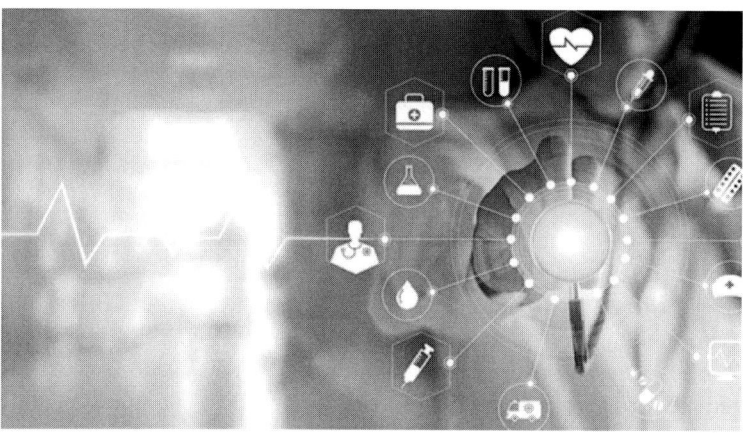

"Digitization promises to make medical care easier and more efficient; instead, doctors feel trapped behind their screens. On a sunny afternoon in May, 2015, I joined a dozen other surgeons at a downtown Boston office building to begin 16 hours of mandatory computer training. We sat in three rows, each of us parked behind a desktop computer. In 1 month, our daily routines would come to depend upon mastery of epic, the new medical software system on the screens in front of us. The upgrade from our home-built software would cost the hospital system where we worked, Partners HealthCare, a staggering $1.6 billion, but it aimed to keep us technologically up to date." Why doctors hate their computers.

Atul Gawande
The New Yorker, November 05, 2018

INTRODUCTION

The 21st century will be known as the century of technology. We are witnessing a march of technology into our homes as well as clinical practice. Thanks to the rapidly evolving communication technology and artificial intelligence

(AI), it is possible to do video consultations in real time with specialists in other countries and robotic surgeries by remote control. With 5G services around the corner in India and smarter smartphones and touchscreen devices already available, we are silent witnesses to a medical revolution which is overtaking both the developed and developing world. Coronavirus disease-2019 (COVID-19) pandemic has hastened the process by the recently issued telemedicine practice guidelines by Government of India on 25 March 2020 wherein patient care can be provided remotely without a need of physical contact between the patient and the doctor.

Medicine has always been taught by the bedside and clinical experience is respected. Advances in technology may be seen to threaten age old practices and may induce reluctance to its usage. Simplification of technological terms and patient consideration of its application may help practitioners overcome the same.

TECHNOLOGY AND MEDICAL PROFESSION

Technology has two components—the hardware and the software. The hardware must be sturdy whereas the software must be user friendly and secure in order to find acceptability in practice. Advances in technology over the past half century have improved patient care, safety, and medical research and teaching. Gadgets like multifunction monitors have not only saved many lives but also act as force multipliers. Remote monitoring devices and automated electrocardiogram (ECG) reporting machines help provide specialist care in remote areas and disaster zones. Introduction of computers has reduced the use of paper but added the burden of typing the data into the systems. This has also resulted in the emergence of a new profession like medical transcription. Availability of internet with smartphones has helped doctors remain in touch with the latest guidelines and provide the best available to their patients **(Fig. 1)**.

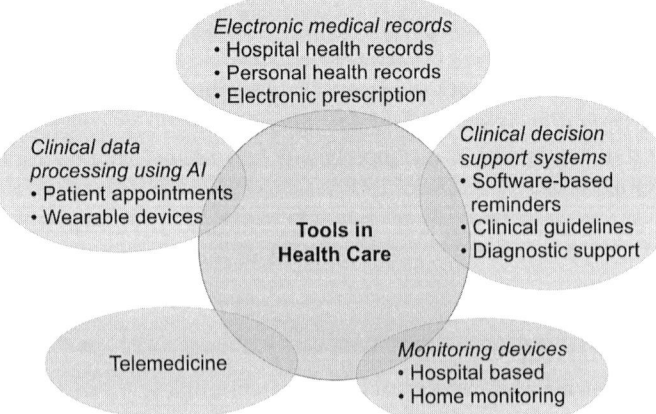

Fig. 1: Tools in health care.

Technology in medicine has improved patient care by digitizing appointments, electronic health records, and limiting access to medical data to authorized personnel. Electronic data has eased the burden of maintaining bulky records and allows easy access to patient records during patient visits as well as assist in medical research. Advances in technology has improved out-of-hospital health care by way of use of universal medical helpline number 108 and connected ambulances where trained paramedical personnel can provide specialist supervised care during transit of patient to hospital.

Health apps are available for android and iOS network smartphone for both medical personnel and general population information search. Medscape, Epocrates, UpToDate, PedOnCall, Totsguide, etc., are some of the popular apps used by healthcare professionals while Netmeds, 1 mg provide patients with tools to find and order their prescriptions online. New age smart phones and smartwatches have the ability to monitor hear rate, blood pressure, and other health-related data such as sleep times, sleep apnea, or calorie intake to help people take control of their health. The Indian Academy of Pediatrics has its own apps such as growth charts, drug formulary as well as other software to assist doctors in their practice while other apps like medical calculators help in calculating right dosage of medication.

With increasing use of technology in healthcare sector, the security and confidentiality of patient data are a major area of concern for both the software developers and the healthcare workers. There is a strong need to introduce the topic of healthcare technology in the undergraduate curriculum as the healthcare sector is likely to be technology driven. The future looks promising for the healthcare sector in the form of sophisticated smartphones capable of performing two-dimensional (2D) echo, ultrasound, and blood analysis in the field as well as wearable devices for monitoring patients and AI which will aid and guide medical practice.

While selecting the appropriate technology for your practice, three points need to be considered:
1. Which technology is right for you? Based on size of your practice.
2. Use software which can be preferably used with existing hardware.
3. Select a reliable vendor with good aftersales service.

CONCLUSION

Computers and technology are here to stay and the healthcare professionals need to learn to adapt and evolve with the changing scenario. At the same time, it is vital to retain the human touch with our patients.

> "We worry about what a child will become tomorrow,
> yet we forget what he is today."
>
> **Stacia Tauscher**

FURTHER READING

1. Bijarnia-Mahay S, Arora V. Next generation clinical practice—it's man versus artificial intelligence! Ind J Pediatr. 2019;56:1007-8.
2. Gulla KM, Sahoo T, Sachdev A. Technology-dependent children. Int J Pediatr Adolesc M. 2020;7:e 64-e69.
3. Dhingra D, Dabas A. Global strategy on digital health. Ind J Pediatr. 2020;57: 356-8.
4. Lehmann CU. Pediatric aspects of inpatient health information technology systems. Pediatrics. 2015;135(3): e756-e768.
5. Santosh MK, Balachander D. Telemedicine—guidance for pediatric practice. Ind J Pract Pediatr. 2020;22(2) :227; 114-7.

Chapter 59

Complementary and Alternative Medicine in Developmental Pediatrics

Shambhavi Seth

INTRODUCTION

Developmental disorders in children are a widely heterogeneous group. The World Health Organization estimates that 15–20% of children worldwide have disabilities; 85% of which are in developing countries. Apart from the variable effect on the child's functioning, these disorders have a significant psychosocial impact on their families. The chronic nature of these disorders need management strategies to continue for years and no single defined treatment option is available for most of them. Families may resort to treatment modalities, which lack evidence but seem to offer quick results. Some of these options are more affordable and avoid use of psychotropic medications, which in itself has limited acceptance with families of children with special needs.

Thus, parents may resort to complementary and alternative medicine (CAM) for the treatment of childhood developmental disorders.

According to the Cochrane Collaboration, CAM is a broad domain of healing resources that encompasses all health systems, modalities, and practices, and their accompanying theories and beliefs, other than those intrinsic to the politically dominant health system of a particular society or culture in a given historical period.

As high as one-third of patients with autism spectrum disorder are treated with CAM. It is reported that 10% of these children would have received a potentially harmful intervention. CAM therapies are considered by as many as 64% of those diagnosed with ADHD.

Complementary and alternative medicine may be broadly divided into: biological and nonbiological.

Biological CAM includes various dietary interventions like gluten-free-casein-free (GFCF) diets, dietary supplementation, hyperbaric oxygen therapy and chelation.

Nonbiological CAM includes mind-body medicine (yoga, meditation, music, dance, and different forms of art), manipulative and body-based practices (massage, sensory integration therapy, auditory integration therapy, chiropractic care, and acupuncture), energy medicine (reiki or homeopathy), and alternative medical systems (homeopathy, traditional Chinese medicine, and Ayurvedic medicine).

RESEARCH IN COMPLEMENTARY AND ALTERNATIVE MEDICINE

Randomized double blind-controlled trials provide the best level of evidence. Most of the trials of CAM are uncontrolled and fall short of evidence for clinical usage. The last decade has seen a few randomized trials but with small study samples. Association of comorbidities and multicomponent interventions has rendered their interpretation difficult.

Biological CAM in the form of elimination diet, particularly GFCF diet is one of the most popular dietary interventions. The rationale for its use is the theory of specific allergen in form of casein or gluten which triggers enhanced immune response in children with autism spectrum disorder (ASD). Children with ASD have been shown to have increased gut permeability and overgrowth of gut microflora. The randomized control trials have not reported significant statistical differences in core symptoms and adherence to diet has been a challenge for most of the families.

Among nutrient supplementation, omega-3-fatty acids are available over the counter and more commonly prescribed. Controlled studies have compared supplementation with placebo and no significant difference is reported between the two groups. Moreover, dosage of omega supplements has not been standardized across different studies. Other nutrient supplementation includes vitamin B12, B6, multivitamins, L-carnosine, probiotics, and herbal remedies. Further research is needed to advocate their clinical usage. Use of hyperbaric oxygen in cerebral palsy, and more recently ASD, has been based on presumption of revival of damaged brain tissue. Few studies have shown promising results but they are not consistent. Hyperbaric oxygen and chelation therapies may have potential to cause harmful effects.

Among nonbiological CAM, music therapy has been more widely studied. Few studies have documented improvement with respect to communication, social reciprocity, and emotion.

Evidence collected under National Standards project launched by National Autism Center has broadly classified available therapies as established, emerging, and unestablished. Interventions such as massage or touch therapy and music therapy are categorized into emerging evidence while interventions like auditory integration therapy, gluten-free/casein-free (GFCF) diet, sensory integration package, animal-assisted therapies, movement-based intervention, and SENSE theater interventions are categorized as unestablished.

As regards stem cell therapies, limited clinical trials have been performed. Several differences (study design, subjects enrolled, cellular types, route of administration, and outcome measures) make comparative reviews difficult. Larger and standardized trials are needed to establish definitive results.

ROLE OF CLINICIANS

While explaining CAM-based interventions, latest research evidence has to be corroborated and explained to the family. Families may try few options available under CAM, which are safe and not burdening in terms of expense but may be advised not to do so at the cost of replacing the conventional evidence-based interventions. Encouraging families to try one option at a time along with monitoring of core symptoms and target effects for a specified time period will rationalize the approach. Families should be clearly discouraged for CAM therapies, which not only lack good clinical evidence but may be potentially harmful by explaining the risks and benefits of the same. These considerations are pertinent from medicolegal point of view as well and clinicians can help families with informed decision making on use of CAM.

FURTHER READING

1. Akins RS, Krakowiak P, Angkustsiri K, Hertz-Picciotto I, Hansen RL. Utilization patterns of conventional and complementary/alternative treatments in children with autism spectrum disorders and developmental disabilities in a population-based study. J Dev Behav Pediatr. 2014;35(1):1-10.
2. Bent S, Bertoglio K, Ashwood P, Bostrom A, Hendren RL. A pilot randomized controlled trial of omega-3 fatty acids for autism spectrum disorder. J Autism Dev Disord. 2011;41(5):545-54.
3. Brondino N, Fusar-Poli L, Rocchetti M, Provenzani U, Barale F, Politi P. Complementary and alternative therapies for autism spectrum disorder. Evid Based Complement Alternat Med. 2015;2015:258589.
4. Challman T. Alternative therapies. Developmental-Behavioral Pediatrics. 2009; 950-6.
5. Chan E. The role of complementary and alternative medicine in attention-deficit hyperactivity disorder. J Dev Behav Pediatr. 2002;23(1 Suppl):S37-45.
6. Committee on Children with Disabilities. American Academy of Pediatrics: Counseling families who choose complementary and alternative medicine for their child with chronic illness or disability. Pediatrics. 2001;107(3):598-601.
7. Will MN, Currans K, Smith J, Weber S, Duncan A, Burton J, et al. Evidence-based interventions for children with autism spectrum disorder. Curr Probl Pediatr Adolesc Heath Care. 2018;48(10):234-49.

Chapter 60

Medicolegal Issues in Developmental and Behavioral Pediatrics

Santhosh Rajagopal

"Dharmasya gahanaaam gathi"   **Mahabharata**
(The pathway of truth is hidden)

Doing the right thing is not always easy! Imagine a child bedridden with spastic quadriplegic cerebral palsy with poor reflexes gets admitted for aspiration pneumonia and the critical care team informs the mother, a single carer, that ventilation is required for survival. The agony of the relatives to consent or withdraw care would be heart breaking.

KEY QUESTIONS

1. Would the caregivers be right in refusing care?
2. Is it right to ask the family for consent to withhold lifesaving treatment?
3. Is it ethical for the team to withhold treatment without any further due process?
4. What is the due process in such cases?

LAWS GOVERNING PEOPLE WITH PHYSICAL AND MENTAL CHALLENGES IN INDIA

There are two kinds of laws in India dealing with children having developmental disabilities. One set that regulates and seeks to control, and the other that enables and fosters support and care. Unfortunately, in India, we do not have a law that mandates multidisciplinary care for young people with developmental concerns, though there are provisions in existing laws to cater to the best interest of these children. Children (<18 years of age) are minors and considered legally less competent than adults when it comes to consent and taking decisions, making it more complex in case of developmentally challenged children.

Apart from fundamental rights and the penal code, the specific legislations affecting children, including those with developmental challenges, are:

- The Persons with Disabilities (PwD) Act
- The Mental Health Act
- The Juvenile Justice Act
- The Child Rights Commissions Act
- The National Trust Act
- The Supreme Court verdict in the passive euthanasia case.

The Persons with Disabilities Act

The PwD Act, enacted in 2016, is the most important legislation affecting children with special needs. The aim is to ensure that the child receives due care and protection and it is the doctor's duty to provide it.

It involves:
- *Education*: The PwD Act actively discourages the practice of conventional schools rejecting these children and sending them to special schools. The law makes it clear that all schools should admit children with disabilities. However, most schools do not have the infrastructure or capacity in Human Resource to attend to these children. So individual cases need specific guidance. Children with cerebral palsy (with mild or moderate cognitive impairment), specific learning disabilities, and specific impairments have a right to inclusive schooling in conventional schools. Children with mild and moderate autism spectrum disorder deserve normal schooling alongside interventions to improve their activities of daily living and behavior.
- *Residential schools and institutions*: It is not uncommon for families of children with disabilities to look for residential care. Under the PwD Act 2016 only a competent court can separate the children from their parents. The PwD Act, Section 9, states:
  - No child with disability shall be separated from his or her parents on the ground of disability; except on an order of a competent court, if required, in the best interest of the child.
  - Where the parents are unable to take care of a child with disability, the competent court shall place such child with his or her near-relatives, and failing that, within the community in a family setting or in exceptional cases in shelter home run by an appropriate government or nongovernmental organization, as may be required.
- *Reproductive rights*: Children with special needs are more prone to fall victims to sexual violence and abuse. Horrifying practices such as compulsory sterilization of the mentally challenged to prevent unwanted pregnancies have fortunately been outlawed, and it is up to a conscientious and law-abiding society to accord protection to these children and adolescents. The caregivers are also faced with issues such as managing sexual needs and reproductive issues of these young people

and developmental pediatricians will be faced with difficult decisions of how to best manage the sexual/reproductive functions of a completely dependent child and the stress of caregivers. The PwD Act, Section 10 states:

- The appropriate government shall ensure that persons with disabilities have access to appropriate information regarding reproductive and family planning.
- No person with disability shall be subject to any medical procedure which leads to infertility without his or her free and informed consent.

As children are minors and especially with disability, consent is a difficult issue to deal with for pediatricians, they should seek legal help and expert opinion in each individual case. The aim should always be the best interest of the child.

- The PwD Act also enumerates punishments for violation of the law.
- It also enjoins the various governments to screen for childhood disabilities and make provisions for their correction. Apart from school level screening, "at risk" screening is also envisaged under Sec 25 (2) as follows:
  - The appropriate government and the local authorities shall take measures and make schemes or programs to promote healthcare and prevent the occurrence of disabilities and for the said purpose shall (a) undertake or cause to be undertaken surveys, investigations, and research concerning the cause of occurrence of disabilities, (b) promote various methods for preventing disabilities, (c) screen all the children at least once in a year for the purpose of identifying "at-risk" cases.

It is clear that there is statutory backing for early screening and intervention.

The Mental Health Act

The Mental Health Act of 2018 does not mention any of the spectrum of neurodevelopmental disorders. However, the PwD Act does mention mental illness as a benchmark disability. Autism has been rightly removed from mental illness but included under intellectual disability (removing it from mental illness is a good step, but going ahead there is a need to separate it from intellectual disability).

The Juvenile Justice Act

The Juvenile Justice Act comes into play if children with serious behavioral issues such as conduct disorder get into situations where they break laws, as these children are likely to do so. The gist of this law is that while it is illegal to detain a child in jail or police custody in India, it is essential to look at the circumstances and to focus on reform rather than punitive measures for the further development of the child.

The Child Rights Commissions Act

The Commissions for Protection of Child Rights (CPCR) Act and its creation, the Child Rights Commissions at the central (National CPCR), and state (State CPCR) levels protect the rights of children with disabilities that are enumerated in the other acts.

The National Trust Act

The National Trust for The Welfare of Persons with Autism, Cerebral Palsy, Mental Retardation and Multiple Disabilities Act, 1999 established the above trust and is engaged in implementing various welfare schemes including health insurance for children with disability.

Medical Care of Children with Disability

It is quite clear that morbidity and mortality of children with disabilities are much higher than their peers without disability. In most circumstances, the medical treatment offered should be no different from that offered to the typically developing peers. However, problems can arise when these children need highly intensive support and decisions need to be taken whether to prolong care or withdraw life support. In most cases of end-of-life care and withdrawal of life support, the decision will be predicated on the irreversibility of the disease and the quality of life in case of survival. In the case of a child with developmental disability who already needed extensive support before the acute illness set in, these formulations are complicated. It is quite natural that caregivers reflect on the baseline health of these children when questions of providing or withdrawing life support arise. The former is a peculiar case in India with its highly privatized and therefore costly tertiary care system. It is not uncommon for hospitals to seek consent from caregivers before instituting invasive support measures such as ventilation even when such interventions have a high probability of reversing the course of the acute disease. But this is legally impermissible since the extant law applies only to withdrawal of care or withholding care when the disease process is irreversible and continuing care is not going to change the final outcome.

The legally safe route is to institute maximum care and then take it forward. It is not open to individual consultants to withhold treatment, especially for a curable condition just because the child or person under care required high degree of support prior to the illness, e.g., GMCFS Level 5 in cerebral palsy. The best interest of the child is paramount.

To answer the questions raised in the example quoted in the beginning of the chapter, it is straightforward that the child should have been ventilated and after optimum treatment, the progress assessed. In case of nonresponse to treatment, the protocol laid down by the highest court of the land should have been followed.

"Nese balasyethi chared adharmam"- Mahabharata

(Just because you have the power to do it, one should not fail to do what is right or do what is wrong by the conscience)

FURTHER READING

1. Bryan C, Melvyn S. The inclusion of students with mental retardation: Theoretical perspectives and implications. Special Services in the Schools. 2000;15(1-2):49-71.
2. Frank B. Making Inclusion Work. Hoboken: Merrill Education/Prentice Hall; 2005.
3. Majer IM, Nusselder WJ, Mackenbach JP, Klijs B, van Baal PH. Mortality risk associated with disability: A population-based record linkage study. Am J Public Health. 2011;101(12):e9-15.
4. The Gazette of India. [online] Available from: http://cara.nic.in/PDF/JJ%20act%202015.pdf. [Last accessed March 2022].
5. The Gazette of India. [online] Available from: https://wcd.nic.in/sites/default/files/TheGazetteofIndia.pdf. [Last accessed March 2022].
6. The National Trust for Welfare of Persons with Autism, Cerebral Palsy, Mental Retardation and Multiple Disabilities Act, 1999. [online] Available from: http://niepid.nic.in/THE%20NATIONAL%20trust.pdf or http://www.swavalamban.info/tifac/national_trust_act1999.pdf. [Last accessed March 2022].
7. Woolfenden SR, Williams K, Peat JK. Family and parenting interventions for conduct disorder and delinquency: A meta-analysis of randomised controlled trials. Arch Dis Child. 2002;86(4):251-6.

Index

Page numbers followed by *b* refer to box, *f* refer to figure, *fc* refer to flowchart, and *t* refer to table.

A

Abuse
  and neglect, types of 253
  impact of 254
  physical 253
  sexual 254, 295
  substance 192, 273
Acupuncture 292
Addictive behaviors 281
ADHD *See* Attention deficit hyperactivity disorder
ADI-R *See* Autism diagnostic interview-revised
ADOS *See* Autism diagnostic observation schedule
Aggressive disorder 272
Agoraphobia 183
Airway and breathing 163
Akinesia 147
Alper's disease 155
Amino acid disorders 49
Ammonia 156
Anemia 68
  management of 263
Aneuploidy 48
Angelman syndrome 92, 123, 152
  clinical features 92
  differential diagnosis 93
  management 93
Angiomyolipomas 106
Anthropometry 56
Antibiotics decisions 35
Antiepileptic drugs 140
Anxiety 68, 82, 177, 180, 212, 233, 239, 272
  clinical features 181
  disorder 183
    treatment of 184
    type of 181, 183
  evaluation for 225
  risk for 282
Aortic stenosis, supravalvular 51
Applied behavior analysis 234, 266
Ariel Tison method 43*t*
Arrhythmias 116

Artificial intelligence 287
Asperger disorder 231
Asperger syndrome 231
Assessing development 42, 42*t*
ASSR *See* Auditory steady-state response
Asthma 120
  chronic 254
Ataxia 147
Athetosis 148, 150
Atomoxetine 174, 194
Attention deficit 239, 258
Attention deficit hyperactivity disorder 55, 82, 86, 107, 123, 129, 149, 160, 169-172, 172*b*, 172*t*, 176, 192-194, 211, 228, 243, 250, 257, 272, 278
  clinical diagnosis 170
  management 173
  subtypes of 170*fc*
  symptoms of 170, 171*fc*
Audible block 221
Audiologic management 197
Audiological tests 198*t*
Auditory 215
  integration therapy 292
  steady-state response 199
Auditory-oral approach 200
Auditory-verbal approach 200
Autism 203, 236, 239, 267
  classic 231
  diagnostic interview-revised 258
  diagnostic observation schedule 258
  early infantile 231
  intervention program for 235*f*
  management of 235*fc*
  social interaction of 237*t*
  spectrum 258
  tools for assessment of 233*t*
Autism spectrum disorder 67, 86, 123, 223, 227, 231, 250, 257, 273, 292
  cause of 81
  clinical diagnosis 228, 232
  clinical features of 232*fc*
  diagnosis of 233
  differential diagnosis 233

learning disabilities 215
management 234
medical comorbidities in 227
symptomatology, prevalence of 67
symptoms of 232
Autistic disorder 231
Autistic spectrum disorder 75, 107, 140
Autoimmune
diseases 156
encephalitis 140
neuropsychiatric disorder 190
Autonomic function, deterioration of 116
Autosomal dominant inheritance
neurocutaneous disorder 99
pattern 49*f*
Autosomal recessive inheritance pattern 49*f*
Azoospermia 85

B

Balance disorders 205
causes of 206*b*
Basal ganglia 190
disorders 149
Bayley's infant neurodevelopmental screen 25
Bayley's scale 31
Behavior and temperament 11
Behavior modification 266
Behavior therapy 278
Behavioral difficulty 155, 258
Behavioral disorders, management of 272
Behavioral issues 65
Behavioral problems 283
range of 89
Behavioral regulation 233
Behavioral screening 27
Behavioral surveillance and screening 26
Behavioral symptoms 82
Behind the ear 197
Benzodiazepines 141
Beta-amyloid precursor protein 63
Binet Kamat test 31
Biological theories 14, 18
Biotinidase deficiency 31
Bipolar disorder 192
Bladder control, absence of 132
Blood pressure 103, 135
Bowel control 132
Bradykinesia 147
Brain
development 261
function 187

pathways 191*f*
structure 187
tissue, damaged 292
tumors 166, 168
Breath-holding spells 138
Breathing disorders, sleep-related 122
Bruxism 116

C

Carbamazepine 141
Cardiac conditions, treatment of 76
Cardiac rhabdomyomas 106
Cardiofaciocutaneous syndrome 76
Cardiovascular disorder 254
CARS *See* Childhood autism rating scale
Cataracts 73
Celiac disease 68
Central disorders 122
Central nervous system 6, 44, 77, 99, 106
infection 191
maturation of 7
Cerebral palsy 123, 143, 145, 257, 258, 269
classification of 143
clinical diagnosis 144
management 144
presentations of 145*t*
risk factors for 144
types of 145
Cerebrospinal fluid 156, 159
Ceruloplasmin 156
Charcot Marie tooth 206
CHARGE syndrome 152
Chemotherapeutic agents 167
Chemotherapy 167
Child abuse 253
incidence 253
risk factors for 254
Child development, theories on 13
Child Rights Commissions Act 295, 297
Child, prematurity of 10
Child's development, measurement of 8
Child's eyes 264
Child's program 58
Childhood autism 231
rating scale 258
Childhood cancer, treatment of 166
Children, development of 261
Children's behavior 3
Chiropractic care 292
Cholesterol metabolism 160
Chorea 148, 149, 153
Chromosomal disorders 248
Chromosomal karyotype,
high-resolution 52

Chromosomal syndrome 29
Chromosome 48, 90
  number of 48
Chronologic age 41
Circadian rhythm sleep-wake disorders 122
Clinical counseling 276
Clonazepam 126, 127
Clonidine 126, 127, 194
CNS *See* Central nervous system
Coagulation defects 75
Cochlear implant 197
Cognition 40
Cognitive ability 54
Cognitive behavior 102
  therapy 135, 188, 247, 278
Cognitive development 16
Cognitive theories 16
Cognitive-adaptive disability, psychotropic management of 273
Cognitive-developmental theory 3, 18
Common movement disorders, characteristics of 147t
Common neurodevelopmental disorders 123t
Communication
  augmentative 118
  behavior, and socialization, red flags for 263
  disorders 220, 245
  nonverbal 221
  technology 287
  verbal 221
Communication-related handicapped children 267
Community-based facilities and care 1
Complex molecules group 159
Consanguinity, history of 30
Constipation 61, 68, 136, 233
  signs of 230
  symptoms of 230
Constraint-induced movement 270
Control one's dysphoric feelings 281
Convulsive disorder 272
Coprolalia 191
Corencephalopathy 154
Cornelia de Lange syndrome 52
Cortical dysplasias 106
Cortical visual impairment 202
Costello syndrome 76
Counseling 276, 277
  behavior therapy 277
COVID-19 4, 288
Cri du chat syndrome 48

D

Daily living, activities of 28
Deaf-blindness 59
Deafness, levels of 196f
Dental enamel pits 105
Deoxyribonucleic acid 82
Depression 68, 177, 82, 185, 187, 189, 192, 233, 239, 272
Depressive disorder 185
  clinical features 185
  major 185, 186
  management 188
Depressive symptoms, chronicity of 186
Desmopressin 135
Development supportive care, implementation of 38
Development, principles of 7
Developmental and behavioral management 59
Developmental behavioral disorders 243
  clinical features 245
  management 246
  treatment of 246
Developmental behavioral paediatrics, history of 1, 2
Developmental context, red flags in 11
Developmental coordination disorder 211
Developmental delay 28
Developmental disorder 25, 98, 291
Developmental dissociation 29
Developmental learning disorder 245
Developmental milestones 10
Developmental problems 25
Developmental quotient 42t
Developmental screening 25
  step-wise approach 26
Developmental surveillance 24
  and screening 24
  program 26
Dietary supplementation 291
Direct observation card 262b
Disability, medical care of 297
Disabled persons 59
Disease manager 21
Disputing thoughts 279
Disruptive behavior 272
  disorders 175
Disruptive mood dysregulation disorder 187
Dix-Hallpike test 208
Dizziness 205
  causes of 206b
  sensation of 205

Down syndrome 48, 51, 62, 63t, 123
   developmental milestones 63
   management 68
   neurobiology of 62
   relative strengths 64
Duchenne muscular dystrophy 206
Dyscalculia 250
Dysgraphia 250
Dyskinesia 147, 274
Dysmorphic facial features 75
Dyspraxias 86
Dysthymia 185, 186
Dystonia 148, 150, 153
   medications for 145
Dystonic tremors 149

Enzyme activity, tests for 156
Epilepsy 93, 137, 139, 155, 206, 258
   drug-resistant 140
   focal 140, 141
   management of 93
   syndrome 139
Epileptic discharges 137
Episodes 133
Episodic ataxia 206
Episodic dyscontrol 82
Eye 101, 106
   almond-shaped 90
   coloboma of 152
   evaluation 45
Eyelids, upper 100

E

Ear, nose and throat 124
Early developmental impairment 28
Early intervention 44, 261
   clinical features 261
   management 263
Echopraxia 192
Eclectic therapy 280
Ecological systems 16
EDS *See* Enveloping distribution sampling
Education 295
Educational considerations 200
EEG *See* Electroencephalogram
Electrocardiogram, automated 288
Electroencephalogram 123
Electronic media and gadgets 281
   clinical features 282
   management 284
Elimination disorders 132, 272
   clinical features 132
   management 134
Emotional neglect 254
Emotional response 11
Empty chair technique 280
Encopresis 132, 134, 272
   classification of 133*f*
Encourage language 222
Endocrine 106
   disorders 75
   dysfunction 156
Endotracheal tubes, displacement of 35
Energy medicine 292
Energy metabolism group 158
ENT *See* Ear, nose and throat
Enuresis 132, 133, 135, 272
   classification of 134*fc*
   treatment of 135
Enveloping distribution sampling 123

F

Facial dysmorphism 96*f*
Faded bedtimes 126
Family-centered care 36
Fatigue, chronic 82
Fatty acid oxidation disorders 50, 158
FDA *See* Food and drug administration
Febrile seizures 137
Feeding behaviors' rating scales 130
Feeding difficulty, prevalence of 128
Feeding disorder 61, 128
   behavioral basis of 130*fc*
   clinical features 128
   management 129
   neurological basis of 129*fc*
Feeding problems 75, 228
Fertility treatments 73
Fibroblasts 159
Fibrous cephalic plaque 104
Fluency disorders 221
Fluoxetine 184, 194
*FMR*1 gene 48
Focal abnormal signal intensity 102
Folate 263
Follicle-stimulating hormone 86
Food and drug administration 194
Fragile X syndrome 50, 81, 123, 151, 152, 239, 248
   clinical features 81
   management 82
   phenotype 81
Freud's theory 2
Friedrich's ataxia 206
Frustration tolerance 67
Fundamental Rights and Penal Code 294

G

Gabapentin 127
Galactosemia 160
Gamma-aminobutyric acid 121
Gastroesophageal reflux 68
  disease 124
Gastrointestinal tract 77
Gaucher disease 155
Gene activity, modification of 49
Generalized anxiety disorder 183
Genetic abnormalities 51
Genetic disorders 25, 48, 54, 229, 233
Genetic influences 248
Genetic predisposition 211
Genetic syndromes 29, 52
Genetic testing 56
Genitalia 135
Genome 48
GERD *See* Gastroesophageal reflux
    disease
Germ cells 70
Gesell's spiral 6*f*
Gesell's work 2
Gestalt therapy 279
GIT *See* Gastrointestinal tract
Global developmental delay 28
  etiology of 29, 29*t*
Glutaric aciduria 155
Gluten-free-casein-free diets 291
Glycogen storage disorders 160
Glycolytic pathway affection 156
Glycosaminoglycans 156
Glycosylation, congenital disorders of 159
GMFM *See* Gross motor function measure
Gross motor function
    classification system 144
    measure 258
Growing children, development in 23
Guanfacine 194
Gustatory 215
Gynecomastia 85, 86

H

Haloperidol 194
Hamartoma tumor syndrome 227
Hand function, early intervention for 265
Handwriting samples 249*f*
Head control, early intervention for 264
Head shaking nystagmus 208
Head thrust test 208
Health
  apps 289
  care, tools in 288*f*
  concept of 21
  provider 21
Hearing 40, 46
  abnormalities, management 195
  aid 197
    types of 197
  assessment 197
  deficits 68
  impairment 67, 195, 269
  loss 143
    profound congenital 195
  monitoring 83
  professionals 201
  screening 196, 262
Heart defects 152
  congenital 71
Hematopoietic stem cell
    transplantation 159
HIE *See* Hypoxic ischemic encephalopathy
High refractive errors 202
High-risk clinic, components of 41
Hormonal replacement therapy 86
Human social behavior 96
Hurler-Scheie syndrome 112
Hyperactivity 233
  disorder 239
Hyperammonemia 49
Hyperbaric oxygen therapy and chelation
    291
Hyperkinetic movement disorders 147
  drug-induced 148*t*
Hyperornithinemia-hyperammonemia-
    homocitrullinemia
    syndrome 155
Hyperphagia 90
Hypersomnolence 122
Hypertelorism 74
Hypertension, pregnancy-induced 30
Hypoglycemia 160
  injury 60
Hypokinetic disorders 151
Hypomelanotic macules 104
Hyponatremia 136
Hypothyroidism, congenital 30
Hypotonia 228
Hypoxic ischemic encephalopathy 41

I

Imipramine 135
Immune disorders 140
Impaired adaptive functioning 56*t*
Individual education plan 269
Infants, high-risk 45*t*

Infection prevention 263
Inflammatory bowel disease 73
Insomnia 82
　disorders 122
　risk for 282
Intellectual ability 54
Intellectual disability 49, 54, 55*t*, 57*t*, 62, 107, 269, 296
Intellectual impairment 57*t*
Intelligence quotient 31, 62, 240, 241
　averages 96
　scores, traditional classification of 57*t*
Intention tremor 149
Interpersonal therapy 188
Interpreting observations 44*t*
Intoxication group 158
Intraoral fibromas 105
Intrauterine
　growth restriction 263
　infections 59
Intraventricular hemorrhage 41
Iodine 263
IQ *See* Intelligence quotient
Iron 263
　deficiency anemia 30
Isotonic saline 163
IVH *See* Intraventricular haemorrhage

J

Juvenile Justice Act 295, 296
Juvenile myoclonic epilepsy 140

K

Kangaroo care 35, 38
Kanner's autism 231
Karyotype detects 48
Ketone body defects 158
Klinefelter syndrome 85, 87*f*, 239, 248
　clinical diagnosis 85
　diagnosis of 86
　management 86
Klinefelter-Reifenstein-Albright syndrome 85
Krabbe's disease 155

L

Lactic acidemias, congenital 158
Lagging behind 54
Language
　development 281
　disorder 220
　　management of 221
　　expressive 64
Laws, kinds of 294
LD *See* Learning disability
Lead poisoning 233
Learning difficulty 258
Learning disability 86, 241, 248, 269
　assessments for 251
　clinical diagnosis 248
　diagnosis of 250
　family history of 248
　functional consequences of 250
　management of 251, 252*fc*
　types of 250
Learning disorders 211, 245
Learning with visual supports 64
Leigh's disease 155
Leopard syndrome 76
Lesch-Nyhan disease 155
Leukocyte 159
Leukodystrophy 154
Leukomalacia, periventricular 41
Life skills modifications 188
Liver
　angiomyolipomas 107
　function tests 156
Low glycemic index treatment 93
Lower limbs 135
Lower urinary tract symptoms 134*t*
Luteinizing hormone 86
Lymphangioleiomyomatosis 106
Lymphatic dysplasias 75
Lysosomal storage disorders 109, 159
Lysosomes 109

M

Maple syrup urine disease 155
Massage 38, 292
Maturational theory 2
Measuring development 8
*MECP*2 gene 48
Medical problems 91
Medically-unexplained symptoms 187
Medicine
　complementary and alternative 291
　technology in 289
Melatonin 121, 126, 127, 229
Menke's disease 155
Menstrual irregularities 141
Mental disorders, diagnostic and statistical manual of 131*b*
Mental Health Act 295, 296
Mental health disorder 25

Mental retardation 54
Metabolic disorders 29
Metabolic syndrome 86
Metabolism
   errors of 154
   group of inborn errors of 109
   inborn errors of 158
Metal disorders 161
Methylphenidate 173
Middle ear disease 67
Migraine, vestibular 207
Minimum developmental screening 23
Miscarriages, history of 30
Mitochondrial diseases 156
Mitochondrial disorders 160, 206
MNE *See* Monosymptomatic enuresis
Monosomy 71*f*
Monosymptomatic enuresis 134
Mood disturbances 67
Moro's reflex 7
Mosaic turner syndrome 72*f*
Motor development 64
Motor disorders, sensory-based 216
Motor tic 193
Mouth 105
Movement disorder 147, 149, 151, 155, 243
   etiology of 148*t*
   management of 152
   sleep-related 122
   treatment of 153*t*
   type of 148
Mucopolysaccharides 109
Mucopolysaccharidosis 50, 110*t*
   clinical features 109
   developmental and behavioral 109
   diagnosis 109
   management 113
Multiple disability 59, 60
   clinical features 60
   management 60
Multiplex ligation-dependent probe amplification 52
Musculoskeletal disorders 75
Mutism
   diagnostic criteria for selective 224*b*
   elective 225
Myelination 121
Myelogenous leukemia, chronic 100
Myeloid leukemia, acute 108
Myoclonic movements 150
Myoclonic seizures 93
Myoclonic spasms 138
Myoclonus 148, 150

N

Narcolepsy 122
National Autism Center 266
National Trust Act 295, 297
NDDs *See* Neurodevelopmental disorders
Neglect, types of 254
Neonatal deaths, history of 30
Neonatal intensive care 10, 35, 40
   unit environment 37
Neoplastic etiology 156
Neurobehavior scoring 262
Neurodegenerative disorder 82, 206
Neurodevelopmental conditions 258*t*, 259*fc*
   evaluation in 256, 257*t*
Neurodevelopmental disability 24, 257
Neurodevelopmental disorders 48, 121, 124, 129, 147, 151, 246
   management of 272
   spectrum of 296
Neurodevelopmental impairment 63
Neurodevelopmental problems 95
Neurodevelopmental profile 96
Neurodevelopmental screening, risk stratification for 40
Neurodevelopmental therapy 270
Neurofibromas 101
Neurofibromatosis 99, 248
   clinical features 100
   management 103
   type 99
   diagnostic criteria of 100*b*
Neurogenetic disorders 243
Neurological disorders 59, 75, 206
Neurometabolic disorders 243
Neuromuscular diseases 206
Neuronal ceroid lipofuscinosis 155
Neuronal migration 121
Neuropsychiatric syndrome, acute-onset 149
Neuroregressive disorders 154
   clinical features 154
   management 156
Neurotransmitter disorders 160
*NF*1 gene 49, 99
Niemann-Pick forms 160
NMNE *See* Nonmonosymptomatic enuresis
No-mobile-phobia 282
Nomophobia 282
Nonketotic hyperglycinemia 160
Nonmonosymptomatic enuresis 134
Nonpharmacologic interventions 169
Non-rapid eye movement 121, 123

Nonverbal skills 72
Noonan syndrome 51, 52, 74, 77*t*
   clinical features 75
   diagnosis and genetics 75
   differential diagnosis 76
   facial features in 76*f*
   growth charts for 79*f*
   management 76
Normal development and behavior 6
   theories of 13
N-REM *See* Non-rapid eye movement
Nystagmus, vibration-induced 208

O

Obesity 283
Obscene gestures 191
Obsessive compulsive
   behavior 193
   disorder 192-194, 272
   symptoms 66
Obstructive sleep apnea 83, 120, 111, 123, 124
Occupational therapy 268
OCD *See* Obsessive compulsive disorder
Olfactory 215
Oligosaccharides 156
Omega-3-fatty acids 292
Oppositional defiant disorder 175
Optic atrophy 202
Optic pathway gliomas 100
Oral motor dysphagia 228
Organ system 109
Organic acids 156
OSA *See* Obstructive sleep apnea
Osteopenia 116
   management of 119
Otitis media, recurrent 73
Ototoxicity 167
Oxcarbazepine 141
Oxybutynin 135

P

Pain, chronic 82
Painful procedures 37
Palilalia 191
Panic attacks 183
Parasomnias 122
Parental sleep education 125
Passive neglect 254
Perinatal brain injury 140
Perinatal causes 29
Perinatal complication 25

Peroxisomal biogenesis disorder 159
Persistent depressive disorder 186
Persons with Disabilities Act 295
Pharmacological interventions 169
Pharmacotherapy 188
   principles of 272
Phelan-McDermid syndrome 227
Phenylalanine 156
Phenytoin 141
Phobia 181
Physical and mental challenges 294
Physical growth 40
Physical neglect 254
Physical problems 283
Physiotherapy 268
Pimozide 194
Pivotal response training 267
Play therapy 267
POCSO Act 255
Poliodystrophy 154
Polypharmacy 274
Polysaccharide 109
Positive bedtime routines 125
Posterior fossa syndrome 167
Postnatal causes 29
Postural tremor 149
Prader-Labhart-Willi syndrome 89
   clinical features 89
   diagnosis of 90
   management 90
Prader-Willi and Angelman syndrome 227
Prader-Willi syndrome 48, 89, 92, 123
Pregnancy, high-risk 73
Prematurity
   complication 25
   correction for 41
Premonitory urges 190
Prenatal causes 29
Pressure-equalization tube 83
Preterm baby 10
   brain 35
Primitive reflexes 7
Protein kinase, mitogen-activated 74
Psychiatric disorders 120
Psychoanalytical theories 13, 16
Psychogenic nonepileptic seizures 138
Psychological problems 91
Psychopharmacologic intervention 236*t*
Psychosexual development 2
Pubertal development 103
Pulmonary arteries 95
PVL *See* Periventricular leukomalacia
Pyramidal dysfunction 155

R

Rational emotive behavior therapy 279
Recklinghausens disease 99
Regular physical activity 24
Rehabilitation problem 259*t*
Renal cysts, multiple 106
Renal disorders 75
Renal malformations 52
Reproductive rights 295
Respiratory chain disorders 158
Respiratory problems, management of 119
Restricted diet 233
Retinal disorders 202
Rett syndrome 93, 115, 123, 151, 153
    clinical features 116
    diagnosis 116
    differential diagnosis 118
    management 118
    medical management 119
    stages of 116
Risperidone 194
Rubella vaccine 263
Russell-Silver syndrome 51

S

Saliva, thick 90
Saudubray's classification 158
Schizophrenias 273
Scholastic backwardness 239, 240, 241*fc*
    clinical features 240
    management 240
School absenteeism 239
Seizure 119, 137, 233
    atypical 93
    classification of 138*f*
    clinical 229
    diaries 141
    disorders 228, 248
    history of 241
    provoked 137
    treatment of 230
    types, classification of 139*f*
Selective mutism 223
    clinical diagnosis 224
    management 225
    prevalence of 223
Selective serotonin reuptake inhibitors 82, 184, 236
Self-injurious behavior 153
Self-injury 273
Sensorimotor stage 3
Sensorineural hearing loss 73
Sensory integration 268
    and praxis tests 258
    disorders 215
    therapy 270, 292
Sensory modulation 216
    disorder 216
Sensory motor approach 270
Sensory processing
    measure 258
    problems 218*t*
Sensory processing disorder 215
    classification of 216*fc*
    clinical features 216
    management 217
Sensory seeking 216
Serotonin norepinephrine reuptake inhibitors 184
Sertraline 184, 194
Sexual violence 295
Shagreen patches 104
Shock, hypovolemic 163
Silent block 221
Single genes 49
Single-family room concept 36
SIPT *See* Sensory integration and praxis tests
Skeletal abnormality 51, 52
Skeletal disease 206
Skilled treatment 268
Skills, part of 5
Skin 104
    disorders 75
    to skin care 38
Sleep 67, 282
    apnea 68
    diary 124
    disturbances 273
    hormone 121
    physiology of 121
    problems 61, 120, 122, 123*t*
    quiet 121
    types of 121
    wake pattern 121
Sleep disorders 120, 124*fc*
    behavioral plan 125
    clinical features 121
    differential diagnosis 125
    drug therapy 126
    management 125
    medications in 127*t*
    miscellaneous drugs 126
    nonpharmacological measures 125
    treatment of 229
Sleep duration 124*t*
    shortened 228

Sleep myoclonus 150
　benign 138
Small lower jaw 71
Small testes 85
Smith-Magenis syndrome 123
Social anxiety disorder 223
Social deficits 82
Social development 64
Social phobia 223
Social skills 19
　training 268
Somatosensory phenomena 190
Spastic quadriplegic cerebral palsy 294
Special educator, role of 268
Speech 40
　and communication, early intervention in 265
　clarity 64
　memory, and learning, delays in 62
　poor expressive 86
　sounds 221
Speech and language
　impairment 143
　pathologists 228
　therapy 269
Speech disorder 220
　management of 221
Spine 135
SPM *See* Sensory processing measure
Stanford Binet test 31
Status epilepticus 138, 140, 141
Stem cell therapies 293
Stereotypy 148, 193*t*
Strabismus 73, 202
Stranger anxiety 22
Streptococcal infections 190
Subependymal giant cell astrocytomas 106
Subependymal nodules 106
Synapse formations 121
Synapse sculpting 121
Syndromic autism 151
Systematic stimulation programme 44
Systems theory 16, 19*f*

T

Target blood pressure 164
Technology and medical profession 288
Testicular sperm extraction 87
Testosterone 86
Thyroid function 68
Tic 148, 149, 153, 190
　clinical features 191
　comparing 193*t*

　disorders 191*f*, 273
　classification of 192*fc*
　medications in 194*t*
　management 193
Tonic-clonic seizures 138
Topiramate 194
Tourette's disorder 192
Tourette's syndrome 147, 190, 192, 193, 248
Traditional therapy 270
Transcutaneous electrical nerve stimulation 136
Traumatic brain injury 162
　management 163
　nonaccidental trauma 202
　pathophysiology of 162
Tremor 148, 149
Trisomy 21 48
TSC1 gene 49
TSC2 gene 49
Tuberous sclerosis 48, 104
　clinical features 104
　complex 104, 107, 108, 151, 248
　learning and behavior 107
　management 107
　treatment of complications 108
Tumor
　factors related to 167
　intracranial 206
Turner phenotype 74
Turner syndrome 51, 70, 71*f*, 248
　clinical features 71
　incidence of 70
　management 73

U

Urinary tract
　diverticula 97
　infection 134
Urine 112
UTI *See* Urinary tract infection

V

Verbal short-term memory 65
Vertigo
　benign positional 207
　duration of 207
Vestibular diseases 206
Vestibular disorders 209
Vestibular function tests 209
Vestibulo-ocular reflex 205
　tests 208
Vestibulospinal pathways 205
Vineland social maturity scale 118

Vision 40, 68, 103, 215
   and hearing, assessing 43
   deficits 143
   functional 203
   problems 213
   screening 262
   therapy 203
Visual acuity
   dynamic 208
   measurements 203
Visual aids, special 204
Visual field defects 202
Visual impairment 202, 203
   causes for 202
   clinical features 202
   management of 203
Visual-spatial perception 250
Visuospatial skills 72
Vitamin B12 deficiency 30
Voice, disorders of 243

W

Well-baby nursery population 195
West syndrome 139, 140

Wide smiling mouth 92
Willful deprivation 254
William syndrome 48, 51, 95, 96f
   clinical features 95
   management 97
Wilson's disease 155
Wood's lamp 229
Writing disabilities 250
Written expression
   difficulties in 249
   disorder of 246

X

X chromosomes 70, 85
   abnormal 85
X-linked inheritance pattern 50f

Z

Zinc 263
Ziprasidone 194
Zolpidem 126